Pulmonary Embolism and Its Complications: Causes, Diagnosis and Treatment

Pulmonary Embolism and Its Complications: Causes, Diagnosis and Treatment

Editor

Brett J. Carroll

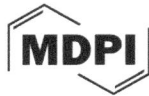

Basel • Beijing • Wuhan • Barcelona • Belgrade • Novi Sad • Cluj • Manchester

Editor
Brett J. Carroll
Harvard Medical School
Boston
USA

Editorial Office
MDPI AG
Grosspeteranlage 5
4052 Basel, Switzerland

This is a reprint of articles from the Special Issue published online in the open access journal *Journal of Clinical Medicine* (ISSN 2077-0383) (available at: https://www.mdpi.com/journal/jcm/special_issues/V34ZG68712).

For citation purposes, cite each article independently as indicated on the article page online and as indicated below:

Lastname, A.A.; Lastname, B.B. Article Title. *Journal Name* **Year**, *Volume Number*, Page Range.

ISBN 978-3-7258-2625-4 (Hbk)
ISBN 978-3-7258-2626-1 (PDF)
doi.org/10.3390/books978-3-7258-2626-1

© 2024 by the authors. Articles in this book are Open Access and distributed under the Creative Commons Attribution (CC BY) license. The book as a whole is distributed by MDPI under the terms and conditions of the Creative Commons Attribution-NonCommercial-NoDerivs (CC BY-NC-ND) license.

Contents

Sneha E. Thomas, Ido Weinberg, Robert M. Schainfeld, Kenneth Rosenfield and Gaurav M. Parmar
Diagnosis of Pulmonary Embolism: A Review of Evidence-Based Approaches
Reprinted from: *J. Clin. Med.* **2024**, *13*, 3722, doi:10.3390/jcm13133722 1

Andrew B. Dicks, Elie Moussallem, Marcus Stanbro, Jay Walls, Sagar Gandhi and Bruce H. Gray
A Comprehensive Review of Risk Factors and Thrombophilia Evaluation in Venous Thromboembolism
Reprinted from: *J. Clin. Med.* **2024**, *13*, 362, doi:10.3390/jcm13020362 17

Nichole Brunton, Robert McBane, Ana I. Casanegra, Damon E. Houghton, Dinu V. Balanescu, Sumera Ahmad, et al.
Risk Stratification and Management of Intermediate-Risk Acute Pulmonary Embolism
Reprinted from: *J. Clin. Med.* **2024**, *13*, 257, doi:10.3390/jcm13010257 37

Aroosa Malik, Nghi B. Ha and Geoffrey D. Barnes
Choice and Duration of Anticoagulation for Venous Thromboembolism
Reprinted from: *J. Clin. Med.* **2024**, *13*, 301, doi:10.3390/jcm13010301 57

Samer Asmar, George Michael, Vincent Gallo and Mitchell D. Weinberg
The Role of IVC Filters in the Management of Acute Pulmonary Embolism
Reprinted from: *J. Clin. Med.* **2024**, *13*, 1494, doi:10.3390/jcm13051494 69

John H. Fountain, Tyler J. Peck and David Furfaro
Sequelae of Acute Pulmonary Embolism: From Post-Pulmonary Embolism Functional Impairment to Chronic Thromboembolic Disease
Reprinted from: *J. Clin. Med.* **2024**, *13*, 6510, doi:10.3390/jcm13216510 83

Marc Righini, Helia Robert-Ebadi and Grégoire Le Gal
Age-Adjusted and Clinical Probability Adapted D-Dimer Cutoffs to Rule Out Pulmonary Embolism: A Narrative Review of Clinical Trials
Reprinted from: *J. Clin. Med.* **2024**, *13*, 3441, doi:10.3390/jcm13123441 95

Ebtisam Bakhsh
The Benefits and Imperative of Venous Thromboembolism Risk Screening for Hospitalized Patients: A Systematic Review
Reprinted from: *J. Clin. Med.* **2023**, *12*, 7009, doi:10.3390/jcm12227009 102

Fahad Alkhalfan, Syed Bukhari, Akiva Rosenzveig, Rohitha Moudgal, Syed Zamrak Khan, Mohamed Ghoweba, et al.
The Obesity Mortality Paradox in Patients with Pulmonary Embolism: Insights from a Tertiary Care Center
Reprinted from: *J. Clin. Med.* **2024**, *13*, 2375, doi:10.3390/jcm13082375 115

Mohamed Rahouma, Shaikha Al-Thani, Haitham Salem, Alzahraa Mahmoud, Sherif Khairallah, David Shenouda, et al.
The Outcomes of Surgical Pulmonary Embolectomy for Pulmonary Embolism: A Meta-Analysis
Reprinted from: *J. Clin. Med.* **2024**, *13*, 4076, doi:10.3390/jcm13144076 123

Truong-An Andrew Ho, Jay Pescatore, Ka U. Lio, Parth Rali, Gerard Criner and Shameek Gayen
Predictors of Residual Pulmonary Vascular Obstruction after Acute Pulmonary Embolism Based on Patient Variables and Treatment Modality
Reprinted from: *J. Clin. Med.* **2024**, *13*, 4248, doi:10.3390/jcm13144248 . . . . **136**

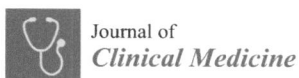 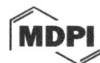

Review

Diagnosis of Pulmonary Embolism: A Review of Evidence-Based Approaches

Sneha E. Thomas, Ido Weinberg, Robert M. Schainfeld *, Kenneth Rosenfield and Gaurav M. Parmar *

Vascular Medicine Section, Massachusetts General Hospital, Boston, MA 02114, USA; sthomas013s@gmail.com (S.E.T.); iweinberg@mgh.harvard.edu (I.W.); krosenfield1@mgh.harvard.edu (K.R.)
* Correspondence: rschainfeld@mgh.harvard.edu (R.M.S.); gmparmar@mgh.harvard.edu (G.M.P.)

Abstract: Venous thromboembolism, commonly presented as pulmonary embolism and deep-vein thrombosis, is a paramount and potentially fatal condition with variable clinical presentation. Diagnosis is key to providing appropriate treatment in a safe and timely fashion. Clinical judgment and assessment using clinical scoring systems should guide diagnostic testing, including laboratory and imaging modalities, for optimal results and to avoid unnecessary testing.

Keywords: pulmonary embolism; venous thromboembolism; deep-vein thrombosis; diagnosis; clinical judgment; blood clots; risk stratification; biomarkers; pulmonary embolism response team; vascular medicine

Citation: Thomas, S.E.; Weinberg, I.; Schainfeld, R.M.; Rosenfield, K.; Parmar, G.M. Diagnosis of Pulmonary Embolism: A Review of Evidence-Based Approaches. *J. Clin. Med.* **2024**, *13*, 3722. https://doi.org/10.3390/jcm13133722

Academic Editor: Francesco Corradi

Received: 13 May 2024
Revised: 10 June 2024
Accepted: 20 June 2024
Published: 26 June 2024

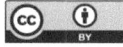

Copyright: © 2024 by the authors. Licensee MDPI, Basel, Switzerland. This article is an open access article distributed under the terms and conditions of the Creative Commons Attribution (CC BY) license (https://creativecommons.org/licenses/by/4.0/).

1. Introduction

Venous thromboembolism (VTE) is a substantial contributor to the burden of non-communicable diseases globally [1]. VTE includes blood clots formed in the venous circulation, deep-vein thrombosis (DVT), along with blood clots that break off and travel to the pulmonary vasculature, leading to pulmonary embolism (PE) [2]. Despite efforts at prevention and prophylactic measures, the incidence of VTE has been rising in the last several decades [3,4]. Studies report annual incidence rates for PE ranging from 39 to 115 per 100,000 people, while the incidence for DVT ranges from 53 to 162 per 100,000 people [5–7]. However, the actual incidence rates are likely significantly higher, as many patients are asymptomatic and many others are underdiagnosed or misdiagnosed. For instance, there are reports of silent PE in 40–50% of patients with proximal DVT and numerous PEs incidentally found upon autopsy [8,9]. Massive PE can lead to elevated physiologic dead space secondary to occlusion in pulmonary vascular flow [10]. Regardless, PE remains a fatal condition with high mortality rates. An epidemiological model created among six countries in the European Union reported an estimated annual total of 465,715 symptomatic DVT cases, 295,982 symptomatic PE cases, and 370,012 VTE-related fatalities [11,12]. Of these deaths, 27,473 (~7%) of the VTE events were identified antemortem, whereas 126,145 (~35%) were deadly PE, and 217,394 (~60%) were undiagnosed PE [13].

The ICOPER study evaluated 2454 patients with acute PE from seven countries in Europe and North America and showed an overall crude mortality rate of 17.4% at 3 months [2]. PE was attributed as the cause of ~45% of deaths, and ~75% of the fatalities transpired during the initial hospitalization for PE [2]. This highlights the importance of timely diagnosis to initiate treatment promptly and reduce the risk of mortality and morbidity. In this article, we hope to summarize a comprehensive approach to the diagnostic evaluation of PE while also avoiding unnecessary testing in appropriate clinical settings.

2. Pretest Probability

2.1. Does Clinical Presentation and Physical Examination Have Any Role in PE Diagnosis in 2024?

Clinical manifestations of acute pulmonary embolism can be very nonspecific, given its various presentations (Table 1), and they often result in a differential diagnosis for numerous typical and atypical presentations. The range of presentation varies from no symptoms to mild–moderate symptoms of shortness of breath to severe cases with hemodynamic collapse [14,15]. PE is typically suspected in patients who present with symptoms such as dyspnea, pleuritic chest discomfort, cough, and hemoptysis, with an incidence of 73%, 66%, 37%, and 13%, respectively, based on PE data from the Prospective Investigation of Pulmonary Embolism Diagnosis (PIOPED) study [14–17]. Syncope is an extensively discussed clinical symptom in PE, given the variable reports of its incidence and prognostic role [16,18,19]. The proposed mechanism for syncope in PE involves pulmonary vascular obstruction by a large embolus, resulting in impaired right ventricular function and consequently impacting left ventricular filling and cardiac output. Hemodynamic instability and circulatory compromise suggestive of right ventricular strain is an infrequent yet significant clinical finding since they may suggest central or widespread pulmonary embolism with a diminished ability to maintain a stable blood flow [16]. Cardiac arrhythmias, the Bezold–Jarisch reflex, hypoxemia, orthostatic dysfunction, and other comorbidities can also precede syncope events [20]. Even though syncope alone may not have a prognostic role, studies have shown elevated risk for early PE-related adverse outcomes such as early mortality (during hospitalization or <30 days) and 30-day negative events in patients with syncope [18]. Common physical examination findings of PE include tachycardia, tachypnea, or pulmonary hypertension/right heart strain, such as jugular venous distension, a loud P2 (pulmonic) component of the second heart, and right ventricular parasternal lift [21]. However, none of these findings are specific enough to diagnose PE, nor does the lack of these findings exclude PE. The presence of clinical symptoms and provoking risk factors for PE enables patients to be classified into distinct pretest probability categories.

Table 1. Common clinical manifestations of pulmonary embolism.

Clinical Features	Physical Examination Findings
Dyspnea	Tachycardia
Pleuritic chest pain	Tachypnea
Cough	Hypotension/Shock
Hemoptysis	Hypoxemia
Syncope	Orthostatic dysfunction
	Cardiac arrythmias
	JVD: Jugular venous distension
	Loud pulmonic heart sound
	Right ventricular parasternal lift

2.2. Role of Clinical Scoring Systems

Pretest probability assessment may be based on clinical judgment alone or clinical prediction scores. The major disadvantage of depending on clinical judgment alone is the subjectivity in the assessment and the lack of standardization. The clinical scoring systems provide objective variables that can allow for a more standardized approach to assess clinical probability and ultimately lead to a more effective diagnostic process. As a result, the clinical prediction rules may become helpful in assessing pretest probability in scenarios where clinical judgment alone is equivocal. The most commonly used and validated systems to assess pretest probability include the simplified and modified Wells Scoring System and the Revised Geneva Scoring System (Table 2) [22,23].

Table 2. Clinical scoring systems.

	Wells Score [22]		Revised Geneva Score [23]	
	Original	Simplified	Original	Simplified
Previous DVT or PE	1.5	1	3	1
Heart rate				
75–94/min			3	1
>=95/min			5	2
>100/min	1.5	1		
Surgery/fracture/immobilization within 4 weeks (1 month)	1.5	1	2	1
Hemoptysis	1	1	2	1
Cancer (active)	1	1	2	1
Clinical signs of DVT	3	1		
One-sided limb pain			3	1
Pain on calf palpation (Homan's positive) and unilateral edema			4	1
Alternative diagnosis less likely than PE	3	1		
Age > 65 years			1	1
PE unlikely	<=4	<=1	<=5	<=2
PE likely	>4	>1	>5	>2

DVT: Deep vein thrombosis; PE: Pulmonary embolism.

2.3. Clinical Judgement versus Decision Rules

Studies have shown a trend toward increasing accuracy with increasing clinical experience, and there is some uncertainty in the accuracy of the clinical gestalt of inexperienced physicians [24–26]. The gestalt of experienced clinicians has demonstrated comparable accuracy in identifying patients with low, moderate, and high pretest probabilities of PE in a few studies [24,25,27]. A retrospective analysis of a prospective cohort of 1038 patients was performed to assess the accuracy of gestalt evaluation compared to the revised Geneva score and the modified Wells score [27]. The area under the curve varied substantially across the three methods. Specifically, the AUC was 0.81 (95% confidence interval (CI) 0.78 to 0.84) for gestalt evaluation while it was 0.71 (95% CI 0.68–0.75) for the Wells score and 0.66 (95% CI, 0.63–0.70) for the revised Geneva score. The study results showed a favorable comparison between gestalt evaluation and clinical decision rules in assessing the clinical probability of PE and especially did better in selecting low- and high-clinical-probability patients [27]. Another meta-analysis of 52 studies involving 55,268 patients compared these different clinical prediction methods and showed comparable results. In 15 studies, gestalt assessment was utilized and showed a sensitivity of 0.85 with a specificity of 0.51. Nineteen studies used Wells scoring with a cutoff < 2, resulting in a sensitivity of 0.84 with a specificity 0.58, while eleven studies used Wells scoring with a cutoff of 4 or less and showed a sensitivity of 0.60 and a specificity of 0.80. Five studies applied the Geneva score and showed a sensitivity of 0.84 and a specificity of 0.50, and finally, four studies adopted the revised Geneva score and showed a sensitivity of 0.91 and a specificity of 0.37 [28]. In summary, it is acceptable to utilize clinical gestalt evaluation (especially by an experienced clinician) or any available scoring systems (Wells or Geneva) to assess the pretest probability of a pulmonary embolism.

3. Ruling out PE

3.1. PERC Rule

Although identifying patients with PE is critical, it is equally important to avoid the overuse of diagnostic tests for PE and lower inappropriate costs and complications of unnecessary testing, especially when clinical suspicion is low. The Pulmonary Embolism Rule-out Criteria (PERC) rule should be utilized for patients who are considered to have a low probability of PE. The PERC includes the following criteria: individuals 50 years of age or older, heart rate of 100 bpm or higher, oxygen saturation level of <95% while on room air, asymmetric lower-extremity swelling, presence of hemoptysis, recent major surgery or traumatic event, history of prior PE or DVT, and use of any type of exogenous hormones [29,30]. If any of the eight criteria are positive, the PERC rule cannot be used to rule out PE, but if all are negative, the risk of testing is greater than the risk for embolism, and PE can be ruled out with no further testing [30–32].

3.2. D-Dimer Testing

3.2.1. Different Techniques of D-Dimer Measurement

D-dimer is a soluble fibrin degradation byproduct of coagulation and fibrinolysis. D-dimer has high sensitivity along with high negative predictive value, though it lacks specificity [33–35]. D-dimer can help to exclude PE in low and intermediate-risk patients. More specifically, the enzyme-linked immunofluorescence assay (ELFA), microplate enzyme-linked immunosorbent assay (ELISA), and latex quantitative assay have lower specificity but higher sensitivity when compared to other D-dimer assays such as whole-blood D-dimer assay, latex semiquantitative assay, and latex qualitative assay (Table 3A) [34,36]. Consequently, it is imperative to note that some individuals with suspected PE may have negative results [37]. In patients with an intermediate pretest probability of PE, low-risk individuals where the PERC rule cannot be applied, or those with a low pretest probability but do not meet all the criteria to rule out PE, it is recommended to obtain a high-sensitivity D-dimer test as the preliminary diagnostic evaluation [38]. In high-risk patients and for patients with elevated D-dimer, advanced imaging, including computed tomography pulmonary angiography (CTPA), should be considered.

Table 3. A: Sensitivity, Specificity, and Negative Predictive Value of commercially available D-dimer assays, Pro-BNP, and Troponin for Detection of Venous Thromboembolism. B: Utility of BNP or NT-Pro-BNP in Prognostication of Pulmonary Embolism. Adapted from two metanalyses where BNP/NT-Pro-BNP was utilized to assess short-term mortality, PE-related mortality, and serious adverse events. C: Associations of Different Troponin Assays with Outcomes. Pooled odds ratio was utilized to assess mortality in acute PE using various troponin assays.

	A				
Biomarker	Sensitivity VTE (%)	Specificity VTE (%)	NPV VTE (%)	Sensitivity DVT (%)	Sensitivity PE (%)
* D-Dimer					
Enzyme-linked immunofluorescence assay (ELFA)	96–97	57	99	96	97
Microplate enzyme-linked immunosorbent assay (ELISA)	95	45	97	94	95
Latex quantitative assay	95	48–61	99	93	95
Whole-blood D-dimer assay	75–87	69–83	89	83	87
Latex qualitative assay	75	99	99	69	75
Pro-BNP	85	80			
Troponin-I	65	42			

Table 3. Cont.

	B				
Outcomes	Sensitivity Study 1/ Study 2 (%)	Specificity Study 1/ Study 2 (%)	PPV Study 1/ Study 2 (%)	NPV Study 1/ Study 2 (%)	OR Study 1/ Study 2
Short-term death	93/96	48/42	14/13	99/99	6.57/7.7
Death resulting from PE	92/97	52/42	13/12	99/97	6.10/6.4
Serious adverse events	89/100	48/36	33/26	94/100	7.47/15.6

	C			
Outcomes	All Troponins	Conventional Troponin-I	Conventional Troponin-T	High-Sensitivity Troponin
	OR (95% CI)	OR (95% CI)	OR (95% CI)	OR (95% CI)
Overall mortality	4.3 (3.3–5.7)	2.8 (2.0–4.0)	7.9 (4.5–13.6)	3.7 (1.2–11.6)
Short-term mortality	5.2 (3.3–8.4)			
PE-related mortality	9.4 (4.1–21.5)			
Adverse outcomes	7.0 (2.4–20.4)			
90-day mortality	4.8 (2.8–8.2)			
Mortality in low-risk PE subgroup				6.9 (1.3–35.8)

A: Adapted from (reference/s): [34,36,39,40]. BNP: brain natriuretic peptide; NPV: negative predictive value. B: Adapted from (reference/s): [39,41,42]. NT-Pro-BNP: N-terminal pro–B-type natriuretic peptide; PE: pulmonary embolism; PPV: positive predictive value, NPV: negative predictive value, OR: odds ratio. C: Adapted from (reference/s): [43–48]. OR: odds ratio; 95% CI: 95% confidence interval; PE: pulmonary embolism. * D-dimer measurement, preferably high-sensitivity assay, with age-adjusted cutoff (age × 10 µg/L in patient with age > 50 yrs) is recommended in outpatient/emergency-room patients with low or intermediate clinical probability/PE unlikely. D-dimer measurement is not recommended in patient with high clinical probability as a negative test does not rule out PE.

3.2.2. Age Adjustment of D-Dimer

The performance of the D-dimer test is significantly influenced by age [49]. In patients who are 50 years of age or older, the age-adjusted D-dimer threshold (age × 10 ng/mL) should be utilized to assess whether imaging is necessary, instead of a generic threshold of 500 ng/mL [50]. Studies have noted that the pretest clinical probability assessment and age-adjusted D-dimer cutoff together yield a greater proportion of individuals in whom PE can be confidently excluded, with a low likelihood of future VTE events, when compared to a set 500 µg/L cutoff [50]. The YEARS diagnostic algorithm looked at D-dimer cutoff adaptations based on clinical probability (three items from the Wells score and D-dimer level). PE was excluded in patients without clinical items (DVT symptoms, hemoptysis, and alternate diagnosis less likely) and D-dimer < 1000 ng/mL vs. one or more clinical items and D-dimer < 500 ng/mL. A study showed a significant reduction of 14% in computed tomography pulmonary angiography (CTPA) tests across all age groups and other relevant subgroups [51].

Certain special populations other than the elderly also need D-dimer modifications. For example, the ELISA D-dimer test appears to be a reliable way to exclude the presence of PE in cancer patients. However, it yields negative results at the standard cutoff value in only 10% of patients. Elevating the threshold of the cutoff value in cancer patients may enhance the use of the test in this particular population; a negative test can still reliably exclude PE diagnosis, nonetheless [52–54]. Similarly, a large proportion of outpatients with suspected pulmonary embolism can be efficiently ruled out by combining D-dimer results with clinical and pretest assessments. For instance, a Wells score of four or lower in conjunction with a negative D-dimer measurement may effectively and safely rule out PE in outpatient settings [55].

D-dimer measurement appears less useful in hospitalized and critically ill patients due to its lower specificity within these specific groups [56]. As such, it is crucial to use clinical judgement and pretest probability in assessing this population. It also remains as a diagnostic challenge in patients with underlying pulmonary etiology such as consolidation or pneumonia [57].

4. Role of Other Laboratory Biomarkers

4.1. Arterial Blood Gas (ABG)

Although few studies in the past have suggested normal (A–a) O_2 gradient as a possible PE exclusion criterion, studies in recent years have revoked these findings [58–60]. Arterial blood gas (ABG) collected from a study of 293 patients showed that ABG, either by itself or in conjunction with other clinical parameters, has little diagnostic utility when PE is suspected [60]. Similarly, PE could not be ruled out in over 30% of cases in patients without preexisting cardiopulmonary disease when the partial pressure of arterial oxygen was 80 mm Hg or higher, the partial pressure of arterial carbon dioxide was 35 mm Hg or higher, and the P(A–a) O_2 gradient was 20 mm Hg or lower [61]. Likewise, PE could not be dismissed as a possibility in over 14% of cases under the same conditions in patients with preexisting cardiopulmonary disease [61]. As a result, blood gas levels do not provide enough information to definitively rule out the possibility of PE.

4.2. Brain Natriuretic Peptide (BNP)

BNP and N-terminal pro BNP (NT-proBNP), its precursor, are neurohormones produced when the myocardium is stretched [62,63]. PE can lead to stretching of the right ventricle from pressure overload. Although both of these biomarkers are not often beneficial for the diagnosis of PE itself, they are frequently useful for prognostication as they can be considered indirect markers of right ventricular dilation and strain (Table 3B) [64–66]. A meta-analysis that reviewed 12 studies noted that higher levels of BNP corresponded with elevated all-cause mortality in the short term (odds ratio, 6.5; 95% CI, 3.1–13.9), mortality-related PE (OR, 6.1; 95% CI, 2.5–14.3), and major adverse events (OR, 7.5; 95% CI, 4.2–13.2) [39,67]. This study has also highlighted that normal BNP is a strong negative predictor in acute PE (Table 3A) [39,43]. However, utility is questionable in patients who may have other etiologies for the elevated BNP/Pro-BNP.

4.3. Troponin

Similar to BNP, troponin is also a great prognostic indicator but has minimal diagnostic value. It is a nonspecific marker of myocardial inflammation or injury. Elevated serum troponin suggests poorer immediate and long-lasting effects in individuals with PE (Table 3C) [40]. It may be utilized as an early and reliable marker of right ventricular dysfunction, especially when an echocardiogram is not immediately available [40,68].

4.4. Lactate

Serum lactate is a marker of tissue hypoxia. Several clinical conditions affecting perfusion and/or oxygen demand and supply, such as sepsis, may affect the serum lactate concentration. It is also a significant prognostic marker in acute pulmonary embolism. In a study of 270 patients, patients with lactate levels (> or =2 mmol/L) showed a mortality rate of 17.3%, (95% CI, 12–20%), while patients with lower lactate levels had a mortality rate of 1.6% (95% CI, 0.8–2%). Serum lactate level had a significant impact on both the overall mortality and composite endpoints in this study. The hazard ratio for overall mortality was 11.7 (95% CI, 3.3–41.0), while the hazard ratio for the composite endpoint was 8.1 (95% CI, 3.8–17.3). These effects were seen irrespective of the occurrence of shock, hypotension, right ventricular failure, or elevated troponin [69]. Another similar study involving 496 normotensive outpatient participants with acute symptomatic PE and an elevated plasma lactate showed that individuals with higher lactate levels had a higher likelihood of PE-related sequelae with an adjusted odds ratio 5.3 (95% CI, 1.9–14.4; $p = 0.001$) in contrast to those with lower lactate levels [69,70]. The positive predictive value of the combination of high plasma lactate with indices of right ventricular dysfunction on echo and myocardial injury such as cardiac troponin was ~18% (95% CI, 6.1–36.9%), making it an exceptionally beneficial prognostic indicator to assess complications associated with PE in <7 days [70].

5. Pulmonary Embolism Severity Index (PESI)

The pulmonary embolism severity index is a prognostic guide that enables the classification of patients with PE into different risk groups based on mortality (Table 4). The PESI rule applies clinical criteria for estimating outcomes within a 30-day period.

Table 4. Comparison of major guidelines on risk stratification and diagnosis of pulmonary embolism.

Guidelines	Categories	Risk Stratification	Diagnosis
ESC 2019 [7]	Low Risk	0 to 3 on revised Geneva or 0 to 1 on modified simplified Geneva score	History + risk assessment PERC rule
	Intermediate Risk	4 to 10 on revised Geneva or 2 to 4 on modified simplified Geneva score	History + risk assessment Age adjusted D-dimer
	High Risk	11 to 25 on revised Geneva or >5 on modified simplified Geneva score	CTPA vs. V/Q SPECT
ACC/AHA 2011 [44]	Non-Massive	Normotensive, normal Biomarkers, and PE unlikely in sPESI (or PESI)	
	Submassive	PESI class III-IV or sPESI $\geq$ 1, echo or CT evidence of RV strain, positive troponin, or elevated BNP or NT-Pro-BNP	
	Massive	Hypotension (systolic blood pressure < 90 mm Hg for $\geq$15 min, drop in systolic blood pressure of $\geq$40 mm Hg or vasopressor), or thrombus in transit, or syncope, or cardiac arrest	

ESC: European Society of Cardiology; ACC: American College of Cardiology; AHA: American Heart Association; CT: computerized tomography; CTPA: CT pulmonary angiogram; V/Q: ventilation- perfusion; SPECT: single-photon emission CT; PE: pulmonary embolism; PERC: PE Rule-out Criteria; PESI: PE severity index; NT-Pro-BNP: N-terminal Pro–B-type natriuretic peptide.

6. Role of PERT (Pulmonary Embolism Response Team)

Currently, there are no guidelines on the timeframe for diagnosis and management, although clinicians understand the critical nature of the diagnosis, especially in hemodynamically unstable patients. Since Massachusetts General Hospital implemented the first pulmonary embolism response team (PERT) in 2012, several other centers have adopted this multidisciplinary initiative to facilitate the diagnosis and treatment of patient with intermediate–high- and high-risk PE over the past decade [71–73]. Although several different structures exist within various small and large institutions, PERT programs generally aim to incorporate team-based multidisciplinary care into PE care by coordinating anticoagulation plans, thrombolytics vs. catheter-directed treatments, surgical options, and follow-ups [74]. The impact of PERT in facilitating multidisciplinary care is crucial, and more data are needed in this area to assess the effect on PE mortality and morbidity [75].

7. Role of EKG/ECG

A 12-lead electrocardiogram (EKG) may provide insights on the PE severity, if any acute changes are present. The six EKG findings including heart rate > 100 bpm (38%), S1Q3T3 (24%), complete right bundle branch block (10%), T-wave inversions in leads V1–V4 (29%), ST segment elevation in aVR (36%), and atrial fibrillation (15%) were found to be predictive of circulatory collapse and 30-day mortality following sudden PE in a systematic review and meta-analysis of 3007 patients [76]. However, these EKG changes alone are not enough to make the diagnosis, and a lack of EKG changes does not reliably reject the possibility of PE diagnosis.

8. Role of Various Imaging Modalities

8.1. Chest X-ray (CXR)

Acute pulmonary embolism is most commonly accompanied by the presence of cardiomegaly on chest radiographs. However, chest radiographs are not helpful in diagnosing pulmonary embolism but rather help exclude other mimickers of PE [77]. Normal CXR is also necessary for accurate and reliable interpretation of the ventilation–perfusion scan.

8.2. CT Pulmonary Angiography vs. Lung Scintigraphy

For patients with suspicion for PE, Multidetector Computed Tomographic Pulmonary Angiography, or CTPA, is the preferred imaging modality [78]. A filling defect that appears following contrast administration in any branch of the pulmonary artery is indicative of PE. The PIOPED II study reported a sensitivity of 83% (95% CI, 76–92%) and a specificity of 96% (95% CI, 93–97%) among 773 patients who had CTPA for the diagnosis of PE [78]. CTA-CTV (CT venogram) was also evaluated in the study and showed a sensitivity of 90% and specificity of 95%. Both CTPA and CTA-CTV had high concordance with clinical assessment. However, if there is discordance between the clinical judgment and the CTPA results, further evaluation should be considered. Motion artifacts, large body habitus, artifacts due to foreign objects, and inadequate contrast enhancement of the pulmonary vasculature can all lead to poor study quality [79]. CTV of the pelvis and lower extremity is not routinely performed in all patients unless there are clinical signs, given the risk of radiation, even though it might improve the diagnostic yield [80].

The detection of smaller emboli has increased with the use of newer scanners with higher resolution. For example, segmental and subsegmental artery visualization and interobserver agreement in the detection of PEs have been substantially enhanced by multi-detector row CT. However, the clinical significance of these smaller embolisms is still unclear [81,82].

For several years, lung scintigraphy/ventilation–perfusion (V-Q) scanning used to be the choice noninvasive imaging for patients with suspected PE. Many have had non-diagnostic evaluations due to the inconclusive results, however. CTPA emerged as the primary imaging technique for suspected pulmonary embolism (PE), effectively replacing V/Q scanning in the United States by 2001 [83]. However, V-Q still has utility in specific situations such as severe contrast allergy, severe renal dysfunction, and low radiation risk in pregnant and even young female patients where scintigraphy provides distinct advantages [84]. A normal chest radiograph is necessary given the risk of false positives due to underlying lung pathologies.

The updated PIOPED criterion, with an area under the ROC curve of 0.753, demonstrated greater accuracy compared to the previous PIOPED criteria [17,85]. However, intermediate probability or indeterminate studies remain a major limitation of V-Q scanning.

In another randomized study involving 1417 patients, the V-Q scan was noted to be non-inferior to CTPA in ruling out PE when used in combination with clinical probability evaluation, D-dimer, and lower-extremity ultrasonography [86]. However, it is important to note that despite achieving statistical significance, the V-Q scan group missed one fatal PE, and CTPA detected more patients with PE [86]. For patients at increased risk of pulmonary embolism (PE), employing a diagnostic approach involving chest X-ray and V-Q scanning based on the PISAPED criteria appears to be less safe compared to using CTPA [87].

8.3. Role of Magnetic Resonance Angiography

Magnetic resonance angiography (MRA) has not yet become a substitute for CTPA in assessing acute PE. However, it has the potential for specific utility in patients who cannot tolerate iodinated contrast and in pregnant or young patients, similar to a V/Q scan. The current MRI technology has a notable level of accuracy and precision in detecting proximal pulmonary embolism (PE), but its ability to detect distal PE is still limited, resulting in a sensitivity shortfall. Additionally, approximately 30% of the results obtained from this technology are inconclusive. While MRI/MRA can be helpful in clinical decision-making, it cannot be relied upon as the sole diagnostic study to rule out PE [88]. For patients with technically satisfactory images, the combination of magnetic resonance pulmonary angiography and magnetic resonance venography demonstrates a higher degree of sensitivity than magnetic resonance pulmonary angiography alone [89]. Regardless, acquiring technically satisfactory images using both methods is more challenging [90].

8.4. Imaging Modalities of the Future

V-Q single-photon emission CT (SPECT) has been reported to provide highly accurate negative and positive predictive values, with just 1% of the results being inconclusive [91]. However, accessibility for this study remains a major limitation, along with varied diagnostic criteria.

V-Q SPECT and low-dose CT without contrast combination has also shown outstanding diagnostic accuracy in a few studies and should be further explored [92]. The utilization of SPECT/low-dose CT can also help distinguish between lung symptoms, leading to a notable enhancement in diagnosing pulmonary embolism or identifying other lung disorders in a substantial number of patients, particularly when anomalies in lung perfusion are observed [93].

8.5. Is Pulmonary Angiography Still a Gold Standard?

Pulmonary angiography is the most accurate examination for detecting embolism and used to be the "gold standard". However, the advancements in noninvasive imaging modalities have changed the criteria for doing angiography. It is rarely performed due to the invasive nature of the test. Conventional pulmonary angiography lacks precision in diagnosing pulmonary embolism that is confined to subsegmental arteries [94]. For instance, one study reported a possibility of misdiagnosis in ~33% of subsegmental emboli and ~33% of solitary subsegmental emboli on pulmonary angiograms initially [95]. Procedure-related complications are also a concern. Among the 1111 patients that underwent angiography in PIOPED, complications of death occurred in five patients, renal dysfunction in thirteen, respiratory distress in four, and hematoma in two patients [77]. However, it is still a justifiable diagnostic technique in the proper clinical context [96].

8.6. Echocardiography

The major utility of an echocardiogram during acute PE is its ability to assess for right ventricular strain and elevated risk for poorer outcomes [97]. Both pulmonary artery enlargement and cardiomegaly do not demonstrate sensitivity or specificity in detecting the echocardiographic manifestation of right ventricular hypokinesis, which is a significant predictor of death in cases of acute pulmonary embolism [98]. Transthoracic echocardiography (TTE) is commonly used to investigate right ventricular (RV) pressure overload in individuals suspected of having acute PE [99]. McConnell's sign, a specific echocardiographic pattern characterized by localized right ventricular failure with the apex being unaffected, can occur in some PEs (77% sensitivity; 94% specificity), but it is not a specific indicator of pulmonary embolism [100–102]. Other findings such as right ventricle/left ventricle size ratio, septal motion abnormality, tricuspid regurgitation, 60/60 sign, hypokinesis of right ventricle, pulmonary hypertension, right ventricular end-diastolic diameter, tricuspid annular plane systolic excursion (TAPSE), and right ventricular systolic pressure can also be evaluated on an echocardiogram [77,103–105].

A meta-analysis of 511 patients with pulmonary embolism and transthoracic echocardiography showed that 71% of patients with PE had no significant abnormalities on TTE [106]. In patients that had TTE findings, ~27% had RV enlargement, ~27% had RV free wall hypokinesis while ~20% had the McConnell sign, 18% had interventricular septal flattening, and 13% had a 60/60 sign [107]. This study also reported that the simultaneous presence of hypokinetic right ventricle along with the 60/60 sign and the McConnell sign to be the most reliable indicator for RV strain [106].

The pulmonary embolism severity index (PESI)-Echo score (PESI + PASP-TAPSE = PESI-Echo) has been reported as an innovative and novel measure to evaluate the risk of mortality in individuals who have acute pulmonary embolism [108]. A multicentric prospective study among 684 patients in 75 academic centers in Argentina showed a PESI-Echo score greater than or equal to 128 as the optimal cutoff point to predict mortality while in the hospital (sensitivity 82%, specificity 69%) [108].

Although very rare, if there is a thrombus within the proximal pulmonary arteries and in the right atrium/right ventricle, this may also be visualized on an echocardiogram. A total of 1.8% of patients in the meta-analysis mentioned earlier had right heart thrombus. The presence of right heart thrombi in patients is mostly associated with the hemodynamic effects of pulmonary embolism rather than the specific characteristics of thrombi. Nevertheless, individuals with right heart thrombi and pulmonary embolism leading to right ventricular dysfunction appear to have a worse outcome compared to controls matched based on propensity scores [109].

8.7. Role of Point-of-Care Ultrasound for Diagnosis of PE in the Modern Era

Point-of-care ultrasound (POCUS) is a fast, safe, effective, and valuable tool that is available at the bedside which can aid in diagnosis if integrated with traditional clinical examination. In acute settings, the POCUS evaluation helps to assess evidence of right heart strain, which is particularly useful if the patient is hemodynamically unstable to travel for imaging or has renal impairment or other contraindications to obtain CTPA urgently. One of the major limitations is operator dependency. Similarly, POCUS cannot distinguish other causes of right heart strain, such as RV infarction, and cannot be used to exclude the diagnosis of PE, as a lack of RV strain does not necessarily rule out PE [110]. More recent studies are also exploring triple point-of-care US (heart, lung, and venous compression ultrasound) for a real-time assessment, which has promising potential but is not yet a formally recommended alternative diagnostic approach [111].

8.8. Compression Ultrasonography

Thrombi are often formed in the lower extremities and embolize to the lungs. As a result, venous compression ultrasound (CUS) is often performed in patients suspected of having DVT/PE. A combination of lower-extremity ultrasound and echocardiography may also offer increased specificity (if positive) or negative predictive value (if negative) in patients who cannot have a CTPA for some reason [112]. However, CUS has low sensitivity (sensitivity, 41%; 95% CI, 36–46%) and, therefore, cannot be used to rule out PE [113]. A retrospective study of 168 patients with acute PE showed that 46.4% of patients had a negative lower-extremity venous compression ultrasound [114]. Negative CUS was more often seen in patients with no history of DVT, low D-dimer levels, PE on V/P-SPECT rather than CT, and peripheral PEs [115].

9. Conclusions

Pulmonary embolism remains a major contributor to cardiovascular mortality despite many advances in diagnostic technologies over the last few decades. Clinical judgment and validated risk assessment tools should be used to guide diagnosis to reduce unnecessary testing. The presence of various clinical and laboratory features in patients can provide hints for diagnosis and indicate characteristics that can reduce the chances of erroneously ruling out the diagnosis of PE. Laboratory testing and imaging may be indicated in patients with intermediate and high risk for PE. Appropriate risk stratification is crucial for both the diagnosis and management of these patients.

Funding: This research received no external funding.

Conflicts of Interest: The authors declare no conflict of interest.

References

1. Raskob, G.E.; Angchaisuksiri, P.; Blanco, A.N.; Buller, H.; Gallus, A.; Hunt, B.J.; Hylek, E.M.; Kakkar, A.; Konstantinides, S.V.; McCumber, M.; et al. ISTH Steering Committee for World Thrombosis Day. Thrombosis: A major contributor to global disease burden. *Arterioscler. Thromb. Vasc. Biol.* **2014**, *34*, 2363–2371. [CrossRef]
2. Goldhaber, S.Z.; Visani, L.; De Rosa, M. Acute pulmonary embolism: Clinical outcomes in the International Cooperative Pulmonary Embolism Registry (ICOPER). *Lancet* **1999**, *353*, 1386–1389. [CrossRef]
3. Mazzolai, L.; Aboyans, V.; Ageno, W.; Agnelli, G.; Alatri, A.; Bauersachs, R.; Brekelmans, M.P.A.; Büller, H.R.; Elias, A.; Farge, D.; et al. Diagnosis and management of acute deep vein thrombosis: A joint consensus document from the European Society of Cardiology working groups of aorta and peripheral vascular diseases and pulmonary circulation and right ventricular function. *Eur. Heart J.* **2018**, *39*, 4208–4218. [CrossRef]
4. Chaar, C.I.O. *Current Management of Venous Diseases*; Springer Science and Business Media LLC: New York, NY, USA, 2018.
5. Kulka, H.C.; Zeller, A.; Fornaro, J.; Wuillemin, W.A.; Konstantinides, S.; Christ, M. Acute Pulmonary Embolism–Its Diagnosis and Treatment from a Multidisciplinary Viewpoint. *Dtsch. Arztebl. Int.* **2021**, *118*, 618–628. [CrossRef]
6. Wendelboe, A.M.; Raskob, G.E. Global Burden of Thrombosis: Epidemiologic Aspects. *Circ. Res.* **2016**, *118*, 1340–1347. [CrossRef]
7. Konstantinides, S.V.; Meyer, G.; Becattini, C.; Bueno, H.; Geersing, G.J.; Harjola, V.P.; Huisman, M.V.; Humbert, M.; Jennings, C.S.; Jiménez, D.; et al. ESC Scientific Document Group, 2019 ESC Guidelines for the Diagnosis and Management of Acute Pulmonary Embolism Developed in Collaboration with the European Respiratory Society (ERS): The Task Force for the Diagnosis and Management of Acute Pulmonary Embolism of the European Society of Cardiology (ESC). Available online: https://academic.oup.com/eurheartj/article/41/4/543/5556136 (accessed on 7 April 2020).
8. Meignan, M.; Rosso, J.; Gauthier, H.; Brunengo, F.; Claudel, S.; Sagnard, L.; d'Azemar, P.; Simonneau, G.; Charbonnier, B. Systematic lung scans reveal a high frequency of silent pulmonary embolism in patients with proximal deep venous thrombosis. *Arch. Intern. Med.* **2000**, *160*, 159–164. [CrossRef]
9. Sweet, P.H., 3rd; Armstrong, T.; Chen, J.; Masliah, E.; Witucki, P. Fatal pulmonary embolism update: 10 years of autopsy experience at an academic medical center. *JRSM Short Rep.* **2013**, *4*, 2042533313489824. [CrossRef]
10. Goldhaber, S.Z.; Elliott, C.G. Acute pulmonary embolism: Part I: Epidemiology, pathophysiology, and diagnosis. *Circulation* **2003**, *108*, 2726–2729. [CrossRef]
11. Cohen, A.T.; Agnelli, G.; Anderson, F.A.; Arcelus, J.I.; Bergqvist, D.; Brecht, J.G.; Greer, I.A.; Heit, J.A.; Hutchinson, J.L.; Kakkar, A.K.; et al. VTE Impact Assessment Group in Europe (VITAE). Venous thromboembolism (VTE) in Europe. The number of VTE events and associated morbidity and mortality. *Thromb. Haemost.* **2007**, *98*, 756–764. [PubMed]
12. Benjamin, E.J.; Muntner, P.; Alonso, A.; Bittencourt, M.S.; Callaway, C.W.; Carson, A.P.; Chamberlain, A.M.; Chang, A.R.; Cheng, S.; Das, S.R.; et al. American Heart Association Council on Epidemiology and Prevention Statistics Committee and Stroke Statistics Subcommittee. Heart Disease and Stroke Statistics-2019 Update: A Report From the American Heart Association. *Circulation* **2019**, *139*, e56–e528, Erratum in *Circulation* **2020**, *141*, e33. [CrossRef]
13. Posadas-Martínez, M.L.; Vázquez, F.J.; Grande-Ratti, M.F.; de Quirós, F.G.; Giunta, D.H. Inhospital mortality among clinical and surgical inpatients recently diagnosed with venous thromboembolic disease. *J. Thromb. Thrombolysis* **2015**, *40*, 225–230. [CrossRef]
14. Pollack, C.V.; Schreiber, D.; Goldhaber, S.Z.; Slattery, D.; Fanikos, J.; O'Neil, B.J.; Thompson, J.R.; Hiestand, B.; Briese, B.A.; Pendleton, R.C.; et al. Clinical characteristics, management, and outcomes of patients diagnosed with acute pulmonary embolism in the emergency department: Initial report of EMPEROR (Multicenter Emergency Medicine Pulmonary Embolism in the Real-World Registry). *J. Am. Coll. Cardiol.* **2011**, *57*, 700–706. [CrossRef]
15. Stein, P.D.; Henry, J.W. Clinical characteristics of patients with acute pulmonary embolism stratified according to their presenting syndromes. *Chest* **1997**, *112*, 974–979. [CrossRef]
16. Prandoni, P.; Lensing, A.W.; Prins, M.H.; Ciammaichella, M.; Perlati, M.; Mumoli, N.; Bucherini, E.; Visonà, A.; Bova, C.; Imberti, D.; et al. PESIT Investigators. Prevalence of Pulmonary Embolism among Patients Hospitalized for Syncope. *N. Engl. J. Med.* **2016**, *375*, 1524–1531. [CrossRef]
17. PIOPED Investigators. Value of the ventilation/perfusion scan in acute pulmonary embolism. Results of the prospective investigation of pulmonary embolism diagnosis (PIOPED). *JAMA* **1990**, *263*, 2753–2759. [CrossRef]
18. Barco, S.; Ende-Verhaar, Y.M.; Becattini, C.; Jimenez, D.; Lankeit, M.; Huisman, M.V.; Konstantinides, S.V.; Klok, F.A. Differential impact of syncope on the prognosis of patients with acute pulmonary embolism: A systematic review and meta-analysis. *Eur. Heart J.* **2018**, *39*, 4186–4195. [CrossRef]
19. Badertscher, P.; du Fay de Lavallaz, J.; Hammerer-Lercher, A.; Nestelberger, T.; Zimmermann, T.; Geiger, M.; Imahorn, O.; Miró, Ò.; Salgado, E.; Christ, M.; et al. Prevalence of Pulmonary Embolism in Patients with Syncope. *J. Am. Coll Cardiol.* **2019**, *74*, 744–754. [CrossRef]
20. Keller, K.; Hobohm, L.; Münzel, T.; Ostad, M.A.; Espinola-Klein, C. Syncope in haemodynamically stable and unstable patients with acute pulmonary embolism—Results of the German nationwide inpatient sample. *Sci. Rep.* **2018**, *8*, 15789. [CrossRef] [PubMed]
21. Morrone, D.; Morrone, V. Acute Pulmonary Embolism: Focus on the Clinical Picture. *Korean Circ. J.* **2018**, *48*, 365–381, Erratum in *Korean Circ. J.* **2018**, *48*, 661–663. [CrossRef] [PubMed]

22. Wells, P.S.; Anderson, D.R.; Rodger, M.; Stiell, I.; Dreyer, J.F.; Barnes, D.; Forgie, M.; Kovacs, G.; Ward, J.; Kovacs, M.J. Excluding pulmonary embolism at the bedside without diagnostic imaging: Management of patients with suspected pulmonary embolism presenting to the emergency department by using a simple clinical model and d-dimer. *Ann. Intern. Med.* **2001**, *135*, 98–107. [CrossRef] [PubMed]
23. Klok, F.A.; Mos, I.C.; Nijkeuter, M.; Righini, M.; Perrier, A.; Le Gal, G.; Huisman, M.V. Simplification of the revised Geneva score for assessing clinical probability of pulmonary embolism. *Arch. Intern. Med.* **2008**, *168*, 2131–2136. [CrossRef]
24. Chunilal, S.D.; Eikelboom, J.W.; Attia, J.; Miniati, M.; Panju, A.A.; Simel, D.L.; Ginsberg, J.S. Does this patient have pulmonary embolism? *JAMA* **2003**, *290*, 2849–2858. [CrossRef]
25. Kabrhel, C.; Camargo, C.A., Jr.; Goldhaber, S.Z. Clinical gestalt and the diagnosis of pulmonary embolism: Does experience matter? *Chest* **2005**, *127*, 1627–1630. [CrossRef]
26. Miniati, M.; Prediletto, R.; Formichi, B.; Marini, C.; Di Ricco, G.; Tonelli, L.; Allescia, G.; Pistolesi, M. Accuracy of clinical assessment in the diagnosis of pulmonary embolism. *Am. J. Respir. Crit. Care Med.* **1999**, *159*, 864–871. [CrossRef]
27. Penaloza, A.; Verschuren, F.; Meyer, G.; Quentin-Georget, S.; Soulie, C.; Thys, F.; Roy, P.M. Comparison of the unstructured clinician gestalt, the wells score, and the revised Geneva score to estimate pretest probability for suspected pulmonary embolism. *Ann. Emerg. Med.* **2013**, *62*, 117–124.e2. [CrossRef]
28. Lucassen, W.; Geersing, G.J.; Erkens, P.M.; Reitsma, J.B.; Moons, K.G.; Büller, H.; van Weert, H.C. Clinical decision rules for excluding pulmonary embolism: A meta-analysis. *Ann. Intern. Med.* **2011**, *155*, 448–460. [CrossRef]
29. Mwansa, H.; Zghouzi, M.; Barnes, G.D. Unprovoked Venous Thromboembolism: The Search for the Cause. *Med. Clin. North Am.* **2023**, *107*, 861–882. [CrossRef]
30. Kline, J.A.; Mitchell, A.M.; Kabrhel, C.; Richman, P.B.; Courtney, D.M. Clinical criteria to prevent unnecessary diagnostic testing in emergency department patients with suspected pulmonary embolism. *J. Thromb. Haemost.* **2004**, *2*, 1247–1255. [CrossRef]
31. Kline, J.A.; Courtney, D.M.; Kabrhel, C.; Moore, C.L.; Smithline, H.A.; Plewa, M.C.; Richman, P.B.; O'Neil, B.J.; Nordenholz, K. Prospective multicenter evaluation of the pulmonary embolism rule-out criteria. *J. Thromb. Haemost.* **2008**, *6*, 772–780. [CrossRef]
32. Freund, Y.; Cachanado, M.; Aubry, A.; Orsini, C.; Raynal, P.A.; Féral-Pierssens, A.L.; Charpentier, S.; Dumas, F.; Baarir, N.; Truchot, J.; et al. Effect of the Pulmonary Embolism Rule-Out Criteria on Subsequent Thromboembolic Events Among Low-Risk Emergency Department Patients: The PROPER Randomized Clinical Trial. *JAMA* **2018**, *319*, 559–566. [CrossRef]
33. Schuetz, P.; Aujesky, D.; Müller, C.; Müller, B. Biomarker-guided personalised emergency medicine for all-hope for another hype? *Swiss. Med. Wkly.* **2015**, *145*, w14079. [CrossRef]
34. Weitz, J.I.; Fredenburgh, J.C.; Eikelboom, J.W. A Test in Context: D-Dimer. *J. Am. Coll. Cardiol.* **2017**, *70*, 2411–2420. [CrossRef]
35. Di Nisio, M.; van Es, N.; Büller, H.R. Deep vein thrombosis and pulmonary embolism. *Lancet* **2016**, *388*, 3060–3073. [CrossRef]
36. Di Nisio, M.; Squizzato, A.; Rutjes, A.W.; Büller, H.R.; Zwinderman, A.H.; Bossuyt, P.M. Diagnostic accuracy of D-dimer test for exclusion of venous thromboembolism: A systematic review. *J. Thromb. Haemost.* **2007**, *5*, 296–304, Erratum in *J. Thromb. Haemost.* **2013**, *11*, 1942. [CrossRef]
37. Salim, A.; Brown, C.; Inaba, K.; Martin, M.J. *Surgical Critical Care Therapy: A Clinically Oriented Practical Approach*, 1st ed.; Surgical Critical Care Therapy; Springer Science and Business Media LLC: New York, NY, USA, 2018.
38. Raja, A.S.; Greenberg, J.O.; Qaseem, A.; Denberg, T.D.; Fitterman, N.; Schuur, J.D. Clinical Guidelines Committee of the American College of Physicians. Evaluation of Patients with Suspected Acute Pulmonary Embolism: Best Practice Advice from the Clinical Guidelines Committee of the American College of Physicians. *Ann. Intern. Med.* **2015**, *163*, 701–711. [CrossRef]
39. Coutance, G.; Le Page, O.; Lo, T.; Hamon, M. Prognostic value of brain natriuretic peptide in acute pulmonary embolism. *Crit. Care* **2008**, *12*, R109. [CrossRef]
40. Horlander, K.T.; Leeper, K.V. Troponin levels as a guide to treatment of pulmonary embolism. *Curr. Opin. Pulm. Med.* **2003**, *9*, 374–377. [CrossRef]
41. Bajaj, A.; Saleeb, M.; Rathor, P.; Sehgal, V.; Kabak, B.; Hosur, S. Prognostic value of troponins in acute nonmassive pulmonary embolism: A meta-analysis. *Heart Lung* **2015**, *44*, 327–334. [CrossRef]
42. Coutance, G.; Cauderlier, E.; Ehtisham, J.; Hamon, M.; Hamon, M. The prognostic value of markers of right ventricular dysfunction in pulmonary embolism: A meta-analysis. *Crit. Care* **2011**, *15*, R103. [CrossRef]
43. Lega, J.C.; Lacasse, Y.; Lakhal, L.; Provencher, S. Natriuretic peptides and troponins in pulmonary embolism: A meta-analysis. *Thorax* **2009**, *64*, 869–875. [CrossRef]
44. Jaff, M.R.; McMurtry, M.S.; Archer, S.L.; Cushman, M.; Goldenberg, N.; Goldhaber, S.Z.; Jenkins, J.S.; Kline, J.A.; Michaels, A.D.; Thistlethwaite, P.; et al. Management of massive and submassive pulmonary embolism, iliofemoral deep vein thrombosis, and chronic thromboembolic pulmonary hypertension: A scientific statement from the American Heart Association. *Circulation* **2011**, *123*, 1788–1830, Erratum in *Circulation* **2012**, *126*, e104; Erratum in *Circulation* **2012**, *125*, e495. [CrossRef]
45. El-Menyar, A.; Sathian, B.; Al-Thani, H. Elevated serum cardiac troponin and mortality in acute pulmonary embolism: Systematic review and meta-analysis. *Respir. Med.* **2019**, *157*, 26–35. [CrossRef]
46. Becattini, C.; Vedovati, M.C.; Agnelli, G. Prognostic value of troponins in acute pulmonary embolism: A meta-analysis. *Circulation* **2007**, *116*, 427–433. [CrossRef]
47. Darwish, O.S.; Mahayni, A.; Patel, M.; Amin, A. Cardiac Troponins in Low-Risk Pulmonary Embolism Patients: A Systematic Review and Meta-Analysis. *J. Hosp. Med.* **2018**, *13*, 509, Erratum in *J. Hosp. Med.* **2018**, *13*, 706–712. [CrossRef]

48. Karolak, B.; Ciurzyński, M.; Skowrońska, M.; Kurnicka, K.; Pływaczewska, M.; Furdyna, A.; Perzanowska-Brzeszkiewicz, K.; Lichodziejewska, B.; Pacho, S.; Machowski, M.; et al. Plasma Troponins Identify Patients with Very Low-Risk Acute Pulmonary Embolism. *J. Clin. Med.* **2023**, *12*, 1276. [CrossRef]
49. Righini, M.; Goehring, C.; Bounameaux, H.; Perrier, A. Effects of age on the performance of common diagnostic tests for pulmonary embolism. *Am. J. Med.* **2000**, *109*, 357–361. [CrossRef]
50. Righini, M.; Van Es, J.; Den Exter, P.L.; Roy, P.M.; Verschuren, F.; Ghuysen, A.; Rutschmann, O.T.; Sanchez, O.; Jaffrelot, M.; Trinh-Duc, A.; et al. Age-adjusted D-dimer cutoff levels to rule out pulmonary embolism: The ADJUST-PE study. *JAMA* **2014**, *311*, 1117–1124, Erratum in *JAMA* **2014**, *311*, 1694. [CrossRef]
51. van der Hulle, T.; Cheung, W.Y.; Kooij, S.; Beenen, L.F.M.; van Bemmel, T.; van Es, J.; Faber, L.M.; Hazelaar, G.M.; Heringhaus, C.; Hofstee, H.; et al. Simplified diagnostic management of suspected pulmonary embolism (the YEARS study): A prospective, multicentre, cohort study. *Lancet* **2017**, *390*, 289–297, Erratum in *Lancet* **2017**, *390*, 230. [CrossRef]
52. Righini, M.; Le Gal, G.; De Lucia, S.; Roy, P.M.; Meyer, G.; Aujesky, D.; Bounameaux, H.; Perrier, A. Clinical usefulness of D-dimer testing in cancer patients with suspected pulmonary embolism. *Thromb. Haemost.* **2006**, *95*, 715–719.
53. Di Nisio, M.; Sohne, M.; Kamphuisen, P.W.; Büller, H.R. D-Dimer test in cancer patients with suspected acute pulmonary embolism. *J. Thromb. Haemost.* **2005**, *3*, 1239–1242. [CrossRef]
54. Sosa Lozano, L.A.; Goodman, L.R.; Shahir, K. Pulmonary embolism: Optimizing the diagnostic imaging approach. *Hosp. Pract.* **2010**, *38*, 153–162. [CrossRef] [PubMed]
55. Geersing, G.J.; Erkens, P.M.; Lucassen, W.A.; Büller, H.R.; Cate, H.T.; Hoes, A.W.; Moons, K.G.; Prins, M.H.; Oudega, R.; van Weert, H.C.; et al. Safe exclusion of pulmonary embolism using the Wells rule and qualitative D-dimer testing in primary care: Prospective cohort study. *BMJ* **2012**, *345*, e6564. [CrossRef]
56. Miron, M.J.; Perrier, A.; Bounameaux, H.; de Moerloose, P.; Slosman, D.O.; Didier, D.; Junod, A. Contribution of noninvasive evaluation to the diagnosis of pulmonary embolism in hospitalized patients. *Eur. Respir. J.* **1999**, *13*, 1365–1370. [CrossRef]
57. Paparoupa, M.; Spineli, L.; Framke, T.; Ho, H.; Schuppert, F.; Gillissen, A. Pulmonary Embolism in Pneumonia: Still a Diagnostic Challenge? Results of a Case-Control Study in 100 Patients. *Dis. Markers* **2016**, *2016*, 8682506. [CrossRef]
58. McFarlane, M.J.; Imperiale, T.F. Use of the alveolar-arterial oxygen gradient in the diagnosis of pulmonary embolism. *Am. J. Med.* **1994**, *96*, 57–62. [CrossRef] [PubMed]
59. Cvitanic, O.; Marino, P.L. Improved use of arterial blood gas analysis in suspected pulmonary embolism. *Chest* **1989**, *95*, 48–51. [CrossRef]
60. Rodger, M.A.; Carrier, M.; Jones, G.N.; Rasuli, P.; Raymond, F.; Djunaedi, H.; Wells, P.S. Diagnostic value of arterial blood gas measurement in suspected pulmonary embolism. *Am. J. Respir. Crit. Care Med.* **2000**, *162*, 2105–2108. [CrossRef]
61. Stein, P.D.; Goldhaber, S.Z.; Henry, J.W.; Miller, A.C. Arterial blood gas analysis in the assessment of suspected acute pulmonary embolism. *Chest* **1996**, *109*, 78–81. [CrossRef]
62. Kiely, D.G.; Kennedy, N.S.; Pirzada, O.; Batchelor, S.A.; Struthers, A.D.; Lipworth, B.J. Elevated levels of natriuretic peptides in patients with pulmonary thromboembolism. *Respir. Med.* **2005**, *99*, 1286–1291. [CrossRef]
63. Henzler, T.; Roeger, S.; Meyer, M.; Schoepf, U.J.; Nance, J.W., Jr.; Haghi, D.; Kaminski, W.E.; Neumaier, M.; Schoenberg, S.O.; Fink, C. Pulmonary embolism: CT signs and cardiac biomarkers for predicting right ventricular dysfunction. *Eur. Respir. J.* **2012**, *39*, 919–926. [CrossRef]
64. Kucher, N.; Printzen, G.; Goldhaber, S.Z. Prognostic role of brain natriuretic peptide in acute pulmonary embolism. *Circulation* **2003**, *107*, 2545–2547. [CrossRef]
65. Bělohlávek, J.; Dytrych, V.; Linhart, A. Pulmonary embolism, part I: Epidemiology, risk factors and risk stratification, pathophysiology, clinical presentation, diagnosis and nonthrombotic pulmonary embolism. *Exp. Clin. Cardiol.* **2013**, *18*, 129–138.
66. Smithline, H. Use of natriuretic peptides in guiding treatment decisions for acute pulmonary embolism. *Circulation* **2003**, *108*, e93. [CrossRef]
67. Ballas, C.; Lakkas, L.; Kardakari, O.; Konstantinidis, A.; Exarchos, K.; Tsiara, S.; Kostikas, K.; Naka, K.K.; Michalis, L.K.; Katsouras, C.S. What is the real incidence of right ventricular affection in patients with acute pulmonary embolism? *Acta Cardiol.* **2023**, *78*, 1089–1098. [CrossRef]
68. Meyer, T.; Binder, L.; Hruska, N.; Luthe, H.; Buchwald, A.B. Cardiac troponin I elevation in acute pulmonary embolism is associated with right ventricular dysfunction. *J. Am. Coll. Cardiol.* **2000**, *36*, 1632–1636. [CrossRef]
69. Vanni, S.; Viviani, G.; Baioni, M.; Pepe, G.; Nazerian, P.; Socci, F.; Bartolucci, M.; Bartolini, M.; Grifoni, S. Prognostic value of plasma lactate levels among patients with acute pulmonary embolism: The thrombo-embolism lactate outcome study. *Ann. Emerg. Med.* **2013**, *61*, 330–338. [CrossRef]
70. Vanni, S.; Jiménez, D.; Nazerian, P.; Morello, F.; Parisi, M.; Daghini, E.; Pratesi, M.; López, R.; Bedate, P.; Lobo, J.L.; et al. Short-term clinical outcome of normotensive patients with acute PE and high plasma lactate. *Thorax* **2015**, *70*, 333–338. [CrossRef]
71. Provias, T.; Dudzinski, D.M.; Jaff, M.R.; Rosenfield, K.; Channick, R.; Baker, J.; Weinberg, I.; Donaldson, C.; Narayan, R.; Rassi, A.N.; et al. The Massachusetts General Hospital Pulmonary Embolism Response Team (MGH PERT): Creation of a multidisciplinary program to improve care of patients with massive and submassive pulmonary embolism. *Hosp. Pract.* **2014**, *42*, 31–37. [CrossRef]

72. Kabrhel, C.; Rosovsky, R.; Channick, R.; Jaff, M.R.; Weinberg, I.; Sundt, T.; Dudzinski, D.M.; Rodriguez-Lopez, J.; Parry, B.A.; Harshbarger, S.; et al. A Multidisciplinary Pulmonary Embolism Response Team: Initial 30-Month Experience with a Novel Approach to Delivery of Care to Patients With Submassive and Massive Pulmonary Embolism. *Chest* **2016**, *150*, 384–393. [CrossRef]
73. Rosovsky, R.; Chang, Y.; Rosenfield, K.; Channick, R.; Jaff, M.R.; Weinberg, I.; Sundt, T.; Witkin, A.; Rodriguez-Lopez, J.; Parry, B.A.; et al. Changes in treatment and outcomes after creation of a pulmonary embolism response team (PERT), a 10-year analysis. *J. Thromb. Thrombolysis* **2018**, *47*, 41, Erratum in *J. Thromb. Thrombolysis* **2019**, *47*, 31–40. [CrossRef]
74. Mahar, J.H.; Haddadin, I.; Sadana, D.; Gadre, A.; Evans, N.; Hornacek, D.; Mahlay, N.F.; Gomes, M.; Joseph, D.; Serhal, M.; et al. A pulmonary embolism response team (PERT) approach: Initial experience from the Cleveland Clinic. *J. Thromb. Thrombolysis* **2018**, *46*, 186–192. [CrossRef] [PubMed]
75. Chaudhury, P.; Gadre, S.K.; Schneider, E.; Renapurkar, R.D.; Gomes, M.; Haddadin, I.; Heresi, G.A.; Tong, M.Z.; Bartholomew, J.R. Impact of Multidisciplinary Pulmonary Embolism Response Team Availability on Management and Outcomes. *Am. J. Cardiol.* **2019**, *124*, 1465–1469. [CrossRef] [PubMed]
76. Shopp, J.D.; Stewart, L.K.; Emmett, T.W.; Kline, J.A. Findings From 12-lead Electrocardiography That Predict Circulatory Shock from Pulmonary Embolism: Systematic Review and Meta-analysis. *Acad. Emerg. Med.* **2015**, *22*, 1127–1137. [CrossRef] [PubMed]
77. Elliott, C.G.; Goldhaber, S.Z.; Visani, L.; DeRosa, M. Chest radiographs in acute pulmonary embolism. Results from the International Cooperative Pulmonary Embolism Registry. *Chest* **2000**, *118*, 33–38. [CrossRef] [PubMed]
78. Stein, P.D.; Fowler, S.E.; Goodman, L.R.; Gottschalk, A.; Hales, C.A.; Hull, R.D.; Leeper, K.V., Jr.; Popovich, J., Jr.; Quinn, D.A.; Sos, T.A.; et al. PIOPED II Investigators. Multidetector computed tomography for acute pulmonary embolism. *N. Engl. J. Med.* **2006**, *354*, 2317–2327. [CrossRef] [PubMed]
79. Wittram, C. How I do it: CT pulmonary angiography. *AJR Am. J. Roentgenol.* **2007**, *188*, 1255–1261. [CrossRef]
80. Hunsaker, A.R.; Zou, K.H.; Poh, A.C.; Trotman-Dickenson, B.; Jacobson, F.L.; Gill, R.R.; Goldhaber, S.Z. Routine pelvic and lower extremity CT venography in patients undergoing pulmonary CT angiography. *AJR Am. J. Roentgenol.* **2008**, *190*, 322–326. [CrossRef]
81. Ghaye, B.; Szapiro, D.; Mastora, I.; Delannoy, V.; Duhamel, A.; Remy, J.; Remy-Jardin, M. Peripheral pulmonary arteries: How far in the lung does multi-detector row spiral CT allow analysis? *Radiology* **2001**, *219*, 629–636. [CrossRef]
82. Carrier, M.; Righini, M.; Wells, P.S.; Perrier, A.; Anderson, D.R.; Rodger, M.A.; Pleasance, S.; Le Gal, G. Subsegmental pulmonary embolism diagnosed by computed tomography: Incidence and clinical implications. A systematic review and meta-analysis of the management outcome studies. *J. Thromb. Haemost.* **2010**, *8*, 1716–1722. [CrossRef]
83. Stein, P.D.; Matta, F.; Gerstner, B.J.; Kakish, E.J.; Hughes, P.G.; Lata, J.; Trigger, C.C.; Jutzy, K.A.; Doyle, M.Q.; Warpinski, M.A.; et al. Ancillary Findings on CT Pulmonary Angiograms that are Negative for Pulmonary Embolism. *Spartan. Med. Res. J.* **2020**, *4*, 11769. [CrossRef]
84. Reid, J.H.; Coche, E.E.; Inoue, T.; Kim, E.E.; Dondi, M.; Watanabe, N.; Mariani, G. International Atomic Energy Agency Consultants' Group. Is the lung scan alive and well? Facts and controversies in defining the role of lung scintigraphy for the diagnosis of pulmonary embolism in the era of MDCT. *Eur. J. Nucl. Med. Mol. Imaging* **2009**, *36*, 505–521. [CrossRef]
85. Sostman, H.D.; Coleman, R.E.; DeLong, D.M.; Newman, G.E.; Paine, S. Evaluation of revised criteria for ventilation-perfusion scintigraphy in patients with suspected pulmonary embolism. *Radiology* **1994**, *193*, 103–107. [CrossRef]
86. Anderson, D.R.; Kahn, S.R.; Rodger, M.A.; Kovacs, M.J.; Morris, T.; Hirsch, A.; Lang, E.; Stiell, I.; Kovacs, G.; Dreyer, J.; et al. Computed tomographic pulmonary angiography vs ventilation-perfusion lung scanning in patients with suspected pulmonary embolism: A randomized controlled trial. *JAMA* **2007**, *298*, 2743–2753. [CrossRef] [PubMed]
87. van Es, J.; Douma, R.A.; Hezemans, R.E.; Penaloza, A.; Motte, S.; Erkens, P.G.; Durian, M.F.; van Eck-Smit, B.L.; Kamphuisen, P.W. Accuracy of X-ray with perfusion scan in young patients with suspected pulmonary embolism. *Thromb. Res.* **2015**, *136*, 221–224. [CrossRef]
88. Bajc, M.; Olsson, B.; Palmer, J.; Jonson, B. Ventilation/Perfusion SPECT for diagnostics of pulmonary embolism in clinical practice. *J. Intern. Med.* **2008**, *264*, 379–387. [CrossRef]
89. Gutte, H.; Mortensen, J.; Jensen, C.V.; Johnbeck, C.B.; von der Recke, P.; Petersen, C.L.; Kjaergaard, J.; Kristoffersen, U.S.; Kjaer, A. Detection of pulmonary embolism with combined ventilation-perfusion SPECT and low-dose CT: Head-to-head comparison with multidetector CT angiography. *J. Nucl. Med.* **2009**, *50*, 1987–1992. [CrossRef]
90. Simanek, M.; Koranda, P. The benefit of personalized hybrid SPECT/CT pulmonary imaging. *Am. J. Nucl. Med. Mol. Imaging* **2016**, *6*, 215–222. [PubMed]
91. Revel, M.P.; Sanchez, O.; Couchon, S.; Planquette, B.; Hernigou, A.; Niarra, R.; Meyer, G.; Chatellier, G. Diagnostic accuracy of magnetic resonance imaging for an acute pulmonary embolism: Results of the 'IRM-EP' study. *J. Thromb. Haemost.* **2012**, *10*, 743–750. [CrossRef] [PubMed]
92. Desai, D.H.; Shah, A.; Shah, H.; Naik, A.A.; Sadat, S.M.; Raval, D. Diagnostic accuracy of MRI compared to CTPA for Pulmonary Embolism: A meta analysis. *medRxiv* **2023**. [CrossRef]

93. Stein, P.D.; Chenevert, T.L.; Fowler, S.E.; Goodman, L.R.; Gottschalk, A.; Hales, C.A.; Hull, R.D.; Jablonski, K.A.; Leeper, K.V., Jr.; Naidich, D.P.; et al. PIOPED III (Prospective Investigation of Pulmonary Embolism Diagnosis III) Investigators. Gadolinium-enhanced magnetic resonance angiography for pulmonary embolism: A multicenter prospective study (PIOPED III). *Ann. Intern. Med.* **2010**, *152*, W142–W143. [CrossRef]
94. Stein, P.D.; Henry, J.W.; Gottschalk, A. Reassessment of pulmonary angiography for the diagnosis of pulmonary embolism: Relation of interpreter agreement to the order of the involved pulmonary arterial branch. *Radiology* **1999**, *210*, 689–691. [CrossRef] [PubMed]
95. Diffin, D.C.; Leyendecker, J.R.; Johnson, S.P.; Zucker, R.J.; Grebe, P.J. Effect of anatomic distribution of pulmonary emboli on interobserver agreement in the interpretation of pulmonary angiography. *AJR Am. J. Roentgenol.* **1998**, *171*, 1085–1089. [CrossRef]
96. Stein, P.D.; Athanasoulis, C.; Alavi, A.; Greenspan, R.H.; Hales, C.A.; Saltzman, H.A.; Vreim, C.E.; Terrin, M.L.; Weg, J.G. Complications and validity of pulmonary angiography in acute pulmonary embolism. *Circulation* **1992**, *85*, 462–468. [CrossRef]
97. Platz, E.; Hassanein, A.H.; Shah, A.; Goldhaber, S.Z.; Solomon, S.D. Regional right ventricular strain pattern in patients with acute pulmonary embolism. *Echocardiography* **2012**, *29*, 464–470. [CrossRef]
98. Pruszczyk, P.; Kostrubiec, M.; Bochowicz, A.; Styczyński, G.; Szulc, M.; Kurzyna, M.; Fijałkowska, A.; Kuch-Wocial, A.; Chlewicka, I.; Torbicki, A. N-terminal pro-brain natriuretic peptide in patients with acute pulmonary embolism. *Eur. Respir. J.* **2003**, *22*, 649–653. [CrossRef]
99. Kurzyna, M.; Torbicki, A.; Pruszczyk, P.; Burakowska, B.; Fijałkowska, A.; Kober, J.; Oniszh, K.; Kuca, P.; Tomkowski, W.; Burakowski, J.; et al. Disturbed right ventricular ejection pattern as a new Doppler echocardiographic sign of acute pulmonary embolism. *Am. J. Cardiol.* **2002**, *90*, 507–511. [CrossRef] [PubMed]
100. Casazza, F.; Bongarzoni, A.; Capozi, A.; Agostoni, O. Regional right ventricular dysfunction in acute pulmonary embolism and right ventricular infarction. *Eur. J. Echocardiogr.* **2005**, *6*, 11–14. [CrossRef]
101. Pruszczyk, P.; Goliszek, S.; Lichodziejewska, B.; Kostrubiec, M.; Ciurzyński, M.; Kurnicka, K.; Dzikowska-Diduch, O.; Palczewski, P.; Wyzgal, A. Prognostic value of echocardiography in normotensive patients with acute pulmonary embolism. *JACC Cardiovasc. Imaging* **2014**, *7*, 553–560. [CrossRef] [PubMed]
102. Takahiro, S. Two-Dimensional and Three-Dimensional Echocardiographic Evaluation of the Right Ventricle. In *Advanced Approaches in Echocardiography*; WB Saunders: Philadelphia, PA, USA, 2012.
103. McConnell, M.V.; Solomon, S.D.; Rayan, M.E.; Come, P.C.; Goldhaber, S.Z.; Lee, R.T. Regional right ventricular dysfunction detected by echocardiography in acute pulmonary embolism. *Am. J. Cardiol.* **1996**, *78*, 469–473. [CrossRef]
104. Fields, J.M.; Davis, J.; Girson, L.; Au, A.; Potts, J.; Morgan, C.J.; Vetter, I.; Riesenberg, L.A. Transthoracic Echocardiography for Diagnosing Pulmonary Embolism: A Systematic Review and Meta-Analysis. *J. Am. Soc. Echocardiogr.* **2017**, *30*, 714–723.e4. [CrossRef]
105. Dresden, S.; Mitchell, P.; Rahimi, L.; Leo, M.; Rubin-Smith, J.; Bibi, S.; White, L.; Langlois, B.; Sullivan, A.; Carmody, K. Right ventricular dilatation on bedside echocardiography performed by emergency physicians aids in the diagnosis of pulmonary embolism. *Ann. Emerg. Med.* **2014**, *63*, 16–24. [CrossRef] [PubMed]
106. Jung, I.H.; Seo, H.S.; Kim, M.J. P569Diastolic dyssynchrony is associated with exercise intolerance in hypertensive patients with left ventricular hypertrophy. *Eur. Heart J. Cardiovasc. Imaging* **2016**, *17* (Suppl. 2), ii102–ii109. [CrossRef] [PubMed]
107. Kurnicka, K.; Lichodziejewska, B.; Goliszek, S.; Dzikowska-Diduch, O.; Zdończyk, O.; Kozłowska, M.; Kostrubiec, M.; Ciurzyński, M.; Palczewski, P.; Grudzka, K.; et al. Echocardiographic Pattern of Acute Pulmonary Embolism: Analysis of 511 Consecutive Patients. *J. Am. Soc. Echocardiogr.* **2016**, *29*, 907–913. [CrossRef] [PubMed]
108. Burgos, L.M.; Scatularo, C.E.; Cigalini, I.M.; Jauregui, J.C.; Bernal, M.I.; Bonorino, J.M.; Thierer, J.; Zaidel, E.J. Argentine Council of Cardiology Residents, Argentina. The addition of echocardiographic parameters to PESI risk score improves mortality prediction in patients with acute pulmonary embolism: PESI-Echo score. *Eur. Heart J Acute Cardiovasc. Care* **2021**, *10*, 250–257. [CrossRef] [PubMed]
109. Koć, M.; Kostrubiec, M.; Elikowski, W.; Meneveau, N.; Lankeit, M.; Grifoni, S.; Kuch-Wocial, A.; Petris, A.; Zaborska, B.; Stefanović, B.S.; et al. RiHTER Investigators. Outcome of patients with right heart thrombi: The Right Heart Thrombi European Registry. *Eur. Respir. J.* **2016**, *47*, 869–875. [CrossRef] [PubMed]
110. Ribeiro, A. The Role of Echocardiography Doppler in Pulmonary Embolism. *Echocardiography* **1998**, *15* Pt 1, 769–778. [CrossRef] [PubMed]
111. Squizzato, A.; Galli, L.; Gerdes, V.E. Point-of-care ultrasound in the diagnosis of pulmonary embolism. *Crit. Ultrasound. J.* **2015**, *7*, 7. [CrossRef] [PubMed]
112. Nazerian, P.; Volpicelli, G.; Gigli, C.; Lamorte, A.; Grifoni, S.; Vanni, S. Diagnostic accuracy of focused cardiac and venous ultrasound examinations in patients with shock and suspected pulmonary embolism. *Intern. Emerg. Med.* **2018**, *13*, 567–574. [CrossRef]
113. Da Costa Rodrigues, J.; Alzuphar, S.; Combescure, C.; Le Gal, G.; Perrier, A. Diagnostic characteristics of lower limb venous compression ultrasonography in suspected pulmonary embolism: A meta-analysis. *J. Thromb. Haemost.* **2016**, *14*, 1765–1772. [CrossRef]

114. Rouleau, S.G.; Casey, S.D.; Kabrhel, C.; Vinson, D.R.; Long, B. Management of high-risk pulmonary embolism in the emergency department: A narrative review. *Am. J. Emerg. Med.* **2024**, *79*, 1–11. [CrossRef]
115. Becher, M.; Heller, T.; Schwarzenböck, S.; Kröger, J.C.; Weber, M.A.; Meinel, F.G. Negative Venous Leg Ultrasound in Acute Pulmonary Embolism: Prevalence, Clinical Characteristics and Predictors. *Diagnostics* **2022**, *12*, 520. [CrossRef] [PubMed]

Disclaimer/Publisher's Note: The statements, opinions and data contained in all publications are solely those of the individual author(s) and contributor(s) and not of MDPI and/or the editor(s). MDPI and/or the editor(s) disclaim responsibility for any injury to people or property resulting from any ideas, methods, instructions or products referred to in the content.

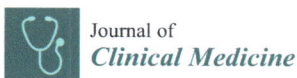 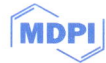

Review

A Comprehensive Review of Risk Factors and Thrombophilia Evaluation in Venous Thromboembolism

Andrew B. Dicks [1,*], Elie Moussallem [1], Marcus Stanbro [1], Jay Walls [2], Sagar Gandhi [1] and Bruce H. Gray [1]

1. Department of Vascular Surgery, Prisma Health, University of South Carolina School of Medicine—Greenville, Greenville, SC 29601, USA; elie.moussallem@prismahealth.org (E.M.); marcus.stanbro@prismahealth.org (M.S.); sagar.gandhi@prismahealth.org (S.G.); bgray71357@gmail.com (B.H.G.)
2. Department of Hematology, Prisma Health, University of South Carolina School of Medicine—Greenville, Greenville, SC 29601, USA; jay.walls@prismahealth.org
* Correspondence: andrew.dicks@prismahealth.org; Tel.: +1-864-454-8272; Fax: +1-864-454-2875

Abstract: Venous thromboembolism (VTE), which encompasses deep vein thrombosis (DVT) and pulmonary embolism (PE), is a significant cause of morbidity and mortality worldwide. There are many factors, both acquired and inherited, known to increase the risk of VTE. Most of these result in increased risk via several common mechanisms including circulatory stasis, endothelial damage, or increased hypercoagulability. Overall, a risk factor can be identified in the majority of patients with VTE; however, not all risk factors carry the same predictive value. It is important for clinicians to understand the potency of each individual risk factor when managing patients who have a VTE or are at risk of developing VTE. With this, many providers consider performing a thrombophilia evaluation to further define a patient's risk. However, guidance on who to test and when to test is controversial and not always clear. This comprehensive review attempts to address these aspects/concerns by providing an overview of the multifaceted risk factors associated with VTE as well as examining the role of performing a thrombophilia evaluation, including the indications and timing of performing such an evaluation.

Keywords: deep vein thrombosis; pulmonary embolism; venous thromboembolism; risk factors; thrombophilia

Citation: Dicks, A.B.; Moussallem, E.; Stanbro, M.; Walls, J.; Gandhi, S.; Gray, B.H. A Comprehensive Review of Risk Factors and Thrombophilia Evaluation in Venous Thromboembolism. *J. Clin. Med.* **2024**, *13*, 362. https://doi.org/10.3390/jcm13020362

Academic Editor: Raimondo De Cristofaro

Received: 15 December 2023
Revised: 29 December 2023
Accepted: 5 January 2024
Published: 9 January 2024

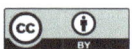

Copyright: © 2024 by the authors. Licensee MDPI, Basel, Switzerland. This article is an open access article distributed under the terms and conditions of the Creative Commons Attribution (CC BY) license (https://creativecommons.org/licenses/by/4.0/).

1. Introduction

Venous thromboembolism (VTE) is a potentially life-threatening condition characterized by the formation of blood clots in deep veins, leading to deep vein thrombosis (DVT) and the potential for pulmonary embolism (PE). VTE is a complex and multifactorial disorder influenced by a wide range of risk factors. A major theory describing the pathogenesis of VTE is Virchow's triad which consists of the stasis of blood flow, vascular endothelial injury, and hypercoagulability [1]. With this, most identified risk factors for the development of VTE have at least one element of Virchow's triad.

Overall, a risk factor can be identified in the majority of patients with VTE, with the most commonly identified factors including age > 40, obesity, a personal history of VTE, and cancer [2]. These risk factors may be permanent, such as related to patients' characteristics, or transient, such as acute clinical condition. Evidence demonstrates that the VTE risk increases proportionally to the number of predisposing risk factors [2]. Understanding the risk factors associated with VTE is important for understanding a patient's risk of VTE development and recurrence, and thus guides providers on the best management strategies moving forward. Importantly, risk factors do not carry an equal risk of VTE development (Table 1) [2,3]. As such, physicians should consider both the strength of each individual risk factor as well as the cumulative impact of all risk factors in determining the type and duration of appropriate prophylaxis. During this evaluation, thrombophilia testing is often considered. Although these tests are readily available, it can be challenging to determine who would benefit from a thrombophilia evaluation and how the testing results will change clinical management.

Table 1. Predisposing risk factors for venous thromboembolism [2,3].

Strong Risk Factors (OR < 10)
• Fracture of lower limb;   • Hospitalization for heart failure or atrial fibrillation/flutter (within previous 3 months);   • Hip or knee replacement;   • Major trauma;   • Myocardial infarction (within previous 3 months);   • Previous VTE;   • Spinal cord injury.
Moderate risk factors (OR 2–9)
• Arthroscopic knee surgery;   • Autoimmune diseases;   • Blood transfusion;   • Central venous lines;   • Intravenous catheters and leads;   • Chemotherapy;   • Congestive heart failure or respiratory failure;   • Erythropoiesis-stimulating agents;   • Hormone replacement therapy (depends on formulation);   • In vitro fertilization;   • Oral contraceptive therapy;   • Post-partum period;   • Infection (specifically pneumonia, urinary tract infection, or HIV);   • Inflammatory bowel disease;   • Cancer (highest risk in metastatic disease);   • Paralytic stroke;   • Superficial vein thrombosis;   • Thrombophilia.
Weak risk factors (OR < 2)
• Bed rest > 3 days;   • Diabetes mellitus;   • Arterial hypertension;   • Immobility due to sitting (i.e., prolonged car or air travel);   • Increasing age;   • Laparoscope surgery (i.e., cholecystectomy);   • Obesity;   • Pregnancy;   • Varicose veins.

VTE—venous thromboembolism; OR—odds ratio; HIV—human immunodeficiency virus.

This review aims to provide an extensive exploration of these risk factors, encompassing both acquired and modifiable risk factors as well as inherited risk factors, as well as review the indications and timing for thrombophilia evaluation.

1.1. Acquired and Modifiable Risk Factors
1.1.1. Previous VTE

Individuals with a history of VTE are at an increased risk of recurrent thrombosis. A prospective cohort of 355 patients reported an incidence of recurrent VTE at 17.5% after two years of follow up, 24.6% after four years, and 30.3% after eight years [4]. Likewise, in a large observational study of 1231 patients with VTE, 19% of the patients reported at least one prior clinically recognized VTE event [5]. However, the risk of recurrence is highly dependent upon patient-specific factors. Patients with a history of VTE in the setting of a transient, reversible risk factor (i.e., immobilization or surgery) have a lower rate of recurrence compared to those with no known risk factors (i.e., unprovoked) or with permanent risk factors (i.e., malignancy). In the study noted above, the presence of cancer was associated with an increased risk of recurrent VTE (hazard ratio (HR) 1.72) while surgery and recent trauma or fracture were associated with a decreased risk of recurrent VTE (HR 0.36) [4]. Similarly, a prospective cohort study of 570 patients followed over 2 years noted zero recurrence of VTE in those whose first VTE occurred within six weeks of surgery compared to 19.4% recurrence in those whose first VTE had no identifiable clinical risk factors [6]. As such, while a previous VTE is a risk factor for a future VTE, the ultimate risk is highly dependent on patient-specific factors, which are further outlined below.

1.1.2. Family History of VTE

Similar to a personal history of VTE, a family history of VTE has also been identified as a risk factor for VTE development. A large national cohort study noted that having a sibling with a history of VTE incurred a relative risk (RR) of 3.08 for developing a VTE event compared to the general population [7]. It appears that the risk increases based on the number of family members with a prior VTE. In a case–control study of 505 patients, a positive family increased the risk of VTE more than 2-fold (odds ratio (OR) 2.2), with the risk increasing up to 4-fold (OR 3.9) when more than one relative has a history of VTE [8]. Interestingly, this study also noted that those with hereditary thrombophilia and a family history of VTE had a higher risk of VTE compared to those with heredity thrombophilia and no family history. Specifically, in those with a factor V Leiden mutation, a positive family history of VTE incurred a 2.9-fold higher risk compared to a negative family history [8]. These findings underscore that there are likely other inherited thrombophilias present that have yet to be discovered.

1.1.3. Immobility

Prolonged periods of immobility, such as postoperative bed rest, paralysis, hospitalization, or long-haul travel, are well-established risk factors for VTE. Immobility leads to venous stasis, particularly in the legs, which promotes thrombosis. A prior autopsy study noted that 15% of patients on bed rest for less than one week before death were found to have a venous thrombosis, with the incidence increasing to 80% for those in bed for a longer period [9]. Likewise, in a large international registry, chronically immobile elderly patients were noted to have an increased risk of recurrent VTE [10]. As immobility can be caused by numerous different factors, the risk of VTE ultimately depends on the cause and length of immobility.

The risk of VTE after an acute cerebrovascular accident (CVA) resulting in paralysis is quite high. The current rates of symptomatic VTE in patients with acute CVA ranges from 1–10%, whereas asymptomatic VTE is even higher, with a report of 11% at 10 days post CVA and 15% at 30 days post CVA [11–13]. Likewise, the rates of DVT within 3 months of paralytic spinal cord injury are also high, with the reported incidence of DVT being greater than 30% in those who are screened for DVT [14,15]. The risk of VTE development after spinal cord injury appears to be greatest during the first two weeks after injury, with fatal PE being rare beyond 3 months after injury [2]. Interestingly, chronic immobility in the setting of CVA or spinal cord injury does not appear to confer the same degree of risk as acute immobility. This difference is likely due to the physiologic changes that occur with chronic immobility, including leg muscle atrophy and changes in venous anatomy [2].

Transient immobility both during hospitalization and upon discharge to home or rehabilitation facility also represents an important risk factor for VTE. In addition to venous stasis due to immobility, acute illness can increase the risk of VTE due to increased alterations in the hypercoagulable state and damage to endothelial cells in the setting of increased inflammation. Common medical illnesses associated with VTE in hospitalized patients include infection, CVA, inflammatory bowel disease, and autoimmune diseases [16]. When compared to patients in the community, those hospitalized for any reason appear to have a 100 times greater incidence of VTE [17]. Likewise, factors associated with institutionalization, defined as current or recent hospitalization within the past three months or being a nursing home resident, independently account for over 50% of all cases of VTE in the community [18].

Prolonged travel, including in the car and by air, also appears to confer an increased risk of VTE. A meta-analysis of 14 studies noted that the pooled RR for VTE in travelers was as high as 2.8 [19]. Additionally, there was a dose–response relationship identified with an 18% higher risk for VTE for each 2 h increase in the duration of travel by any mode and a 26% higher risk for every 2 h of air travel.

Lastly, prolonged sitting such as at a computer for a prolonged period also appears to confer an increased risk. In a series of patients admitted for DVT/PE, 34% reported seated immobility for a prolonged period of time (8–12 h) at work [20].

1.1.4. Surgery

Surgical procedures have long been associated with an increased risk of VTE, as surgery can result in damage to blood vessels, activation of the coagulation cascade, and venous stasis due to immobility, both during the surgery and in the post-operative period. However, not all surgery carries the same risk of VTE, with thrombotic risk being the highest amongst orthopedic, major vascular, neurosurgery, and cancer surgery. Hip and knee arthroplasty are considered amongst the highest-risk surgeries for VTE development. Initial reports have demonstrated that the VTE incidence is as high as 30% in patients undergoing major orthopedic surgery who were not receiving thromboprophylaxis [21]. However, during more recent studies, where anticoagulation was used for VTE prophylaxis, the incidence is much lower, typically less than 5% [22,23]. The American College of Chest Physicians (ACCP) estimates the baseline perioperative, 35-day risk at 4.3% after major orthopedic surgery, with the risk highest within the first 7–14 days [24]. As such, several guidelines, including the International Consensus Meeting on VTE in 2022 (Strength of Recommendation: Strong), the American Society of Hematology in 2019 (conditional recommendation based on very low certainty), and the National Institute for Health and Care Excellence (NICE) in 2018, recommend the use of chemoprophylaxis for the prevention of VTE in this patient population [25–27].

In non-orthopedic surgery, open abdominal and open pelvic surgery, particularly for those associated with cancer, are also considered high risk [28,29]. Neurosurgical interventions have also reported increased rates of VTE, with a meta-analysis reporting approximately one in four patients developing VTE after neurosurgery [30,31]. Other surgeries reporting an elevated risk of VTE in the post-operative setting include coronary artery bypass, major urologic surgery, thoracic surgery, and bariatric surgery [32–34].

In contrast, laparoscopic surgery does not appear to confer the same degree of risk compared to open surgery. A retrospective study of 750,159 patients demonstrated an incidence of VTE of 0.32% within 30 days of abdominal laparoscopic surgery, with the highest incidence among patients undergoing colorectal surgery at 1.12% [35]. Similarly, another retrospective study of over 138,595 patients demonstrated that the incidence of VTE among patients undergoing laparoscopic surgery was lower compared to those undergoing open surgery (0.28% versus 0.59%, respectively) [36].

1.1.5. Trauma

Trauma resulting in fracture and severe injury elevates the risk of VTE, often due to blood stasis in the setting of immobilization and via endothelial activation in the setting of injury, resulting in the activation of the clotting cascade. Like surgery, not all trauma confers the same degree of risk of thrombosis. Major trauma is associated with a significantly increased risk of VTE. A study of 716 patients with major trauma, defined as an Injury Severity Score of at least 9, who underwent screening evaluation for DVT reported a DVT incidence of 58%, with 18% occurring in the proximal veins [37,38]. Of note, these patients did not receive prophylactic anticoagulation. Interestingly, while the use of prophylactic anticoagulation does reduce the risk of VTE in patients with major trauma, the reported rates of VTE in this patient population remain high, with a reported incidence of VTE of 44% with the use of low-dose heparin and of 31% with the use of low-molecular-weight heparin [39]. Trauma resulting in fracture, particularly those involving the lower limb, is a strong VTE risk factor. The incidence differs based on the location of the fracture, with the highest risk locations including the hip (16.6%), tibial plateau (16.3%), and tibial shaft (13.3%) [1].

In contrast, minor trauma does not appear to confer the same degree of risk. In a cohort of 294 cancer-free patients with VTE admitted to hospital, the adjusted incidence rate ratio (IRR) for VTE for open wounds was 0.46 (95% CI, 0.15–1.39), for sprains 1.15 (95% CI, 0.44–3.04), and for dislocations 1.54 (95% CI, 0.37–6.48). In contrast, the adjusted IRR in the same cohort was elevated for fractures (2.45, 95% CI 1.29–4.68) and immobility (3.84, 95% CI 2.39–6.15) [40]. Likewise, a systematic review of 15 studies demonstrated an incidence of VTE of 4.8% in patients undergoing temporary lower limb immobilization due to isolated trauma [41].

1.1.6. Cancer

Malignancy is a well-established risk factor for the development of VTE. Cancer is known to create a hypercoagulable state via the expression of hemostatic proteins on tumor cells, the release of inflammatory cytokines, and the activation of the clotting system [42]. Additionally, depending on the location and size of the tumor, the local mass effect can lead to the compression of veins with the stasis of venous flow. Amongst patients with symptomatic DVT, approximately 20% will have a known active malignancy [18,43]. The risk of cancer-associated thrombosis (CAT) varies due to several factors, including cancer site and stage, malignancy treatment, and other patient-specific factors. The risk of VTE varies broadly by cancer type. In a large registry study, the cancers associated with the highest 6-month cumulative VTE incidence were pancreatic cancer (4.4%), ovarian cancer (3.1%), Hodgkin lymphoma (2.9%), and non-Hodgkin lymphoma (2.7%); in contrast, melanoma (0.36%) and breast cancer (0.64%) were amongst the malignancies with the lowest risk [44]. Other significant risk factors for VTE development included a prior history of VTE (subdistribution HR (SHR) 7.6), distant metastasis (SHR 3.2), and the use of chemotherapy (SHR 3.4). These findings have been confirmed elsewhere with metastatic disease and the use of high-risk treatment, including surgery, radiotherapy, and chemotherapy, being associated with an increased risk of VTE [45].

The risk of VTE is highest in the first 3 months after cancer diagnosis [44,46,47]. This increased risk is likely related to cancer treatments, as several treatments, including chemotherapy, protein kinase inhibitors, antiangiogenic therapy, and immunotherapy, as well as the use of central venous catheters, have been associated with an increased risk of thrombosis [44,48]. Aside from the increased morbidity associated with VTE, CAT is reported to be the second leading cause of death after disease progression amongst patients with cancer [49].

Given the clear association of malignancy as a risk factor for VTE, the question often arises about screening for malignancy in a patient with VTE without other identified risk factors with the goal of the earlier detection of malignancy and thus decreasing the cancer-related mortality and improving the quality of life. Of note, the majority of cancers associated with thromboembolic events have previously been diagnosed at the time of VTE diagnosis [50]. In those without a known history of malignancy, the rate of occult cancer detection for unprovoked VTE was ~5% within 12 months of VTE diagnosis [51–53]. Despite this, there has been no data demonstrating improved patient-specific outcomes [53]. As such, the 2017 International Society on Thrombosis and Haemostasis recommend performing age- and gender-specific cancer screening (breast, cervical, colon, and prostate) while more intensive screening with whole-body CT or PET scan is not routinely recommended [54].

1.1.7. Pregnancy and Postpartum

Pregnancy and the postpartum period are associated with an increased risk of VTE via several different mechanisms. Venous stasis frequently occurs in pregnancy due to the compression of the pelvic vein by the gravid uterus and due to pregnancy-associated changes in venous capacitance. Additionally, pregnancy can result in an alteration in several coagulation factors, resulting in a hypercoagulable state, as well as result in vascular injury at the time of delivery [55]. The overall incidence of VTE in pregnancy is relatively low with reports of VTE diagnosis during 1 in 1000 to 2000 pregnancies [56,57]. The incidence of DVT is reported to be three times higher than that of PE and the majority of VTE events occur in the postpartum period [56,57]. Compared to non-pregnant patients, pregnant patients have a 5-fold increased risk of VTE during pregnancy, with the risk increasing substantially to 60-fold during the first three months after delivery [58]. Additional reported risk factors associated with pregnancy-related VTE include increasing age (age > 40) and the use of assisted reproductive technology [59–61].

1.1.8. Hormone-Based Contraception and Hormone Replacement Therapy

Estrogen-containing contraceptives and hormone replacement therapy (HRT) have been associated with an increased risk of both arterial and venous thrombosis. The mechanism is not fully understood but appears to be related to the effect that estrogen has on inducing prothrombotic and fibrinolytic changes in hemostatic factors as well as impacting the regulation of endothelial function [62]. Given their widespread use, oral contraceptives (OCPs) are one of the most important causes of thrombosis in young women. It is reported that OCPs increase the relative risk of VTE by approximately threefold [61,63,64]. The risk of VTE development with the use of OCPs appears to be highest in the first 6–12 months after the initiation of OCPs [65]. At the time of cessation of OCPs, the risk of VTE is felt to return to the level prior to OCP initiation within one to three months. Overall, the risk of VTE is considerably lower with the use of OCPs compared to the risk seen in pregnancy and the postpartum period. Additional factors that are felt to increase the risk of VTE during OCP use include smoking, obesity, polycystic ovary syndrome, older age, venous compression, and immobilization [66–68].

HRT is also associated with increased risk; however, this risk appears to be lower than that of OCPs, potentially due to the lower estrogen doses used in HRT compared to OCPs. Studies suggest that HRT causes an approximate twofold increase in the VTE risk [69–71]. Similar to OCPs, the risk of VTE development appears to be highest in the first year of HRT treatment [71]. Other risk factors associated with VTE in the setting of HRT use include older age, overweight/obesity, and factor V Leiden mutation [72].

1.1.9. Obesity

Obesity is a recognized risk factor for VTE, likely due to its association with inflammation and the enhanced production of clotting factors. There are numerous studies demonstrating that obesity is associated with an increased risk of DVT and PE, and conversely, that underweight patients are at a reduced risk. In a study of 19,293 patients evaluating cardiovascular risk factors and venous thromboembolism, a body mass index (BMI) of greater than 40 had a sex-adjusted HR of 2.7 [73]. Likewise, a national database study demonstrated an RR of 2.5 for DVT and 2.21 for PE when comparing obese patients to non-obese patients [74]. Conversely, results from the EDITH study demonstrated underweight patients had a statistically significant reduction in risk for VTE compared with normal weight (OR 0.55) [75].

1.1.10. Smoking

Cigarette smoking is linked to endothelial damage and inflammation and thus a heightened risk of VTE, especially in combination with other risk factors. Smoking is a well-established risk factor for atherosclerosis but has a less established link with VTE. There are several studies that have demonstrated no significant relationship between smoking and

VTE [73,76]. However, others have demonstrated a link between smoking and VTE, with several demonstrating a dose-dependent link between smoking and non-smoking, with those having a higher pack year and currently smoking being at the highest risk [77,78].

1.1.11. Age

Advancing age has been demonstrated in numerous studies to be associated with VTE, with proposed mechanisms including changes within the venous system and less effective inherent anticoagulation mechanisms. A prior study has demonstrated an exponential increase in VTE risk with age, with the annual incidence rate for DVT increasing from 17 per 100,000 persons/years for patients between the ages of 40 to 49 to 232 per 100,000 persons/year for those between the ages of 70 and 79 [79]. Similarly, it has been noted that the risk of VTE approximately doubles with each decade, starting at age 40 [2]. With this, VTEs in children and young adults are rare. When they do occur, they are usually associated with a strong predisposing risk factor, such as trauma/fracture or surgery.

1.1.12. Male Sex

Male sex has been demonstrated in several studies to be a risk factor for VTE recurrence; however, there is no reported sex differences in the risk of the first VTE event. In a meta-analysis of 2554 patients with a first VTE, the incidence of recurrence was higher in men than women, both at one year (9.5% vs. 5.3%) and at three years (11.3% vs. 7.3%) [80]. Likewise, another large meta-analysis of over 2185 demonstrated a 2.8-fold higher risk of VTE recurrence in men compared to women [81]. The mechanism behind this difference is unclear but has been reported to be due to differences in other VTE risk factors between the sexes. One prior study noted a factor V Leiden mutation as a risk factor for VTE recurrence in male patients, while the age at the first event and obesity were noted as risk factors for female patients [82].

1.1.13. SARS-CoV-2 Disease (COVID-19)

Since the start of the COVID-19 pandemic, there have been numerous reports demonstrating an increased risk of VTE. Mechanistically, SARS-CoV-2 is felt to increase the risk of VTE via the release of proinflammatory cytokines which activate platelet aggregation, tissue factor, and the coagulation cascade, as well as via the interaction with the angiotensin converting enzyme (ACE)-2 receptor on endothelial cells, resulting in endothelial dysfunction as well as the release of vasoconstrictor angiotensin-II [83,84]. With this, numerous studies have reported increased rates of VTE in patients hospitalized with COVID-19. A large meta-analysis demonstrated that the overall prevalence of PE/DVT in hospitalized patients with COVID-19 who underwent a screening assessment for VTE was approximately 30% [85]. Moreover, a meta-analysis of twelve studies demonstrated a VTE prevalence of 31% among ICU patients, despite the use of prophylactic or therapeutic anticoagulation [86]. In contrast, the incidence of VTE in non-hospitalized patients with COVID-19 does not appear to be increased. In a large cohort of 398,000 patients, the overall incidence of VTE in non-hospitalized patients with COVID-19 was reported to be 0.1%. Likewise, in a retrospective cohort comparing COVID-19-positive patients with COVID-19-negative controls, the 30-day prevalence of VTE events was not different between the two groups (1.4% vs. 1.3%, respectively) [87]. Interestingly, it appears that the risk of VTE also differs by the strain of SARS-CoV-2 virus [88]. While there is still much left to understand about the role of COVID-19 in the VTE risk, it does appear that both the severity of COVID-19 illness and the strain of COVID-19 virus do impact the risk.

1.1.14. Superficial Vein Thrombosis

As the name implies, superficial vein thrombosis (SVT) results in the thrombosis of a superficial vein. While often considered to not be as severe as DVT, studies have demonstrated that patients with SVT do have an increased risk of developing DVT. As the superficial venous system connects with the deep systems, the location of SVT does confer some risk as thrombosis near the saphenofemoral or saphenopopiteal junction is associated with an increased risk of DVT and PE development. With this, a meta-analysis of 21 studies noted that 18.1% of patients have concomitant DVT at the time of SVT diagnosis; in 11 studies, 6.9% of patients were found to have concomitant PE [89]. Longitudinally, a history of SVT also appears to carry a risk of developing DVT, with a study demonstrating that approximately one third of patients developed a DVT in four years of follow up after SVT [90]. The increased risk of developing a DVT or PE in patients with a history of SVT is likely due to shared risk factors between superficial and deep thrombosis.

1.1.15. Central Vein Catheters

Intravenous catheters can lead to VTE development due to endothelial trauma and inflammation associated with catheter insertion and maintenance. The majority of SVT and DVT occurring in the upper extremities occurs in the setting of intravenous catheters [91,92]. Due to the nature of intravenous catheters, any catheter has the potential to cause venous thrombosis. In prior reports, there is a wide variation in the incidence of venous thrombosis associated with central access, ranging from 0 to 28% [93]. The risk of VTE appears to be higher with the use of peripherally inserted central catheters (PICCs) compared to a central port. Additional risk factors include active malignancy, a history of DVT, the improper positioning of catheter tip, and a subclavian venipuncture insertion site [94,95].

1.1.16. Anatomic Risk Factors

There are several anatomic risk factors for the development of DVT. Venous compression due to anatomic variations can occur in both the upper and lower extremities, increasing the risk of VTE. In the lower extremity, May–Thurner syndrome is a common anatomic variant, resulting in the hemodynamically significant compression of the left common iliac vein between the overlying right common iliac artery and the underlying vertebral body [96]. In the upper extremity, venous thoracic outlet syndrome, also known as Paget–Schroetter syndrome, results in the compression of the subclavian vein between the first rib and a hypertrophied scalene or subclavius tendon or between the tendons themselves [97]. Compression often occurs in the setting of repetitive overhead movements, such as with weightlifting and certain sports. Both anatomic variants can lead to venous stasis and endothelial injury from repetitive compression, resulting in an increased risk of thrombosis.

Varicose veins also appear to confer increased risk for VTE. In a large cohort of patients in Taiwan, patients with varicose veins were at an increased risk of both DVT (HR 5.30) and PE (HR 1.73) [98]. Interestingly, a population-based case–control study demonstrated that the risk of VTE associated with varicose veins appears to decrease with age: OR 4.2 at age 45, 1.9 at age 60, and 0.9 at age 75 [99].

1.1.17. Other Medical Conditions

There are reports of an increased risk of VTE in patients with renal, liver, cardiovascular, and hematologic diseases. Amongst patients with renal dysfunction, chronic kidney disease, the use of hemodialysis, nephrotic syndrome, and renal transplantation have been associated with an increased risk of VTE [100–103]. As for cardiovascular disease, myocardial infarction and heart failure have been reported to be independent risk factors for VTE development [104,105]. Diabetes has also been reported as causing an increased risk of VTE, with a large meta-analysis reporting an HR of 1.35 [106]. The data on liver disease is mixed, with both increased and decreased VTE risk reported [99,107]. Myeloproliferative neoplasms, including polycythemia vera and essential thrombocythemia, are associated with both arterial and venous thrombosis [108]. Additionally, paroxysmal nocturnal hemoglobinuria (PNH) is associated with an increased risk of intrabdominal and cerebral venous thrombosis [109].

1.1.18. Antiphospholipid Syndrome

Antiphospholipid syndrome (APS) is an acquired thrombophilia characterized by the presence of antiphospholipid antibodies, including lupus anticoagulant (LAC), beta-2 glycoprotein 1 antibodies (B2GPI), and anticardiolipin antibodies, which are directed against plasma proteins bound to anionic phospholipids [110]. These antibodies result in numerous clinical manifestations, including venous, arterial, and microcirculation thrombosis, recurrent fetal loss, and thrombocytopenia. The mechanism behind the hypercoagulability of this syndrome is multifaceted and includes inhibitions of the natural anticoagulation system, activation of procoagulant and proinflammatory effects, and activation of endothelial cells, immune cells, and the complement cascade [111–115]. APS may be primary or associated with systemic lupus erythematosus or other rheumatic diseases. VTE in APS typically occurs as DVT in the lower extremities; however, VTE in unusual locations, including hepatic veins, mesenteric veins, and cerebral veins are also common [116]. Amongst the antibodies, LAC is associated with this highest risk of VTE, with increasing risk with each subsequent positive antibody [117]. The risk of first VTE among asymptomatic patients with triple positive APS (positive for LAC, anticardiolipin, and anti-B2GPI) is 5.3% per year and the risk of recurrent thrombosis without anticoagulation therapy is 44% over a 10-year follow-up period [118].

Making a diagnosis of APS is not always straightforward. It is reported that between 2 and 5% of people in the general population have antiphospholipid antibodies without clinical sequelae [119]. Additionally, antiphospholipid antibody levels may be transiently elevated for several different reasons, including autoimmune disorders, acute infection, or chronic disease. The Sapporo criteria is useful for making the diagnosis of APS; it requires one clinical criteria and one laboratory test result that is positive on two occasions at least 12 weeks apart [120].

1.2. Inherited Thrombophilia

1.2.1. Factor V Leiden Mutation

Factor V plays a role in the conversion of prothrombin to thrombin, a crucial step in the formation of blood clots. Factor V Leiden (FVL) mutation results in a point mutation in the F5 gene which encodes the factor V protein in the coagulation cascade [121]. The mutation makes factor V resistant to inactivation by activated protein C (aPC), a protein that normally helps regulate blood clotting and prevent excessive clot formation, resulting in an increased risk of VTE. Heterozygosity for FVL is the most common inherited thrombophilia in White individuals. A series of over 4000 individuals in the United States reported frequencies for FVL heterozygosity in White Americans at 5.3%, Hispanic Americans at 2.2%, Native Americans at 1.2%, African Americans at 1.2%, and Asian Americans at 0.45% [122].

Transmission is autosomal dominant and the risk of VTE differs based on patients who are heterozygous versus homozygous for the variant. Individuals with heterozygous FVL mutations infer a three- to fourfold increased risk of VTE [123,124]. In comparison, those with homozygous FVL mutations have a substantially higher risk, with reported ORs ranging from 11.5 to 79.4 [123,125]. With regards to the risk of recurrent VTE, a systematic review demonstrated that the presence of a heterozygous FVL mutation does confer only a modest increase in recurrence (OR 1.4, 95% CI 1.1–1.8) [126]. As such, most providers do not alter the long-term anticoagulation plan for a patient with heterozygous FVL. In contrast, those with a homozygous FVL mutation are typically placed on indefinite anticoagulation due to concerns for the risk of recurrent VTE.

1.2.2. Prothrombin G20210A Gene Mutation

The prothrombin G20210A gene mutation (PGM) is a gain-of-function mutation that leads to higher levels of prothrombin, and thus elevated thrombin formation, resulting in an increased risk of VTE. The G20210A point mutation in the prothrombin gene is a substitution of guanine to adenine at position 20,210 in the 3-untranslated region [127]. PGM is the second most common inherited thrombophilia after factor V Leiden, with an overall prevalence estimate of 2.0% [128]. There are geographic differences in prevalence, with prevalence being higher in individuals of European descent and very rare in individuals of Asian and African descent.

Similar to FVL, the transmission of PGM is autosomal dominant. Individuals who are heterozygous for PGM have a three- to fourfold increased risk of VTE compared to those without the variant [127,129,130]. The data on the risk of VTE in patients who are homozygous for PGM is more limited; a small study of 36 patients with homozygous PGM reported that 33% of the patients developed VTE [131]. Interestingly, despite the increased risk associated with VTE, a systematic review of 18 articles noted that PGM heterozygosity did not confer a significant increased risk of recurrent VTE (OR 1.45, 95% CI 0.96–2.2) [132]. As such, the presence of PGM generally does not impact the decision making with regards to the duration of anticoagulation management. However, similar to homozygous FVL mutations, patients with homozygous PGM are typically recommended for indefinite anticoagulation to reduce the risk of recurrent VTE.

1.2.3. Protein C Deficiency

Protein C (PC) is an anticoagulant protein synthesized in the liver. Upon activation (aPC), the primary role of aPC is to inactive the coagulation factors Va and VIIIa, which are required for thrombin generation and factor X activation [133]. PC deficiency results in the reduced inactivation of factors Va and VIIIa, thus increasing the risk of VTE. The incidence of PC deficiency in the general population is estimated at 1 in 200 to 300 individuals [134]. In contrast, PC deficiency amongst individuals with VTE is higher, typically between 3 and 4% [135,136]. It is estimated that PC deficiency confers an approximate sevenfold increased risk of VTE [137,138]. As for VTE recurrence, a study of 130 patients with hereditary deficiencies of PC, PS, or antithrombin reported the annual incidence of recurrent VTE was 6.0% for PC deficiency [139]. The management of acute VTE in patients with inherited PC deficiency does not differ from patients without inherited thrombophilia.

1.2.4. Protein S Deficiency

Protein S (PS) is a cofactor for aPC, which inactivates the procoagulant factors Va and VIIIa, reducing thrombin generation [140]. PS deficiency impairs the normal control of this mechanism, resulting in an increased risk of VTE. The prevalence of PS deficiency is difficult to interpret due to the variability in PS levels; in a cohort of 2331 adults with a personal history of VTE without a strong family history, the frequency of PS deficiency, defined as <33 units/dL, was 0.9% [141]. It is estimated the PS deficiency confers a two- to elevenfold increased risk of VTE [142]. With regards to VTE recurrence, a study of 130 patients with hereditary deficiencies of PC, PS, or antithrombin reported the annual incidence of recurrent VTE was 8.4% for PS deficiency [139]. Similar to PC deficiency, the management of acute VTE in patients with inherited PS deficiency does not differ from patients without inherited thrombophilia.

1.2.5. Antithrombin Deficiency

Antithrombin III (AT) deficiency, defined as an AT activity level consistently less than 80%, is associated with a significantly increased risk of VTE. Antithrombin is a natural anticoagulant which inhibits thrombin, factor Xa, and other serine proteases in the coagulation cascade [143]. AT deficiency can either be inherited or acquired, with acquired causes included impaired production, nephrotic losses, or accelerated consumption. Hereditary AT deficiency is relatively uncommon, with an estimated prevalence of approximately 0.2 per 1000 [144]. Compared to other thrombophilias, hereditary AT deficiency confers a much higher risk of VTE, with a prior meta-analysis demonstrating an odds ratio of VTE of 16.3 [145]. Given this increased risk, most experts recommend an indefinite course of anticoagulation to reduce the risk of recurrent thrombosis.

1.2.6. Hyperhomocysteinemia

Hyperhomocysteinemia can occur by both genetic and acquired abnormality. The most common genetic defect resulting in hyperhomocysteinemia is a mutation of the enzyme methylenetetrahydrofolate reductase (MTHFR). Acquired causes include deficiencies in vitamin B6, B12, or folic acid. While older studies have reported a two- to threefold increased risk of VTE, a recent large cohort study demonstrated no increased risk of VTE in patients with elevated homocysteine concentrations [146]. Likewise, another cohort study of 478 patients reported an adjusted RR 1.6 (CI, 0.6–4.5) in patients with elevated homocysteine levels compared to those with normal levels. Additionally, the use of B vitamins to lower homocysteine levels has not been shown to reduce the recurrence of DVT or PE [147]. Consequently, measuring homocysteine levels and testing for MTHFR mutations are not recommended in patients with VTE.

1.3. Thrombophilia Evaluation

Performing a thrombophilia evaluation for a patient with VTE remains a controversial issue. While these tests are readily available and typically easy to order, it can be challenging to determine who should undergo a thrombophilia evaluation and how to interpret the results. Patients with inherited thrombophilia can often be identified without testing due to several risk factors, including VTE at a young age (less than 40–50 years), a strong family history of VTE, VTE in conjunction with weak provoking factors at a young age, recurrent VTE events, and VTE in unusual sites, such as cerebral and splanchnic veins [148]. As noted in the prior sections, there are numerous acquired and inherited thrombophilias that increase the risk of VTE. Despite the associated increased risk of VTE, many studies have demonstrated that the clinical usefulness and benefits of evaluating these thrombophilias are limited, specifically as it pertains to VTE outcomes including death [148]. With this, the results of thrombophilia testing rarely impact the treatment strategy for VTE. Additionally, the significance of a positive or negative test result is often misinterpreted by clinicians. A positive test often leads to overtreatment with indefinite anticoagulation despite studies demonstrating a low risk of recurrent VTE in patients with inherited thrombophilia; in contrast, those with negative results might be missing a yet-to-be-determined thrombophilia that is not present on standard testing panels, and as such, a negative test does not always equate with low risk. With this, it is generally agreed upon that routine thrombophilia evaluation in all patients with a diagnosis of VTE is not warranted. However, there are specific patients with whom a thrombophilia evaluation might be beneficial, which are outlined below.

1.3.1. Unprovoked VTE

For patients with unprovoked VTE, the risk of recurrence is known to be high, especially compared to patients with provoked VTE. The estimated rate of recurrence is approximately 10% in the first year after anticoagulation therapy is discontinued and increases to more than 50% at 10 years [149]. Interestingly, studies evaluating the risk of VTE recurrence based on thrombophilia status in patients with VTE have demonstrated no significant difference between those with and without thrombophilia. A prospective study of 474 patients without malignancy with a first VTE reported no increased risk of recurrent thrombosis in those with thrombophilia (HR 1.4; 95% CI, 0.9–2.2) [150]. Likewise, another prospective study of 570 patients with a first VTE noted that recurrence rates were not related to the presence or absence of an inherited thrombophilia (HR 1.5; 95% CI, 0.82–2.77) [6]. Lastly, the thrombophilia status of patients is unlikely to change the long-term management in those with unprovoked VTE, as guidelines recommend indefinite anticoagulation, regardless of thrombophilia status. As such, the majority of guidelines recommend against performing a thrombophilia evaluation in patients with a first unprovoked VTE event [151–155].

1.3.2. Provoked VTE

Patients with VTE due to a strong, modifiable provoking risk factor, such as major surgery, trauma, hospitalization, or immobility, have a low risk of VTE recurrence, regardless of the thrombophilia status. As noted in the Surgery section above, the risk of VTE recurrence after a surgically provoked VTE is very low, with two studies demonstrating a less than 1% recurrence over a two-year period [6,156]. Given the low risk of recurrence, the presence or absence of an inherited thrombophilia is unlikely to change the anticoagulation management in these patients with recommendations for treatment for 3–6 months. As such, guidelines recommend against performing a thrombophilia evaluation in patients with a first provoked VTE event in the setting of surgery [152–155].

Aside from surgery, there are numerous other modifiable provoking risk factors for the development of VTE, including trauma, immobility, pregnancy, the use of OCPs, and hospitalization for acute medical illness. In general, while these factors are not considered to be as strongly associated with VTE risk as surgery, they do a have clear association with the development of VTE. With this, patients with provoked VTE by nonsurgical risk factors still have low rates of recurrent VTE, regardless of the thrombophilia status [157]. Similar to the recommendations for provoked VTE events in the setting of surgery, the majority of guidelines recommend against performing a thrombophilia evaluation in patients with a first provoked VTE event in the setting of a non-surgery major risk factor [152–154]. However, this is not agreed upon in all societal recommendations; for instance, the recently published 2023 American Society of Hematology (ASH) guidelines now recommends a thrombophilia evaluation for this with VTE provoked by a nonsurgical major transient risk factor, pregnancy or postpartum, and the use of OCP with recommendations for indefinite anticoagulation treatments in those patients with thrombophilia [155]. Of note, this is a significant change from the prior ASH recommendations published in 2013, which previously recommended against this testing. It should be noted that these are conditional recommendations based on a low level of evidence. As such, the consideration of thrombophilia testing in these patient populations should ultimately be done on an individual basis, with patients being educated on the risk/benefit of thrombophilia testing and taking into account the patient's values and preferences.

1.3.3. VTE in Unusual Sites

Cerebral and splanchnic (portal, hepatic, splenic, or mesenteric) vein thromboses are rare compared to lower extremity VTE. Thromboses in these locales have been associated with inherited thrombophilias, including FVL, PGM, and deficiencies in PC, PS, and AT [158]. The role for screening for thrombophilia in this patient population is less straightforward given the limited data and concerns for increased morbidity associated with thrombosis at these sites. As such, in those who are planning to discontinue anticoagulation after primary short-term treatment (i.e., 3–6 months), thrombophilia evaluation might be helpful to understand the risk of VTE recurrence [155]. In contrast, for those who would otherwise remain on anticoagulation indefinitely, guidelines do not recommend obtaining thrombophilia testing [155].

1.3.4. Other Clinical Considerations

In patients with recurrent VTE, thrombophilia testing is often not necessary as it rarely changes the long-term management, given these patients have an indication for indefinite anticoagulation. However, many of these patients worry about the possibility of having an inherited thrombophilia and thus the potential risk of their offspring inheriting their thrombophilia. In this situation, a thrombophilia evaluation could be considered after properly educating the patient on the risk/benefits and implications of testing.

In young patients (age < 40) with unprovoked VTE or VTE provoked by weak risk factors, performing a thrombophilia evaluation can be considered to better understand the long-term risk of VTE recurrence. Most of these patients have an indication for an indefinite anticoagulation course; however, many young patients are not keen on being on anticoagulation for a prolonged period. With this, a thrombophilia evaluation can add further clarification to the ultimate risk of VTE recurrence, and a positive result can be used to reiterate a commitment to anticoagulation. However, it should be noted that a negative panel does not necessarily confer a lower risk of VTE recurrence and as such, long-term anticoagulation management ultimately depends on the perceived risk of VTE recurrence based on the cumulative impact of other risk factors.

1.3.5. Timing of Testing

For those undergoing thrombophilia evaluation, typical testing includes evaluation for Factor V Leiden, Prothrombin gene mutation, Protein C deficiency, Protein S deficiency, Antithrombin deficiency, and evaluation for antiphospholipid antibody syndrome. For those who are undergoing thrombophilia evaluation, the timing of the testing and the presence of anticoagulation are important considerations. Acute thrombosis can impact the levels of protein S and antithrombin, resulting in low levels which are difficult to interpret. As such, it is recommended that testing occurs outside of the acute VTE window (typically after 3 months of anticoagulation therapy). Additionally, many of the commonly used anticoagulants are known to impact the interpretability of test results, and thus it is recommended that thrombophilia testing occurs at a time when the patient is able to stop his/her anticoagulation [159]. Specifically, it is recommended to hold direct oral anticoagulants (DOACs) for 48 h and vitamin K antagonists for two weeks prior to performing thrombophilia testing [148].

2. Conclusions

VTE is a multifaceted condition influenced by a wide array of risk factors. There are many factors, both acquired and inherited, known to increase the risk of VTE. A risk factor can be identified in the majority of patients with VTE. However, there is heterogeneity amongst the risk factors with regards to their predictive value. As such, it is important for clinicians to understand the potency of each individual risk factor when managing patients who have a VTE or are at risk of developing VTE as this will guide counseling and management, both of the patient and their family.

Funding: The research received no external funding.

Data Availability Statement: Not applicable.

Conflicts of Interest: The authors declare no conflicts of interest.

References

1. Pastori, D.; Cormaci, V.M.; Marucci, S.; Franchino, G.; Del Sole, F.; Capozza, A.; Fallarino, A.; Corso, C.; Valeriani, E.; Menichelli, D.; et al. A Comprehensive Review of Risk Factors for Venous Thromboembolism: From Epidemiology to Pathophysiology. *Int. J. Mol. Sci.* **2023**, *24*, 3169. [CrossRef] [PubMed]
2. Anderson, F.A.; Spencer, F.A. Risk factors for venous thromboembolism. *Circulation* **2003**, *107* (Suppl. S1), I9–I16. [CrossRef] [PubMed]
3. Konstantinides, S.V.; Meyer, G.; Becattini, C.; Bueno, H.; Geersing, G.-J.; Harjola, V.-P.; Huisman, M.V.; Humbert, M.; Jennings, C.S.; Jiménez, D.; et al. 2019 ESC Guidelines for the diagnosis and management of acute pulmonary embolism developed in collaboration with the European Respiratory Society (ERS). *Eur. Heart J.* **2020**, *41*, 543–603. [CrossRef] [PubMed]
4. Prandoni, P.; Lensing, A.W.; Cogo, A.; Cuppini, S.; Villalta, S.; Carta, M.; Cattelan, A.M.; Polistena, P.; Bernardi, E.; Prins, M.H. The long-term clinical course of acute deep venous thrombosis. *Ann. Intern. Med.* **1996**, *125*, 1–7. [CrossRef] [PubMed]
5. Anderson, F.A.; Wheeler, H.B. Physician practices in the management of venous thromboembolism: A community-wide survey. *J. Vasc. Surg.* **1992**, *16*, 707–714. [CrossRef] [PubMed]
6. Baglin, T.; Luddington, R.; Brown, K.; Baglin, C. Incidence of recurrent venous thromboembolism in relation to clinical and thrombophilic risk factors: Prospective cohort study. *Lancet* **2003**, *362*, 523–526. [CrossRef] [PubMed]
7. Sørensen, H.T.; Riis, A.H.; Diaz, L.J.; Andersen, E.W.; Baron, J.A.; Andersen, P.K. Familial risk of venous thromboembolism: A nationwide cohort study. *J. Thromb. Haemost.* **2011**, *9*, 320–324. [CrossRef] [PubMed]
8. Bezemer, I.D.; van der Meer, F.J.M.; Eikenboom, J.C.J.; Rosendaal, F.R.; Doggen, C.J.M. The value of family history as a risk indicator for venous thrombosis. *Arch. Intern. Med.* **2009**, *169*, 610–615. [CrossRef]
9. Gibbs, N.M. Venous thrombosis of the lower limbs with particular reference to bed-rest. *Br. J. Surg.* **1957**, *45*, 209–236. [CrossRef]

10. Weinberg, I.; Elgendy, I.Y.; Dicks, A.B.; Marchena, P.J.; Malý, R.; Francisco, I.; Pedrajas, J.M.; Font, C.; Hernández-Blasco, L.; Monreal, M.; et al. Comparison of Presentation, Treatment, and Outcomes of Venous Thromboembolism in Long-Term Immobile Patients Based on Age. *J. Gen. Intern. Med.* **2023**, *38*, 1877–1886. [CrossRef]
11. Dennis, M.; Mordi, N.; Graham, C.; Sandercock, P.; CLOTS trials collaboration. The timing, extent, progression and regression of deep vein thrombosis in immobile stroke patients: Observational data from the CLOTS multicenter randomized trials. *J. Thromb. Haemost.* **2011**, *9*, 2193–2200. [CrossRef]
12. Kamran, S.I.; Downey, D.; Ruff, R.L. Pneumatic sequential compression reduces the risk of deep vein thrombosis in stroke patients. *Neurology* **1998**, *50*, 1683–1688. [CrossRef] [PubMed]
13. Amin, A.N.; Lin, J.; Thompson, S.; Wiederkehr, D. Rate of deep-vein thrombosis and pulmonary embolism during the care continuum in patients with acute ischemic stroke in the United States. *BMC Neurol.* **2013**, *13*, 17. [CrossRef] [PubMed]
14. Waring, W.P.; Karunas, R.S. Acute spinal cord injuries and the incidence of clinically occurring thromboembolic disease. *Paraplegia* **1991**, *29*, 8–16. [CrossRef] [PubMed]
15. Green, D.; Lee, M.Y.; Ito, V.Y.; Cohn, T.; Press, J.; Filbrandt, P.R.; VandenBerg, W.C.; Yarkony, G.M.; Meyer, P.R. Fixed- vs. adjusted-dose heparin in the prophylaxis of thromboembolism in spinal cord injury. *JAMA* **1988**, *260*, 1255–1258. [CrossRef] [PubMed]
16. Henke, P.K.; Kahn, S.R.; Pannucci, C.J.; Secemksy, E.A.; Evans, N.S.; Khorana, A.A.; Creager, M.A.; Pradhan, A.D.; American Heart Association Advocacy Coordinating Committee. Call to Action to Prevent Venous Thromboembolism in Hospitalized Patients: A Policy Statement From the American Heart Association. *Circulation* **2020**, *141*, e914–e931. [CrossRef]
17. Heit, J.A.; Melton, L.J.; Lohse, C.M.; Petterson, T.M.; Silverstein, M.D.; Mohr, D.N.; O'Fallon, W.M. Incidence of venous thromboembolism in hospitalized patients vs. community residents. *Mayo Clin. Proc.* **2001**, *76*, 1102–1110. [CrossRef] [PubMed]
18. Heit, J.A.; O'Fallon, W.M.; Petterson, T.M.; Lohse, C.M.; Silverstein, M.D.; Mohr, D.N.; Melton, L.J. Relative impact of risk factors for deep vein thrombosis and pulmonary embolism: A population-based study. *Arch. Intern. Med.* **2002**, *162*, 1245–1248. [CrossRef]
19. Chandra, D.; Parisini, E.; Mozaffarian, D. Meta-analysis: Travel and risk for venous thromboembolism. *Ann. Intern. Med.* **2009**, *151*, 180–190. [CrossRef]
20. Aldington, S.; Pritchard, A.; Perrin, K.; James, K.; Wijesinghe, M.; Beasley, R. Prolonged seated immobility at work is a common risk factor for venous thromboembolism leading to hospital admission. *Intern. Med. J.* **2008**, *38*, 133–135. [CrossRef]
21. Lee, A.Y.Y.; Gent, M.; Julian, J.A.; Bauer, K.A.; Eriksson, B.I.; Lassen, M.R.; Turpie, A.G.G. Bilateral vs. ipsilateral venography as the primary efficacy outcome measure in thromboprophylaxis clinical trials: A systematic review. *J. Thromb. Haemost.* **2004**, *2*, 1752–1759. [CrossRef] [PubMed]
22. Bjørnarå, B.T.; Gudmundsen, T.E.; Dahl, O.E. Frequency and timing of clinical venous thromboembolism after major joint surgery. *J. Bone Joint Surg. Br.* **2006**, *88*, 386–391. [CrossRef] [PubMed]
23. Januel, J.-M.; Chen, G.; Ruffieux, C.; Quan, H.; Douketis, J.D.; Crowther, M.A.; Colin, C.; Ghali, W.A.; Burnand, B.; IMECCHI Group. Symptomatic in-hospital deep vein thrombosis and pulmonary embolism following hip and knee arthroplasty among patients receiving recommended prophylaxis: A systematic review. *JAMA* **2012**, *307*, 294–303. [CrossRef] [PubMed]
24. Falck-Ytter, Y.; Francis, C.W.; Johanson, N.A.; Curley, C.; Dahl, O.E.; Schulman, S.; Ortel, T.L.; Pauker, S.G.; Colwell, C.W. Prevention of VTE in orthopedic surgery patients: Antithrombotic Therapy and Prevention of Thrombosis, 9th ed: American College of Chest Physicians Evidence-Based Clinical Practice Guidelines. *Chest* **2012**, *141* (Suppl. S2), e278S–e325S. [CrossRef] [PubMed]
25. Recommendations from the ICM-VTE: Hip & Knee. *J. Bone Joint Surg. Am.* **2022**, *104* (Suppl. S1), 180–231. [CrossRef]
26. Anderson, D.R.; Morgano, G.P.; Bennett, C.; Dentali, F.; Francis, C.W.; Garcia, D.A.; Kahn, S.R.; Rahman, M.; Rajasekhar, A.; Rogers, F.B.; et al. American Society of Hematology 2019 guidelines for management of venous thromboembolism: Prevention of venous thromboembolism in surgical hospitalized patients. *Blood Adv.* **2019**, *3*, 3898–3944. [CrossRef] [PubMed]
27. Venous Thromboembolism in over 16s: Reducing the Risk of Hospital-Acquired Deep Vein Thrombosis or Pulmonary Embolism; National Institute for Health and Care Excellence (NICE): London, UK. 2019. Available online: http://www.ncbi.nlm.nih.gov/books/NBK561646/ (accessed on 29 December 2023).
28. White, R.H.; Zhou, H.; Romano, P.S. Incidence of symptomatic venous thromboembolism after different elective or urgent surgical procedures. *Thromb. Haemost.* **2003**, *90*, 446–455. [CrossRef] [PubMed]
29. Nemeth, B.; Lijfering, W.M.; Nelissen, R.G.H.H.; Schipper, I.B.; Rosendaal, F.R.; le Cessie, S.; Cannegieter, S.C. Risk and Risk Factors Associated with Recurrent Venous Thromboembolism Following Surgery in Patients with History of Venous Thromboembolism. *JAMA Netw. Open* **2019**, *2*, e193690. [CrossRef]
30. Iorio, A.; Agnelli, G. Low-molecular-weight and unfractionated heparin for prevention of venous thromboembolism in neurosurgery: A meta-analysis. *Arch. Intern. Med.* **2000**, *160*, 2327–2332. [CrossRef]
31. Joffe, S.N. Incidence of postoperative deep vein thrombosis in neurosurgical patients. *J. Neurosurg.* **1975**, *42*, 201–203. [CrossRef]
32. Collins, R.; Scrimgeour, A.; Yusuf, S.; Peto, R. Reduction in fatal pulmonary embolism and venous thrombosis by perioperative administration of subcutaneous heparin. Overview of results of randomized trials in general, orthopedic, and urologic surgery. *N. Engl. J. Med.* **1988**, *318*, 1162–1173. [CrossRef] [PubMed]
33. Reis, S.E.; Polak, J.F.; Hirsch, D.R.; Cohn, L.H.; Creager, M.A.; Donovan, B.C.; Goldhaber, S.Z. Frequency of deep venous thrombosis in asymptomatic patients with coronary artery bypass grafts. *Am. Heart J.* **1991**, *122*, 478–482. [CrossRef] [PubMed]

34. Rocha, A.T.; de Vasconcellos, A.G.; da Luz Neto, E.R.; Araújo, D.M.A.; Alves, E.S.; Lopes, A.A. Risk of venous thromboembolism and efficacy of thromboprophylaxis in hospitalized obese medical patients and in obese patients undergoing bariatric surgery. *Obes. Surg.* **2006**, *16*, 1645–1655. [CrossRef] [PubMed]
35. Alizadeh, R.F.; Sujatha-Bhaskar, S.; Li, S.; Stamos, M.J.; Nguyen, N.T. Venous thromboembolism in common laparoscopic abdominal surgical operations. *Am. J. Surg.* **2017**, *214*, 1127–1132. [CrossRef] [PubMed]
36. Nguyen, N.T.; Hinojosa, M.W.; Fayad, C.; Varela, E.; Konyalian, V.; Stamos, M.J.; Wilson, S.E. Laparoscopic surgery is associated with a lower incidence of venous thromboembolism compared with open surgery. *Ann. Surg.* **2007**, *246*, 1021–1027. [CrossRef] [PubMed]
37. Baker, S.P.; O'Neill, B.; Haddon, W.; Long, W.B. The injury severity score: A method for describing patients with multiple injuries and evaluating emergency care. *J. Trauma* **1974**, *14*, 187–196. [CrossRef] [PubMed]
38. Geerts, W.H.; Code, K.I.; Jay, R.M.; Chen, E.; Szalai, J.P. A prospective study of venous thromboembolism after major trauma. *N. Engl. J. Med.* **1994**, *331*, 1601–1606. [CrossRef] [PubMed]
39. Geerts, W.H.; Jay, R.M.; Code, K.I.; Chen, E.; Szalai, J.P.; Saibil, E.A.; Hamilton, P.A. A comparison of low-dose heparin with low-molecular-weight heparin as prophylaxis against venous thromboembolism after major trauma. *N. Engl. J. Med.* **1996**, *335*, 701–707. [CrossRef]
40. Rogers, M.A.M.; Levine, D.A.; Blumberg, N.; Flanders, S.A.; Chopra, V.; Langa, K.M. Triggers of hospitalization for venous thromboembolism. *Circulation* **2012**, *125*, 2092–2099. [CrossRef]
41. Horner, D.; Pandor, A.; Goodacre, S.; Clowes, M.; Hunt, B.J. Individual risk factors predictive of venous thromboembolism in patients with temporary lower limb immobilization due to injury: A systematic review. *J. Thromb. Haemost.* **2019**, *17*, 329–344. [CrossRef]
42. Hisada, Y.; Mackman, N. Cancer-associated pathways and biomarkers of venous thrombosis. *Blood* **2017**, *130*, 1499–1506. [CrossRef] [PubMed]
43. Bauer, K.A. Venous thromboembolism in malignancy. *J. Clin. Oncol.* **2000**, *18*, 3065–3067. [CrossRef] [PubMed]
44. Mulder, F.I.; Horváth-Puhó, E.; van Es, N.; van Laarhoven, H.W.M.; Pedersen, L.; Moik, F.; Ay, C.; Büller, H.R.; Sørensen, H.T. Venous thromboembolism in cancer patients: A population-based cohort study. *Blood* **2021**, *137*, 1959–1969. [CrossRef] [PubMed]
45. Horsted, F.; West, J.; Grainge, M.J. Risk of venous thromboembolism in patients with cancer: A systematic review and meta-analysis. *PLoS Med.* **2012**, *9*, e1001275. [CrossRef] [PubMed]
46. Imberti, D.; Agnelli, G.; Ageno, W.; Moia, M.; Palareti, G.; Pistelli, R.; Rossi, R.; Verso, M. Clinical characteristics and management of cancer-associated acute venous thromboembolism: Findings from the MASTER Registry. *Haematologica* **2008**, *93*, 273–278. [CrossRef] [PubMed]
47. Lyman, G.H. Venous thromboembolism in the patient with cancer: Focus on burden of disease and benefits of thromboprophylaxis. *Cancer* **2011**, *117*, 1334–1349. [CrossRef] [PubMed]
48. Cortelezzi, A.; Moia, M.; Falanga, A.; Pogliani, E.M.; Agnelli, G.; Bonizzoni, E.; Gussoni, G.; Barbui, T.; Mannucci, P.M.; CATHEM Study Group. Incidence of thrombotic complications in patients with haematological malignancies with central venous catheters: A prospective multicentre study. *Br. J. Haematol.* **2005**, *129*, 811–817. [CrossRef] [PubMed]
49. Khorana, A.A.; Francis, C.W.; Culakova, E.; Kuderer, N.M.; Lyman, G.H. Thromboembolism is a leading cause of death in cancer patients receiving outpatient chemotherapy. *J. Thromb. Haemost.* **2007**, *5*, 632–634. [CrossRef]
50. Sørensen, H.T.; Mellemkjaer, L.; Olsen, J.H.; Baron, J.A. Prognosis of cancers associated with venous thromboembolism. *N. Engl. J. Med.* **2000**, *343*, 1846–1850. [CrossRef]
51. Prandoni, P.; Lensing, A.W.; Büller, H.R.; Cogo, A.; Prins, M.H.; Cattelan, A.M.; Cuppini, S.; Noventa, F.; ten Cate, J.W. Deep-vein thrombosis and the incidence of subsequent symptomatic cancer. *N. Engl. J. Med.* **1992**, *327*, 1128–1133. [CrossRef]
52. Carrier, M.; Le Gal, G.; Wells, P.S.; Fergusson, D.; Ramsay, T.; Rodger, M.A. Systematic review: The Trousseau syndrome revisited: Should we screen extensively for cancer in patients with venous thromboembolism? *Ann. Intern. Med.* **2008**, *149*, 323–333. [CrossRef]
53. D'Astous, J.; Carrier, M. Screening for Occult Cancer in Patients with Venous Thromboembolism. *J. Clin. Med.* **2020**, *9*, 2389. [CrossRef] [PubMed]
54. Delluc, A.; Antic, D.; Lecumberri, R.; Ay, C.; Meyer, G.; Carrier, M. Occult cancer screening in patients with venous thromboembolism: Guidance from the SSC of the ISTH. *J. Thromb. Haemost.* **2017**, *15*, 2076–2079. [CrossRef] [PubMed]
55. Marik, P.E.; Plante, L.A. Venous thromboembolic disease and pregnancy. *N. Engl. J. Med.* **2008**, *359*, 2025–2033. [CrossRef] [PubMed]
56. Morris, J.M.; Algert, C.S.; Roberts, C.L. Incidence and risk factors for pulmonary embolism in the postpartum period. *J. Thromb. Haemost.* **2010**, *8*, 998–1003. [CrossRef] [PubMed]
57. Heit, J.A.; Kobbervig, C.E.; James, A.H.; Petterson, T.M.; Bailey, K.R.; Melton, L.J. Trends in the incidence of venous thromboembolism during pregnancy or postpartum: A 30-year population-based study. *Ann. Intern. Med.* **2005**, *143*, 697–706. [CrossRef]
58. Raia-Barjat, T.; Edebiri, O.; Chauleur, C. Venous Thromboembolism Risk Score and Pregnancy. *Front. Cardiovasc. Med.* **2022**, *9*, 863612. [CrossRef] [PubMed]
59. Hwang, H.-G.; Lee, J.H.; Bang, S.-M. Incidence of Pregnancy-Associated Venous Thromboembolism: Second Nationwide Study. *Thromb. Haemost.* **2023**, *123*, 904–910. [CrossRef] [PubMed]

60. Goualou, M.; Noumegni, S.; de Moreuil, C.; Le Guillou, M.; De Coninck, G.; Hoffmann, C.; Robin, S.; Morcel, K.; Le Moigne, E.; Tremouilhac, C.; et al. Venous Thromboembolism Associated with Assisted Reproductive Technology: A Systematic Review and Meta-analysis. *Thromb. Haemost.* **2023**, *123*, 283–294. [CrossRef]
61. Thachil, R.; Nagraj, S.; Kharawala, A.; Sokol, S.I. Pulmonary Embolism in Women: A Systematic Review of the Current Literature. *J. Cardiovasc. Dev. Dis.* **2022**, *9*, 234. [CrossRef]
62. Godsland, I.F.; Winkler, U.; Lidegaard, O.; Crook, D. Occlusive vascular diseases in oral contraceptive users. Epidemiology, pathology and mechanisms. *Drugs* **2000**, *60*, 721–869. [CrossRef]
63. Peragallo Urrutia, R.; Coeytaux, R.R.; McBroom, A.J.; Gierisch, J.M.; Havrilesky, L.J.; Moorman, P.G.; Lowery, W.J.; Dinan, M.; Hasselblad, V.; Sanders, G.D.; et al. Risk of acute thromboembolic events with oral contraceptive use: A systematic review and meta-analysis. *Obstet. Gynecol.* **2013**, *122 Pt 1*, 380–389. [CrossRef] [PubMed]
64. Stegeman, B.H.; de Bastos, M.; Rosendaal, F.R.; van Hylckama Vlieg, A.; Helmerhorst, F.M.; Stijnen, T.; Dekkers, O.M. Different combined oral contraceptives and the risk of venous thrombosis: Systematic review and network meta-analysis. *BMJ* **2013**, *347*, f5298. [CrossRef] [PubMed]
65. Bloemenkamp, K.W.; Rosendaal, F.R.; Helmerhorst, F.M.; Vandenbroucke, J.P. Higher risk of venous thrombosis during early use of oral contraceptives in women with inherited clotting defects. *Arch. Intern. Med.* **2000**, *160*, 49–52. [CrossRef]
66. Farley, T.M.; Meirik, O.; Chang, C.L.; Poulter, N.R. Combined oral contraceptives, smoking, and cardiovascular risk. *J. Epidemiol. Community Health* **1998**, *52*, 775–785. [CrossRef] [PubMed]
67. Bird, S.T.; Hartzema, A.G.; Brophy, J.M.; Etminan, M.; Delaney, J.A.C. Risk of venous thromboembolism in women with polycystic ovary syndrome: A population-based matched cohort analysis. *CMAJ* **2013**, *185*, E115–E120. [CrossRef] [PubMed]
68. Dulicek, P.; Ivanova, E.; Kostal, M.; Sadilek, P.; Beranek, M.; Zak, P.; Hirmerova, J. Analysis of Risk Factors of Stroke and Venous Thromboembolism in Females with Oral Contraceptives Use. *Clin. Appl. Thromb. Hemost.* **2018**, *24*, 797–802. [CrossRef]
69. Miller, J.; Chan, B.K.S.; Nelson, H.D. Postmenopausal estrogen replacement and risk for venous thromboembolism: A systematic review and meta-analysis for the U.S. Preventive Services Task Force. *Ann. Intern. Med.* **2002**, *136*, 680–690. [CrossRef]
70. Grodstein, F.; Stampfer, M.J.; Goldhaber, S.Z.; Manson, J.E.; Colditz, G.A.; Speizer, F.E.; Willett, W.C.; Hennekens, C.H. Prospective study of exogenous hormones and risk of pulmonary embolism in women. *Lancet* **1996**, *348*, 983–987. [CrossRef]
71. Pérez Gutthann, S.; García Rodríguez, L.A.; Castellsague, J.; Duque Oliart, A. Hormone replacement therapy and risk of venous thromboembolism: Population based case-control study. *BMJ* **1997**, *314*, 796–800. [CrossRef]
72. Cushman, M.; Kuller, L.H.; Prentice, R.; Rodabough, R.J.; Psaty, B.M.; Stafford, R.S.; Sidney, S.; Rosendaal, F.R.; Women's Health Initiative. Investigators Estrogen plus progestin and risk of venous thrombosis. *JAMA* **2004**, *292*, 1573–1580. [CrossRef] [PubMed]
73. Tsai, A.W.; Cushman, M.; Rosamond, W.D.; Heckbert, S.R.; Polak, J.F.; Folsom, A.R. Cardiovascular risk factors and venous thromboembolism incidence: The longitudinal investigation of thromboembolism etiology. *Arch. Intern. Med.* **2002**, *162*, 1182–1189. [CrossRef] [PubMed]
74. Stein, P.D.; Beemath, A.; Olson, R.E. Obesity as a risk factor in venous thromboembolism. *Am. J. Med.* **2005**, *118*, 978–980. [CrossRef] [PubMed]
75. Delluc, A.; Mottier, D.; Le Gal, G.; Oger, E.; Lacut, K. Underweight is associated with a reduced risk of venous thromboembolism. Results from the EDITH case-control study. *J. Thromb. Haemost.* **2009**, *7*, 728–729. [CrossRef] [PubMed]
76. Braekkan, S.K.; Mathiesen, E.B.; Njølstad, I.; Wilsgaard, T.; Størmer, J.; Hansen, J.B. Family history of myocardial infarction is an independent risk factor for venous thromboembolism: The Tromsø study. *J. Thromb. Haemost.* **2008**, *6*, 1851–1857. [CrossRef] [PubMed]
77. Cheng, Y.-J.; Liu, Z.-H.; Yao, F.-J.; Zeng, W.-T.; Zheng, D.-D.; Dong, Y.-G.; Wu, S.-H. Current and former smoking and risk for venous thromboembolism: A systematic review and meta-analysis. *PLoS Med.* **2013**, *10*, e1001515. [CrossRef] [PubMed]
78. Pomp, E.R.; Rosendaal, F.R.; Doggen, C.J.M. Smoking increases the risk of venous thrombosis and acts synergistically with oral contraceptive use. *Am. J. Hematol.* **2008**, *83*, 97–102. [CrossRef]
79. Anderson, F.A.; Wheeler, H.B.; Goldberg, R.J.; Hosmer, D.W.; Patwardhan, N.A.; Jovanovic, B.; Forcier, A.; Dalen, J.E. A population-based perspective of the hospital incidence and case-fatality rates of deep vein thrombosis and pulmonary embolism. The Worcester DVT Study. *Arch. Intern. Med.* **1991**, *151*, 933–938. [CrossRef]
80. Douketis, J.; Tosetto, A.; Marcucci, M.; Baglin, T.; Cosmi, B.; Cushman, M.; Kyrle, P.; Poli, D.; Tait, R.C.; Iorio, A. Risk of recurrence after venous thromboembolism in men and women: Patient level meta-analysis. *BMJ* **2011**, *342*, d813. [CrossRef]
81. Roach, R.E.J.; Lijfering, W.M.; Tait, R.C.; Baglin, T.; Kyrle, P.A.; Cannegieter, S.C.; Rosendaal, F.R. Sex difference in the risk of recurrent venous thrombosis: A detailed analysis in four European cohorts. *J. Thromb. Haemost.* **2015**, *13*, 1815–1822. [CrossRef]
82. Olié, V.; Zhu, T.; Martinez, I.; Scarabin, P.-Y.; Emmerich, J. Sex-specific risk factors for recurrent venous thromboembolism. *Thromb. Res.* **2012**, *130*, 16–20. [CrossRef] [PubMed]
83. Varga, Z.; Flammer, A.J.; Steiger, P.; Haberecker, M.; Andermatt, R.; Zinkernagel, A.S.; Mehra, M.R.; Schuepbach, R.A.; Ruschitzka, F.; Moch, H. Endothelial cell infection and endotheliitis in COVID-19. *Lancet* **2020**, *395*, 1417–1418. [CrossRef] [PubMed]
84. Gianni, P.; Goldin, M.; Ngu, S.; Zafeiropoulos, S.; Geropoulos, G.; Giannis, D. Complement-mediated microvascular injury and thrombosis in the pathogenesis of severe COVID-19: A review. *World J. Exp. Med.* **2022**, *12*, 53–67. [CrossRef] [PubMed]
85. Kollias, A.; Kyriakoulis, K.G.; Lagou, S.; Kontopantelis, E.; Stergiou, G.S.; Syrigos, K. Venous thromboembolism in COVID-19: A systematic review and meta-analysis. *Vasc. Med.* **2021**, *26*, 415–425. [CrossRef] [PubMed]

86. Hasan, S.S.; Radford, S.; Kow, C.S.; Zaidi, S.T.R. Venous thromboembolism in critically ill COVID-19 patients receiving prophylactic or therapeutic anticoagulation: A systematic review and meta-analysis. *J. Thromb. Thrombolysis* **2020**, *50*, 814–821. [CrossRef] [PubMed]
87. Thoppil, J.J.; Courtney, D.M.; McDonald, S.; Kabrhel, C.; Nordenholz, K.E.; Camargo, C.A.; Kline, J.A. SARS-CoV-2 Positivity in Ambulatory Symptomatic Patients Is Not Associated with Increased Venous or Arterial Thrombotic Events in the Subsequent 30 Days. *J. Emerg. Med.* **2022**, *62*, 716–724. [CrossRef] [PubMed]
88. Roubinian, N.H.; Vinson, D.R.; Knudson-Fitzpatrick, T.; Mark, D.G.; Skarbinski, J.; Lee, C.; Liu, V.X.; Pai, A.P. Risk of posthospital venous thromboembolism in patients with COVID-19 varies by SARS-CoV-2 period and vaccination status. *Blood Adv.* **2023**, *7*, 141–144. [CrossRef]
89. Di Minno, M.N.D.; Ambrosino, P.; Ambrosini, F.; Tremoli, E.; Di Minno, G.; Dentali, F. Prevalence of deep vein thrombosis and pulmonary embolism in patients with superficial vein thrombosis: A systematic review and meta-analysis. *J. Thromb. Haemost.* **2016**, *14*, 964–972. [CrossRef]
90. Martinelli, I.; Cattaneo, M.; Taioli, E.; De Stefano, V.; Chiusolo, P.; Mannucci, P.M. Genetic risk factors for superficial vein thrombosis. *Thromb. Haemost.* **1999**, *82*, 1215–1217.
91. Mustafa, S.; Stein, P.D.; Patel, K.C.; Otten, T.R.; Holmes, R.; Silbergleit, A. Upper extremity deep venous thrombosis. *Chest* **2003**, *123*, 1953–1956. [CrossRef]
92. Flinterman, L.E.; Van Der Meer, F.J.M.; Rosendaal, F.R.; Doggen, C.J.M. Current perspective of venous thrombosis in the upper extremity. *J. Thromb. Haemost.* **2008**, *6*, 1262–1266. [CrossRef]
93. Rooden, C.J.; Tesselaar, M.E.T.; Osanto, S.; Rosendaal, F.R.; Huisman, M.V. Deep vein thrombosis associated with central venous catheters—A review. *J. Thromb. Haemost.* **2005**, *3*, 2409–2419. [CrossRef] [PubMed]
94. Saber, W.; Moua, T.; Williams, E.C.; Verso, M.; Agnelli, G.; Couban, S.; Young, A.; De Cicco, M.; Biffi, R.; van Rooden, C.J.; et al. Risk factors for catheter-related thrombosis (CRT) in cancer patients: A patient-level data (IPD) meta-analysis of clinical trials and prospective studies. *J. Thromb. Haemost.* **2011**, *9*, 312–319. [CrossRef] [PubMed]
95. Decousus, H.; Bourmaud, A.; Fournel, P.; Bertoletti, L.; Labruyère, C.; Presles, E.; Merah, A.; Laporte, S.; Stefani, L.; Piano, F.D.; et al. Cancer-associated thrombosis in patients with implanted ports: A prospective multicenter French cohort study (ONCOCIP). *Blood* **2018**, *132*, 707–716. [CrossRef] [PubMed]
96. Peters, M.; Syed, R.K.; Katz, M.; Moscona, J.; Press, C.; Nijjar, V.; Bisharat, M.; Baldwin, D. May-Thurner syndrome: A not so uncommon cause of a common condition. *Proc. (Bayl. Univ. Med. Cent.)* **2012**, *25*, 231–233. [CrossRef] [PubMed]
97. Alla, V.M.; Natarajan, N.; Kaushik, M.; Warrier, R.; Nair, C.K. Paget-Schroetter Syndrome: Review of Pathogenesis and Treatment of Effort Thrombosis. *West. J. Emerg. Med.* **2010**, *11*, 358–362. [PubMed]
98. Chang, S.-L.; Huang, Y.-L.; Lee, M.-C.; Hu, S.; Hsiao, Y.-C.; Chang, S.-W.; Chang, C.J.; Chen, P.-C. Association of Varicose Veins with Incident Venous Thromboembolism and Peripheral Artery Disease. *JAMA* **2018**, *319*, 807–817. [CrossRef] [PubMed]
99. Heit, J.A.; Silverstein, M.D.; Mohr, D.N.; Petterson, T.M.; O'Fallon, W.M.; Melton, L.J., III. Risk Factors for Deep Vein Thrombosis and Pulmonary Embolism: A Population-Based Case-Control Study. *Arch. Intern. Med.* **2000**, *160*, 809–815. [CrossRef]
100. Tveit, D.P.; Hypolite, I.O.; Hshieh, P.; Cruess, D.; Agodoa, L.Y.; Welch, P.G.; Abbott, K.C. Chronic dialysis patients have high risk for pulmonary embolism. *Am. J. Kidney Dis.* **2002**, *39*, 1011–1017. [CrossRef]
101. Wattanakit, K.; Cushman, M.; Stehman-Breen, C.; Heckbert, S.R.; Folsom, A.R. Chronic kidney disease increases risk for venous thromboembolism. *J. Am. Soc. Nephrol.* **2008**, *19*, 135–140. [CrossRef]
102. Schlegel, N. Thromboembolic risks and complications in nephrotic children. *Semin. Thromb. Hemost.* **1997**, *23*, 271–280. [CrossRef]
103. Poli, D.; Zanazzi, M.; Antonucci, E.; Marcucci, R.; Rosati, A.; Bertoni, E.; Salvadori, M.; Liotta, A.A.; Abbate, R.; Prisco, D.; et al. High rate of recurrence in renal transplant recipients after a first episode of venous thromboembolism. *Transplantation* **2005**, *80*, 789–793. [CrossRef]
104. Fanola, C.L.; Norby, F.L.; Shah, A.M.; Chang, P.P.; Lutsey, P.L.; Rosamond, W.D.; Cushman, M.; Folsom, A.R. Incident Heart Failure and Long-Term Risk for Venous Thromboembolism. *J. Am. Coll. Cardiol.* **2020**, *75*, 148–158. [CrossRef] [PubMed]
105. Sørensen, H.T.; Horvath-Puho, E.; Søgaard, K.K.; Christensen, S.; Johnsen, S.P.; Thomsen, R.W.; Prandoni, P.; Baron, J.A. Arterial cardiovascular events, statins, low-dose aspirin and subsequent risk of venous thromboembolism: A population-based case-control study. *J. Thromb. Haemost.* **2009**, *7*, 521–528. [CrossRef] [PubMed]
106. Bai, J.; Ding, X.; Du, X.; Zhao, X.; Wang, Z.; Ma, Z. Diabetes is associated with increased risk of venous thromboembolism: A systematic review and meta-analysis. *Thromb. Res.* **2015**, *135*, 90–95. [CrossRef] [PubMed]
107. Dabbagh, O.; Oza, A.; Prakash, S.; Sunna, R.; Saettele, T.M. Coagulopathy does not protect against venous thromboembolism in hospitalized patients with chronic liver disease. *Chest* **2010**, *137*, 1145–1149. [CrossRef] [PubMed]
108. Landolfi, R.; Marchioli, R.; Patrono, C. Mechanisms of bleeding and thrombosis in myeloproliferative disorders. *Thromb. Haemost.* **1997**, *78*, 617–621. [CrossRef] [PubMed]
109. Hillmen, P.; Lewis, S.M.; Bessler, M.; Luzzatto, L.; Dacie, J.V. Natural history of paroxysmal nocturnal hemoglobinuria. *N. Engl. J. Med.* **1995**, *333*, 1253–1258. [CrossRef] [PubMed]
110. Garcia, D.; Erkan, D. Diagnosis and Management of the Antiphospholipid Syndrome. *N. Engl. J. Med.* **2018**, *378*, 2010–2021. [CrossRef]
111. Simantov, R.; LaSala, J.M.; Lo, S.K.; Gharavi, A.E.; Sammaritano, L.R.; Salmon, J.E.; Silverstein, R.L. Activation of cultured vascular endothelial cells by antiphospholipid antibodies. *J. Clin. Investig.* **1995**, *96*, 2211–2219. [CrossRef]

112. Marciniak, E.; Romond, E.H. Impaired catalytic function of activated protein C: A new in vitro manifestation of lupus anticoagulant. *Blood* **1989**, *74*, 2426–2432. [CrossRef] [PubMed]
113. Arvieux, J.; Jacob, M.C.; Roussel, B.; Bensa, J.C.; Colomb, M.G. Neutrophil activation by anti-beta 2 glycoprotein I monoclonal antibodies via Fc gamma receptor II. *J. Leukoc. Biol.* **1995**, *57*, 387–394. [CrossRef] [PubMed]
114. Fischetti, F.; Durigutto, P.; Pellis, V.; Debeus, A.; Macor, P.; Bulla, R.; Bossi, F.; Ziller, F.; Sblattero, D.; Meroni, P.; et al. Thrombus formation induced by antibodies to beta2-glycoprotein I is complement dependent and requires a priming factor. *Blood* **2005**, *106*, 2340–2346. [CrossRef] [PubMed]
115. Wahl, D.; Membre, A.; Perret-Guillaume, C.; Regnault, V.; Lecompte, T. Mechanisms of antiphospholipid-induced thrombosis: Effects on the protein C system. *Curr. Rheumatol. Rep.* **2009**, *11*, 77–81. [CrossRef] [PubMed]
116. Bucci, T.; Ames, P.R.J.; Triggiani, M.; Parente, R.; Ciampa, A.; Pignatelli, P.; Pastori, D.; Multicenter ATHERO-APS Study group. Cardiac and vascular features of arterial and venous primary antiphospholipid syndrome. The multicenter ATHERO-APS study. *Thromb. Res.* **2022**, *209*, 69–74. [CrossRef] [PubMed]
117. Galli, M.; Luciani, D.; Bertolini, G.; Barbui, T. Lupus anticoagulants are stronger risk factors for thrombosis than anticardiolipin antibodies in the antiphospholipid syndrome: A systematic review of the literature. *Blood* **2003**, *101*, 1827–1832. [CrossRef] [PubMed]
118. Pengo, V.; Ruffatti, A.; Legnani, C.; Gresele, P.; Barcellona, D.; Erba, N.; Testa, S.; Marongiu, F.; Bison, E.; Denas, G.; et al. Clinical course of high-risk patients diagnosed with antiphospholipid syndrome. *J. Thromb. Haemost.* **2010**, *8*, 237–242. [CrossRef] [PubMed]
119. Petri, M. Epidemiology of the Antiphospholipid Antibody Syndrome. *J. Autoimmun.* **2000**, *15*, 145–151. [CrossRef]
120. Miyakis, S.; Lockshin, M.D.; Atsumi, T.; Branch, D.W.; Brey, R.L.; Cervera, R.; Derksen, R.H.W.M.; Groot, P.G.D.; Koike, T.; Meroni, P.L.; et al. International consensus statement on an update of the classification criteria for definite antiphospholipid syndrome (APS). *J. Thromb. Haemost.* **2006**, *4*, 295–306. [CrossRef]
121. Bertina, R.M.; Koeleman, B.P.C.; Koster, T.; Rosendaal, F.R.; Dirven, R.J.; de Ronde, H.; van der Velden, P.A.; Reitsma, P.H. Mutation in blood coagulation factor V associated with resistance to activated protein C. *Nature* **1994**, *369*, 64–67. [CrossRef]
122. Ridker, P.M.; Miletich, J.P.; Hennekens, C.H.; Buring, J.E. Ethnic distribution of factor V Leiden in 4047 men and women. Implications for venous thromboembolism screening. *JAMA* **1997**, *277*, 1305–1307. [CrossRef]
123. Simone, B.; De Stefano, V.; Leoncini, E.; Zacho, J.; Martinelli, I.; Emmerich, J.; Rossi, E.; Folsom, A.R.; Almawi, W.Y.; Scarabin, P.Y.; et al. Risk of venous thromboembolism associated with single and combined effects of Factor V Leiden, Prothrombin 20210A and Methylenetethraydrofolate reductase C677T: A meta-analysis involving over 11,000 cases and 21,000 controls. *Eur. J. Epidemiol.* **2013**, *28*, 621–647. [CrossRef] [PubMed]
124. Ridker, P.M.; Hennekens, C.H.; Lindpaintner, K.; Stampfer, M.J.; Eisenberg, P.R.; Miletich, J.P. Mutation in the gene coding for coagulation factor V and the risk of myocardial infarction, stroke, and venous thrombosis in apparently healthy men. *N. Engl. J. Med.* **1995**, *332*, 912–917. [CrossRef] [PubMed]
125. Rosendaal, F.R.; Koster, T.; Vandenbroucke, J.P.; Reitsma, P.H. High risk of thrombosis in patients homozygous for factor V Leiden (activated protein C resistance). *Blood* **1995**, *85*, 1504–1508. [CrossRef] [PubMed]
126. Ho, W.K.; Hankey, G.J.; Quinlan, D.J.; Eikelboom, J.W. Risk of recurrent venous thromboembolism in patients with common thrombophilia: A systematic review. *Arch. Intern. Med.* **2006**, *166*, 729–736. [CrossRef] [PubMed]
127. Poort, S.; Rosendaal, F.; Reitsma, P.; Bertina, R. A common genetic variation in the 3′-untranslated region of the prothrombin gene is associated with elevated plasma prothrombin levels and an increase in venous thrombosis. *Blood* **1996**, *88*, 3698–3703. [CrossRef] [PubMed]
128. Rosendaal, F.R.; Doggen, C.J.; Zivelin, A.; Arruda, V.R.; Aiach, M.; Siscovick, D.S.; Hillarp, A.; Watzke, H.H.; Bernardi, F.; Cumming, A.M.; et al. Geographic distribution of the 20210 G to A prothrombin variant. *Thromb. Haemost.* **1998**, *79*, 706–708. [PubMed]
129. Margaglione, M.; Brancaccio, V.; Giuliani, N.; D'Andrea, G.; Cappucci, G.; Iannaccone, L.; Vecchione, G.; Grandone, E.; Di Minno, G. Increased risk for venous thrombosis in carriers of the prothrombin G-->A20210 gene variant. *Ann. Intern. Med.* **1998**, *129*, 89–93. [CrossRef]
130. Leroyer, C.; Mercier, B.; Oger, E.; Chenu, E.; Abgrall, J.F.; Férec, C.; Mottier, D. Prevalence of 20210 A allele of the prothrombin gene in venous thromboembolism patients. *Thromb. Haemost.* **1998**, *80*, 49–51.
131. Girolami, A.; Scarano, L.; Tormene, D.; Cella, G. Homozygous patients with the 20210 G to A prothrombin polymorphism remain often asymptomatic in spite of the presence of associated risk factors. *Clin. Appl. Thromb. Hemost.* **2001**, *7*, 122–125. [CrossRef]
132. Segal, J.B.; Brotman, D.J.; Necochea, A.J.; Emadi, A.; Samal, L.; Wilson, L.M.; Crim, M.T.; Bass, E.B. Predictive value of factor V Leiden and prothrombin G20210A in adults with venous thromboembolism and in family members of those with a mutation: A systematic review. *JAMA* **2009**, *301*, 2472–2485. [CrossRef] [PubMed]
133. Clouse, L.H.; Comp, P.C. The regulation of hemostasis: The protein C system. *N. Engl. J. Med.* **1986**, *314*, 1298–1304. [CrossRef] [PubMed]
134. Miletich, J.; Sherman, L.; Broze, G. Absence of thrombosis in subjects with heterozygous protein C deficiency. *N. Engl. J. Med.* **1987**, *317*, 991–996. [CrossRef] [PubMed]

135. Mateo, J.; Oliver, A.; Borrell, M.; Sala, N.; Fontcuberta, J. Laboratory evaluation and clinical characteristics of 2132 consecutive unselected patients with venous thromboembolism—Results of the Spanish Multicentric Study on Thrombophilia (EMET-Study). *Thromb. Haemost.* **1997**, *77*, 444–451. [CrossRef] [PubMed]
136. Gladson, C.L.; Scharrer, I.; Hach, V.; Beck, K.H.; Griffin, J.H. The frequency of type I heterozygous protein S and protein C deficiency in 141 unrelated young patients with venous thrombosis. *Thromb. Haemost.* **1988**, *59*, 18–22. [CrossRef] [PubMed]
137. Martinelli, I.; Mannucci, P.M.; De Stefano, V.; Taioli, E.; Rossi, V.; Crosti, F.; Paciaroni, K.; Leone, G.; Faioni, E.M. Different risks of thrombosis in four coagulation defects associated with inherited thrombophilia: A study of 150 families. *Blood* **1998**, *92*, 2353–2358. [CrossRef] [PubMed]
138. Koster, T.; Rosendaal, F.R.; Briët, E.; van der Meer, F.J.; Colly, L.P.; Trienekens, P.H.; Poort, S.R.; Reitsma, P.H.; Vandenbroucke, J.P. Protein C deficiency in a controlled series of unselected outpatients: An infrequent but clear risk factor for venous thrombosis (Leiden Thrombophilia Study). *Blood* **1995**, *85*, 2756–2761. [CrossRef] [PubMed]
139. Brouwer, J.-L.P.; Lijfering, W.M.; Ten Kate, M.K.; Kluin-Nelemans, H.C.; Veeger, N.J.G.M.; van der Meer, J. High long-term absolute risk of recurrent venous thromboembolism in patients with hereditary deficiencies of protein S, protein C or antithrombin. *Thromb. Haemost.* **2009**, *101*, 93–99. [CrossRef]
140. Esmon, C.T. Protein S and protein C Biochemistry, physiology, and clinical manifestation of deficiencies. *Trends Cardiovasc. Med.* **1992**, *2*, 214–219. [CrossRef]
141. Pintao, M.C.; Ribeiro, D.D.; Bezemer, I.D.; Garcia, A.A.; de Visser, M.C.H.; Doggen, C.J.M.; Lijfering, W.M.; Reitsma, P.H.; Rosendaal, F.R. Protein S levels and the risk of venous thrombosis: Results from the MEGA case-control study. *Blood* **2013**, *122*, 3210–3219. [CrossRef]
142. Lipe, B.; Ornstein, D.L. Deficiencies of natural anticoagulants, protein C, protein S, and antithrombin. *Circulation* **2011**, *124*, e365–e368. [CrossRef]
143. Khor, B.; Van Cott, E.M. Laboratory tests for antithrombin deficiency. *Am. J. Hematol.* **2010**, *85*, 947–950. [CrossRef] [PubMed]
144. Wells, P.S.; Blajchman, M.A.; Henderson, P.; Wells, M.J.; Demers, C.; Bourque, R.; McAvoy, A. Prevalence of antithrombin deficiency in healthy blood donors: A cross-sectional study. *Am. J. Hematol.* **1994**, *45*, 321–324. [CrossRef] [PubMed]
145. Di Minno, M.N.D.; Ambrosino, P.; Ageno, W.; Rosendaal, F.; Di Minno, G.; Dentali, F. Natural anticoagulants deficiency and the risk of venous thromboembolism: A meta-analysis of observational studies. *Thromb. Res.* **2015**, *135*, 923–932. [CrossRef] [PubMed]
146. Ospina-Romero, M.; Cannegieter, S.C.; den Heijer, M.; Doggen, C.J.M.; Rosendaal, F.R.; Lijfering, W.M. Hyperhomocysteinemia and Risk of First Venous Thrombosis: The Influence of (Unmeasured) Confounding Factors. *Am. J. Epidemiol.* **2018**, *187*, 1392–1400. [CrossRef] [PubMed]
147. den Heijer, M.; Willems, H.P.J.; Blom, H.J.; Gerrits, W.B.J.; Cattaneo, M.; Eichinger, S.; Rosendaal, F.R.; Bos, G.M.J. Homocysteine lowering by B vitamins and the secondary prevention of deep vein thrombosis and pulmonary embolism: A randomized, placebo-controlled, double-blind trial. *Blood* **2007**, *109*, 139–144. [CrossRef] [PubMed]
148. Connors, J.M. Thrombophilia Testing and Venous Thrombosis. *N. Engl. J. Med.* **2017**, *377*, 1177–1187. [CrossRef] [PubMed]
149. Prandoni, P.; Noventa, F.; Ghirarduzzi, A.; Pengo, V.; Bernardi, E.; Pesavento, R.; Iotti, M.; Tormene, D.; Simioni, P.; Pagnan, A. The risk of recurrent venous thromboembolism after discontinuing anticoagulation in patients with acute proximal deep vein thrombosis or pulmonary embolism. A prospective cohort study in 1626 patients. *Haematologica* **2007**, *92*, 199–205. [CrossRef]
150. Christiansen, S.C.; Cannegieter, S.C.; Koster, T.; Vandenbroucke, J.P.; Rosendaal, F.R. Thrombophilia, clinical factors, and recurrent venous thrombotic events. *JAMA* **2005**, *293*, 2352–2361. [CrossRef]
151. Evaluation of Genomic Applications in Practice and Prevention (EGAPP) Working Group Recommendations from the EGAPP Working Group: Routine testing for Factor V Leiden (R506Q) and prothrombin (20210G>A) mutations in adults with a history of idiopathic venous thromboembolism and their adult family members. *Genet. Med.* **2011**, *13*, 67–76. [CrossRef]
152. National Clinical Guideline Centre (UK). *Venous Thromboembolic Diseases: The Management of Venous Thromboembolic Diseases and the Role of Thrombophilia Testing*; Royal College of Physicians (UK): London, UK, 2012. Available online: http://www.ncbi.nlm.nih.gov/books/NBK132796/ (accessed on 4 December 2023).
153. Stevens, S.M.; Woller, S.C.; Bauer, K.A.; Kasthuri, R.; Cushman, M.; Streiff, M.; Lim, W.; Douketis, J.D. Guidance for the evaluation and treatment of hereditary and acquired thrombophilia. *J. Thromb. Thrombolysis* **2016**, *41*, 154–164. [CrossRef]
154. Hicks, L.K.; Bering, H.; Carson, K.R.; Kleinerman, J.; Kukreti, V.; Ma, A.; Mueller, B.U.; O'Brien, S.H.; Pasquini, M.; Sarode, R.; et al. The ASH Choosing Wisely®campaign: Five hematologic tests and treatments to question. *Blood* **2013**, *122*, 3879–3883. [CrossRef] [PubMed]
155. Middeldorp, S.; Nieuwlaat, R.; Baumann Kreuziger, L.; Coppens, M.; Houghton, D.; James, A.H.; Lang, E.; Moll, S.; Myers, T.; Bhatt, M.; et al. American Society of Hematology 2023 guidelines for management of venous thromboembolism: Thrombophilia testing. *Blood Adv.* **2023**, *7*, 7101–7138. [CrossRef] [PubMed]
156. Iorio, A.; Kearon, C.; Filippucci, E.; Marcucci, M.; Macura, A.; Pengo, V.; Siragusa, S.; Palareti, G. Risk of recurrence after a first episode of symptomatic venous thromboembolism provoked by a transient risk factor: A systematic review. *Arch. Intern. Med.* **2010**, *170*, 1710–1716. [CrossRef] [PubMed]
157. Lijfering, W.M.; Middeldorp, S.; Veeger, N.J.G.M.; Hamulyák, K.; Prins, M.H.; Büller, H.R.; van der Meer, J. Risk of recurrent venous thrombosis in homozygous carriers and double heterozygous carriers of factor V Leiden and prothrombin G20210A. *Circulation* **2010**, *121*, 1706–1712. [CrossRef] [PubMed]

158. Shatzel, J.J.; O'Donnell, M.; Olson, S.R.; Kearney, M.R.; Daughety, M.M.; Hum, J.; Nguyen, K.P.; DeLoughery, T.G. Venous thrombosis in unusual sites: A practical review for the hematologist. *Eur. J. Haematol.* **2019**, *102*, 53–62. [CrossRef] [PubMed]
159. Goodwin, A.J.; Adcock, D.M. Thrombophilia Testing and Venous Thrombosis. *N. Engl. J. Med.* **2017**, *377*, 2297–2298. [CrossRef] [PubMed]

Disclaimer/Publisher's Note: The statements, opinions and data contained in all publications are solely those of the individual author(s) and contributor(s) and not of MDPI and/or the editor(s). MDPI and/or the editor(s) disclaim responsibility for any injury to people or property resulting from any ideas, methods, instructions or products referred to in the content.

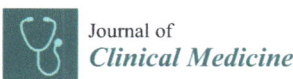

Review

Risk Stratification and Management of Intermediate-Risk Acute Pulmonary Embolism

Nichole Brunton [1], Robert McBane [1], Ana I. Casanegra [1], Damon E. Houghton [1], Dinu V. Balanescu [2], Sumera Ahmad [3], Sean Caples [3], Arashk Motiei [1] and Stanislav Henkin [1,*]

[1] Gonda Vascular Center, Mayo Clinic, Rochester, MN 55901, USA; brunton.nichole@mayo.edu (N.B.)
[2] Department of Cardiovascular Medicine, Mayo Clinic, Rochester, MN 55901, USA
[3] Division of Pulmonary and Critical Care Medicine, Mayo Clinic, Rochester, MN 55901, USA
* Correspondence: henkin.stanislav@mayo.edu

Abstract: Pulmonary embolism (PE) is the third most common cause of cardiovascular death and necessitates prompt, accurate risk assessment at initial diagnosis to guide treatment and reduce associated mortality. Intermediate-risk PE, defined as the presence of right ventricular (RV) dysfunction in the absence of hemodynamic compromise, carries a significant risk for adverse clinical outcomes and represents a unique diagnostic challenge. While small clinical trials have evaluated advanced treatment strategies beyond standard anticoagulation, such as thrombolytic or endovascular therapy, there remains continued debate on the optimal care for this patient population. Here, we review the most recent risk stratification models, highlighting differences between prediction scores and their limitations, and discuss the utility of serologic biomarkers and imaging modalities to detect right ventricular dysfunction. Additionally, we examine current treatment recommendations including anticoagulation strategies, use of thrombolytics at full and reduced doses, and utilization of invasive treatment options. Current knowledge gaps and ongoing studies are highlighted.

Keywords: intermediate-risk pulmonary embolism; risk stratification; right ventricular dysfunction; thrombolytic therapy

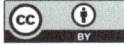

1. Introduction

Acute venous thromboembolism (VTE), presenting as pulmonary embolism (PE) or deep venous thrombosis (DVT), is a frequent cause of cardiovascular death worldwide, ranking third after myocardial infarction and stroke [1]. In longitudinal studies from the early 2000s to 2010s, the incidence of PE increased over time, with a concurrent increase in PE-related hospitalizations [2–4]. During this same timeframe, the case-fatality rates decreased in the United States and other developed countries. PE-related mortality is estimated from 19.4 to 32.3 per 100,000 individuals, with an in-hospital mortality rate of approximately 7% [5,6]. In patients with hemodynamic compromise due to PE, the reported mortality reaches 33%, often occurring suddenly or before therapy can be initiated [5].

Risk factors for the development of VTE include hospitalization, major surgery, fracture of the lower limb, trauma, spinal cord injury, cancer, hormonal therapy, pregnancy, autoimmune disease, presence of invasive lines, severe coronavirus disease (COVID-19), obesity, and thrombophilia [4,7,8]. It is well established that the incidence of VTE also increases with advancing age, with an estimated eight-fold increase for patients in the eighth decade of life compared to those in the fifth decade [4,6].

Due to the high morbidity and mortality associated with PE, early diagnosis and accurate risk assessment for hemodynamic compromise is vital to guide appropriate patient care. However, there is a vast spectrum of clinical presentations in acute PE, ranging from asymptomatic to obstructive shock with circulatory collapse. For this reason, acute PE has been further subdivided into classifications ranging from low-risk to high-risk, though these categories vary by societal guideline [4,9]. A growing body of literature has emerged in recent years investigating metrics, including serologic biomarkers and imaging parameters, to predict impending hemodynamic compromise. Studies have also focused on potential adjunctive therapies, such as mechanical thrombectomy and systemic or catheter-directed thrombolysis, to reduce mortality in this population.

Right ventricular (RV) failure is the main driver of mortality in PE, occurring as a consequence of acute RV pressure overload. In patients with high-risk PE, intervention with thrombolytics is essential, while those with low-risk PE can safely be managed conservatively with anticoagulation alone. However, an intermediate-risk (previously known as "submassive") group demonstrates RV dysfunction without hemodynamic collapse, indicating increased risk for PE-related mortality. Accurately identifying this cohort is difficult due to the heterogeneous nature of patient symptoms, which may range from asymptomatic to dyspnea or chest pain. Recent studies have focused on identifying objective clinical markers and imaging parameters to quickly and accurately risk-stratify patients. In this review, we focus on current definitions of intermediate-risk PE, highlighting the benefits and limitations of available risk prediction models and discussing the utility of serologic biomarkers and imaging metrics of RV dysfunction, along with invasive hemodynamic assessment in this population. We also discuss escalation of care (EOC) therapies and the most recent results from thrombolytic trials, reviewing the controversial role of mechanical thrombectomy and alternative invasive procedures, as well as current knowledge gaps.

2. Acute Pulmonary Embolism Definitions and Classification

Acute pulmonary embolism may be classified based on the presence or absence of a provoking factor, symptoms, or acute hemodynamic instability, as well as the embolized material (e.g., thrombus, air, fat, tumor), its anatomic location and extent, and the risk of mortality. This review will focus on acute pulmonary embolism due to VTE and its classification based on risk models.

In 2011, the American Heart Association (AHA) published a scientific statement on the management of PE which outlined the classification of PE in three groups: low-risk, submassive, and massive [9]. Low-risk PE was defined as normotensive patients without biomarker elevation and normal RV function, while massive PE encompassed patients with sustained hypotension (systolic blood pressure < 90 mm Hg for 15 min), pulselessness, or profound bradycardia as a direct consequence of PE. Another group, deemed submassive, was defined as normotensive patients at an increased risk for adverse mortality outcomes. This patient population, while hemodynamically stable, had evidence of RV injury by serologic biomarker (troponin or natriuretic peptide), or RV dysfunction by imaging (RV dilatation on CT or echocardiography with an RV: LV ratio of >0.9), or new electrocardiographic changes (new right-bundle branch block, anteroseptal ST elevation depression, or anteroseptal T-wave inversion). These criteria were established from a body of studies conducted between 1999 to 2009 [4,10–15]. Simultaneously, two main clinical predictive scores were developed: the Geneva and the Pulmonary Embolism Severity Index (PESI), which supported these metrics as predictive for adverse outcomes in PE [9,11].

The European Society of Cardiology (ESC) released their guidelines, which remain the most frequently utilized for defining PE classifications, in 2019. As the understanding of RV dysfunction evolved, these updated guidelines aimed to accurately define metrics indicative of acute RV failure and identify additional risk factors that could predispose patients to poor clinical outcomes. The most notable difference in these guidelines when compared to the AHA 2011 definitions is the further subclassification of intermediate-risk to either intermediate-low or intermediate-high-risk (Table 1). This stratification developed from the realization that patients with submassive PE were still representative of a large and diverse patient group with a persistently high mortality rate, reportedly as high as 12.3% to 14.4% despite modern interventions [16,17].

Table 1. Guidelines for classification of pulmonary embolism severity by society [4,9].

Guideline/ Statement	Classification	Hemodynamic Status	Cardiac Biomarkers	RV Dysfunction on Imaging	Risk Score
American Heart Association (2011) [9]	Low	Stable	Negative	Negative	Not incorporated
	Intermediate	Stable	BNP > 90 pg/mL N-terminal pro-BNP > 500 pg/mL Troponin I > 0.4 ng/mL Troponin T > 0.1 ng/mL	RV dilatation (4-chamber RV/LV diameter > 0.9) on CT or ECHO RV systolic dysfunction on ECHO	
	High	Sustained hypotension (systolic BP of <90 mm Hg) for 15 min or requiring iatrogenic support. Pulselessness Persistent bradycardia (HR < 40)	Present	Present	
European Society of Cardiology (2019) [4]	Low	Stable	Negative	Negative	PESI I-II
	Intermediate-Low	Stable	Requires EITHER positive biomarkers OR RV dysfunction imaging. *(definitions below)*		Meets classification of PESI III-IV or sPESI ≥ 1 (see Table 2)
	Intermediate-High	Stable	N-terminal pro-BNP > 600 pg/mL Troponin I or T elevation, consider age-adjusted high-sensitivity cut-off values.	RV/LV diameter ratio ≥ 1.0 on CT or ECHO RV systolic dysfunction on ECHO (ex TAPSE < 16 mm)	
	High	Cardiac arrest Obstructive shock with end-organ hypoperfusion (systolic BP < 90 mmHg or vasopressors despite adequate filling status) Persistent hypotension (systolic BP < 90 mmHg or a systolic BP drop ≥ 40 mmHg for >15 min)	Present	Present	

Blood pressure (BP), brain natriuretic peptide (BNP), computed tomography (CT), echocardiogram (ECHO), heart rate (HR), Pulmonary Embolism Severity Index (PESI), tricuspid annular plane systolic excursion (TAPSE), right ventricle (RV).

In 2019, the AHA released an updated scientific statement specifically focused on interventions for PE. In this document, the differences between the ESC/AHA risk classification model were highlighted as inherently different due to the creation of the risk models for different purposes. However, for simplicity, the AHA adopted the classification of patients previously classified as "submassive" as an intermediate-risk group and patients previously classified as "massive" as a high-risk group. The 2019 AHA intermediate-risk group included all patients in the ESC intermediate-risk group (both intermediate-low-risk and intermediate-high-risk) [18].

Table 2. Pulmonary Embolism Severity Index scores: original and simplified [19,20].

Parameter	Original PESI Score	Simplified PESI Score (sPESI)
Demographics - Age - Male sex	 + Age in years + 10 points	 1 point if >80 years old -
Medical Comorbidities - Cancer - Congestive Heart Failure - Chronic Pulmonary Disease	 + 30 points + 10 points + 10 points	 1 point *1 point for chronic lung or heart disease*
Initial Clinical Assessment - Pulse: >110 bpm - Respiratory rate: >30 bpm - Systolic BP: <100 mmHg - Temperature: <36 °C - Altered mentation - Arterial oxygen saturation < 90%	 + 20 points + 20 points + 30 points + 20 points + 60 points + 20 points	 1 point - 1 point - - -
Interpretation of PESI vs. sPESI Risk Calculations		
Low-Risk Categories: Outpatient Management to be Considered	Class I (very low): <65 points Class II: 66–85 points	0 Points
Moderate to Very High-Risk Categories: Inpatient Management Recommended	Class III (moderate): 86–105 points Class IV (high): 106–125 points Class V (very high): >125 points	≥1 point: estimated 30-day mortality risk 10.9%

In the ESC risk model, the Pulmonary Embolism Severity Index (PESI), either the original or simplified model (Table 2), is employed to distill clinical information, including vital signs and medical comorbidities, into a risk score. The PESI score was developed in 2005 and utilized 11 patient characteristics independently associated with increased mortality. These were used to stratify patients into five severity classes (I–V) ranging from very low-risk to very high-risk [19]. For patients in class I, the risk of inpatient death and complications was found to be <1%, and it ranged from 10–24.5% in class V. This is useful for rapidly identifying patients at risk for all-cause mortality at 30 days after PE diagnosis and was validated using both an internal and external validation cohort in the initial study [19]. In 2010, Jiménez et al. completed a derivation study simplifying this score (sPESI) to help quickly identify patients at an increased risk for 30-day mortality [10]. This is helpful for quick assessment of patient disposition but is not useful for nuanced risk category placement or analysis. It is worth remaining mindful of clinical characteristics influencing PESI variables, such as sepsis for example, and that sPESI has limited specificity in predicting mortality in high-risk patients.

Patients scoring as PESI I–II or with an sPESI of ≤1 are considered low-risk, and selected cases could be managed in the outpatient setting. This has been validated by additional studies demonstrating the safety of this strategy [21]. In patients with PESI class III–V or with an sPESI score of ≥1, further evaluation is necessary. Imaging parameters and cardiac serologic biomarkers are utilized to further classify these patients to predict PE-related mortality at 30 days (Table 2). Patients with both evidence of RV dysfunction by imaging and serologic biomarkers were defined as intermediate-high-risk, while patients with only one or neither metric fulfilled are classified as intermediate-low-risk. This was an important update from prior AHA statements because it served to identify a PE population at risk for hemodynamic compromise while also attempting to limit confounders such as chronic RV dysfunction from other causes.

The latest release of societal guidelines on the management of PE is the 2021 guidelines on Antithrombotic Therapy for VTE Disease from the American College of Chest Physicians (ACCP). These guidelines more broadly categorize PE on the basis of 'associated with hypotension' or 'not associated with hypotension' to guide next treatment steps [22]. However, a limitation of this model is its lack of inclusion of RV hemodynamic parameters. As such, the guidelines potentially exclude a population of PE patients at risk for hemodynamic compromise and place a higher burden on the clinician to differentiate between hypotension due to PE or due to other causes (e.g., cardiogenic shock, sepsis, etc.).

3. Indicators of Risk in Pulmonary Embolism

3.1. Serologic Biomarkers

It is crucial to highlight that any single serologic marker is not sufficient to detect risk for hemodynamic collapse and must be considered within the context of clinical history, baseline comorbid conditions, physical examination, and imaging parameters. Therefore, serologic markers of myocardial injury and right ventricular dysfunction can be useful in identifying patients at high risk for circulatory collapse when interpreted in the appropriate clinical setting.

The most widely used marker for myocardial injury is plasma troponin (T or I) level. In hemodynamically stable patients with PE, an elevated troponin level on presentation is associated with higher risk of mortality when compared to those with negative troponin (T or I) values [23,24]. Similar findings are reported with the employment of high-sensitivity troponin T (hsTnT) assays [17,23,24]. In small prospective trials, patients with higher baseline hsTnT values on presentation were noted to experience higher rates of adverse 30-day outcomes compared to those with low hsTnT values (defined as <14 pg/mL). Furthermore, the increased sensitivity of this assay led to the re-classification of nearly 50% of patients who otherwise would have been classified as low-risk by traditional AHA guidelines [17]. A post-hoc analysis from the Prognostic Value of Computed Tomography (PROTECT) trial compared outcomes of PE patients with conventional troponin elevation to patients with hsTnT elevation. When evaluating troponin as a binary metric, only conventional troponin elevation was associated with increased odds for hemodynamic collapse or all-cause death within 30 days of PE. Moreover, there were no reported adverse outcomes in patients with normal conventional troponin and elevated hsTNT [25]. This supports the addition of the intermediate-low-risk ESC classification, where subtle signs of myocardial injury can be detected but may not necessarily translate to the need for more aggressive interventions.

Serologic evaluation for ventricular dysfunction, due to increased RV pressure and myocardial stretch, includes B-type natriuretic peptide (BNP) and N-terminal (NT)-BNP. Again, prior meta-analyses support the prognostic value of elevated BNP and/or NT-proBNP, with elevated values conferring a higher risk for adverse clinical outcomes, including death [4,26]. Conversely, patients with low troponin values, BNP, or NT-proBNP levels are useful for identifying low-risk PE events with a high negative predictive value [4].

The difficulty with all of the aforementioned biomarkers is the lack of specificity for PE. While prognostically helpful for identifying higher-risk PE patients, these biomarkers can also be elevated independently from the presence of concurrent medical conditions such as chronic pulmonary hypertension, left-sided heart failure, volume overload in the context of renal failure, etc. A classic example of this confounding is the patient with left ventricular failure with volume overload with high NT-pro BNP, but who is incidentally found to have a single, subsegmental pulmonary embolism. However, in patients with known baseline values of these markers, in the absence of new clinical scenarios that may be associated with abnormal serologic markers, it is reasonable to attribute elevations to PE.

To summarize, troponin and BNP or NT-pro BNP are generally reliable parameters of acute RV dysfunction due to PE; however, interpretation of these values is difficult in the medically complex patient and makes curating an algorithm for the management of PE patients challenging. This is particularly true when attempting to identify intermediate-high-risk patients for invasive therapy strategies. Further studies are needed to understand the appropriate utilization of biomarkers in this population and if threshold values or delta from baseline values could be useful to provide additional insight.

3.2. Imaging: Use of Echocardiography, Computed Tomography Pulmonary Angiography, and Invasive Hemodynamic Assessment

Under normal physiologic circumstances, the RV functions with a low pulmonary vascular resistance (PVR) and, therefore, low afterload. In acute PE, the PVR increases quickly and results in a rapid increase in RV systolic pressure, causing pressure and volume overload and RV dysfunction. This can lead to overt RV failure in severe cases [27]. Increased pulmonary artery pressure (PAP) occurs when at least 30% to 50% of the pulmonary arterial vasculature is occluded from thromboemboli [4]. RV dysfunction and volume overload can be appreciated on imaging by echocardiography or computed tomography pulmonary angiography (CTPA) in at least half of patients hospitalized for PE [28]. These imaging findings serve as important prognostic markers for patients with intermediate-risk PE but can be challenging to quantify due to the irregular shape of the RV, which limits the utility of a single metric to quantify severity of dysfunction. When carefully utilized, echocardiography (ECHO) parameters of RV dysfunction can provide helpful insight into cardiac function to help prognosticate mortality in patients with intermediate-risk PE [29]. It is important to note that signs of RV dysfunction on imaging are not specific to acute PE alone and may be present in patients without PE. Therefore, these must be evaluated in the context of the patient's baseline cardiac function, other medical comorbidities, and interpreted with caution due to variations in techniques.

Standardization of RV function on echocardiography by the American Society of Echocardiography (ASE) did not occur until 2010. As a result, early echocardiography studies utilized an array of measurements to define RV dysfunction [30]. Despite this challenge, early meta-analyses did show a 2.29-fold increase (95% CI 1.61–3.26) in short-term mortality for hemodynamically stable patients with evidence of RV dysfunction on echocardiography [30]. Frequently utilized measures include RV cavity dilatation, diminished inspiratory phase of a distended inferior vena cava (IVC), and elevated RV to left ventricle (LV) ratio (>1.0). RV dilatation is considered a hallmark for PE and has been reported in >25% of PE cases [27,31,32].

Frequently on both CTPA and ECHO assessment, a comparison of RV to LV size is made on imaging, with a ratio of ≥ 0.9 accompanied by an underfilling LV being suggestive of PE. While the RV:LV ratio remains one of the most frequently cited metrics for RV dysfunction in the medical literature, there are significant variations in calculation that impact the diagnostic accuracy of this measurement. This occurs due to different methods of measurement, utilizing the epicardial border (outer edge-to-outer edge) or endocardial border (inner edge-to-inner edge), timing of the measurement (end-diastole versus end-systole), and use of a gated image. For this reason, the RV:LV ratio may not always be a reliable metric of RV dysfunction. One study demonstrated that when studied in isolation in patients with low-risk PE, an RV:LV ratio of >1.0 on imaging did not carry significant risk for mortality, recurrent PE, or total adverse events at 3 months [32].

For CTPA, the simplest and accepted way to identify RV dysfunction is by assessing the axial plane where ventricular cavities are maximally visualized, typically at the plane of the mitral valve. RV dysfunction is considered dilated if the RV cavity is wider than the LV cavity. Another CTA finding consistent with RV dysfunction is the deviation of the interventricular septum to the LV (Figure 1) [33]. Again, it is important to note that this method carries limitations in patients with pre-existing lung conditions or pulmonary hypertension with baseline RV enlargement. Other findings suggestive of RV dysfunction on CTPA include reflux of contrast into the IVC, interventricular septal deviation, assessment of pulmonary artery size, and presence of RV dilatation [34,35].

Echocardiographic metrics of RV dysfunction include the McConnell sign, whereby the free RV midwall becomes hypokinetic with hyperkinetic apical segment; a decreased RV tricuspid annular plan systolic excursion (TAPSE) of <16 mm; decreased peak systolic velocity of the tricuspid annulus (<9.5 cm/s); and the presence of interventricular septal bowing, which occurs in severe RV dysfunction near the point of hemodynamic collapse [27,34]. However, due to the asymmetric shape of the RV, basal segments and TAPSE may remain normal in cases of dysfunctional RV. Additionally, in individuals with baseline pulmonary hypertension with elevated PVR, RV hypertrophy can develop, reducing the sensitivity and predictive value of these measures [4,27,28]. For this reason, recent studies have attempted to develop a combination of echocardiographic findings to achieve a high positive predictive value for PE that can be utilized even in those with pre-existing cardiopulmonary pathology [4,31]. One proposed method is the "60/60" sign, defined as the presence of both a shortened pulmonary ejection acceleration time (AcT) of <60 ms with a "notched" midsystolic velocity deceleration in the RV outflow tract (RVOT) and reduced (<60 mmHg) tricuspid regurgitation peak systolic gradient (TRPG) (Figure 1). A single center analysis of 511 consecutive patients with PE reviewed echocardiograms in acute PE (all subtypes) for presence of the McConnell sign, the "60/60" sign, and the presence of right heart thrombus, occurring in 19.8%, 12.9%, and 1.8% of patients, respectively. These rates increased dramatically in a subgroup analysis for high-risk PE patients, with a reported prevalence of 75% with the McConnell sign and 31.2% with the 60/60 sign. Conventional metrics of RV dysfunction (RV:LV ratio of ≥ 0.9) were identified in only 20% of all patients included in the study [31]. It is important to note that studies utilize varying definitions of RV dysfunction, commonly using either an RV:LV ratio of ≥ 0.9 or ≥ 1.0. Prior meta-analyses have demonstrated an association between higher cut-offs of RV:LV ventricle ratio with a higher risk of death [36]. It is unclear which ratio should be employed routinely, though our group utilizes RV:LV > 0.9 to increase sensitivity and in accordance with previously published guidelines [9].

Additional studies have demonstrated the RVOT velocity time integral (VTI), an echocardiographic surrogate for stroke volume, as a significant predictor for invasively derived low cardiac index (CI) and risk of mortality related to PE [29,36]. Specifically, in a small study, an RVOT VTI of <9.5 cm was associated with higher PE-related mortality (13.6%) when compared to patients with an RVOT > 9.5 cm (1.28%), though all-cause mortality between the groups was not significantly differently [29]. Three-dimensional echocardiographic assessment of global and regional RV strain in patients with intermediate-risk PE may provide additive fidelity for patients at risk for hemodynamic compromise, though further studies are needed to explore this [37].

For patients with intermediate-risk PE undergoing endovascular intervention, hemodynamic assessment by right heart catheterization can further provide insights about mortality risk. A CI < 2.2 L/min/m^2 has been associated with increased risk for PE-related mortality [29]. In small studies, approximately half of patients undergoing endovascular intervention are noted to have reduced CI on hemodynamic assessment despite being normotensive [29,38]. However, this metric was not utilized in the early interventional trials for risk stratification. Future studies may be helpful to fully ascertain if this cohort derives additive benefit from more aggressive management strategies.

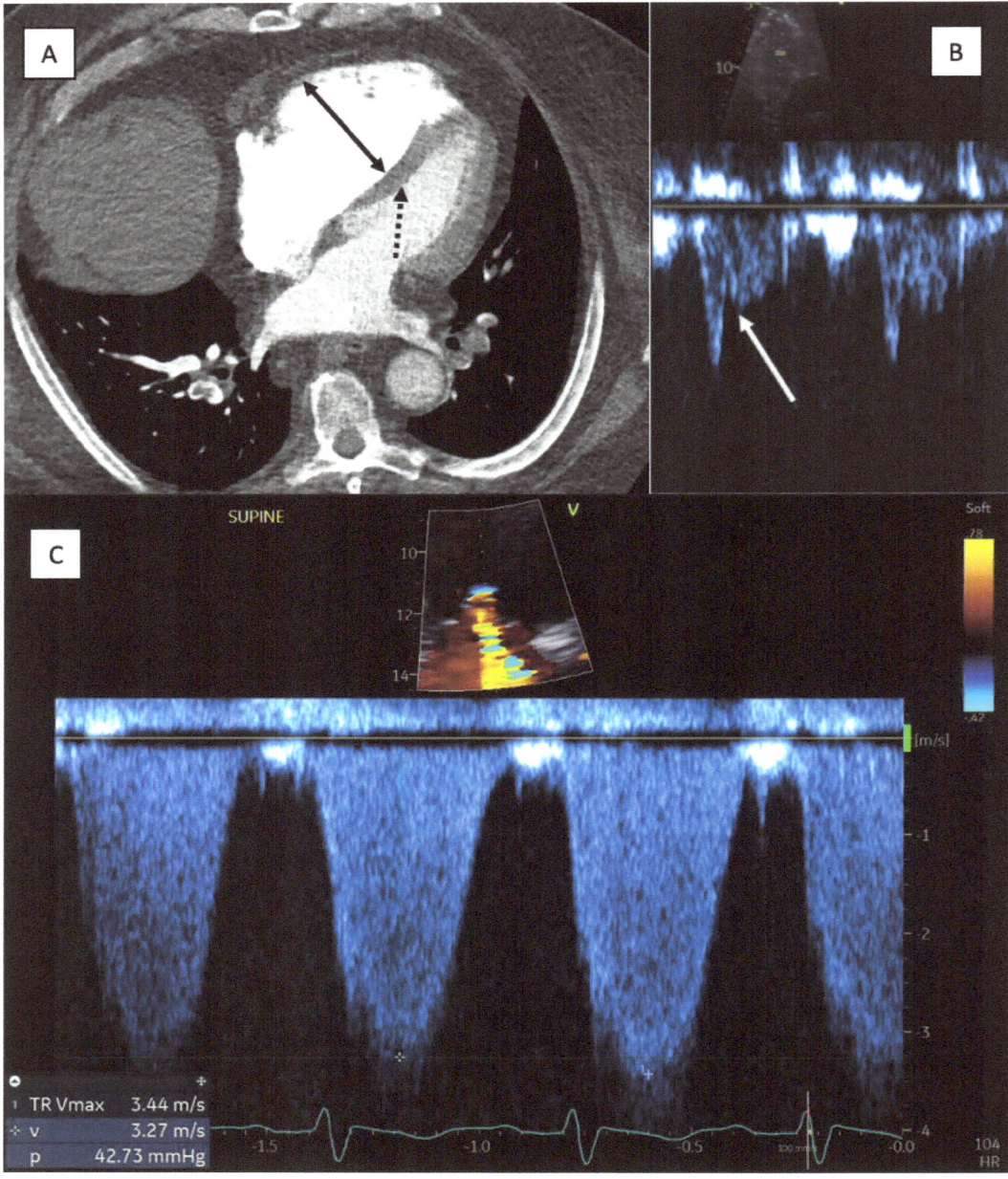

Figure 1. Computed tomography angiography findings consistent with right ventricular dysfunction [32]. (**A**) CTA chest: Axial image at the level of the mitral valve. Solid arrow demonstrating enlargement of the right ventricle compared to the left ventricular cavity. Dashed arrow highlights the deviation of the interventricular septum towards the left ventricle. (**B**) Transthoracic ECHO (same patient): shortened pulmonary ejection acceleration time (AcT) with a "notched" midsystolic velocity deceleration in the RV outflow track (white arrow). (**C**) Transthoracic ECHO (same patient): demonstrating tricuspid regurgitation (TR) peak systolic gradient (TRPG) of less than 60 mm Hg (42.7 mm Hg), consistent with the proposed 60/60 sign.

When invasive hemodynamic assessment is pursued, a clearer understanding of the hemodynamic consequences of a PE can be obtained through evaluation of right ventricle to pulmonary artery (RV-PA) coupling [39]. Simply stated, the RV is able to accommodate for increased afterload from the pulmonary artery (PA) to a certain degree; however, there is a point in which adaptive mechanisms are no longer able to compensate. This leads to an 'uncoupling' between the RV-PA, which signals RV decompensation [40,41]. The gold standard for RV-PA assessment is by invasive catheterization and is calculated by the ratio between the RV end-systolic elastance (Ees) and the pulmonary arterial elastance (Ea). When the RV begins to decompensate, a decline is noted in the Ees, resulting in a decline in the Ees/Ea, implying uncoupling of the RV-PA [39,40]. There has been recent effort to derive this metric non-invasively by echocardiography. Examples include using surrogate markers of the tricuspid annular plane systolic excursion (TAPSE) to systolic pulmonary artery pressure (PASP) ratio, right ventricular ejection fraction (RVEF) to PASP, or right ventricular fractional area change (RVFAC) to right ventricular systolic pressure (RVSP) [39]. Further studies are required to fully understand the reproducibility and feasibility of these metrics, since good-quality images are essential for calculation. Further trials are also needed to determine clinically significant Ees/Ea values and thresholds for intervention.

4. Management of Intermediate-Risk Pulmonary Embolism

Medical Management: Anticoagulation

The cornerstone of acute medical management for PE is anticoagulation [42]. Initial parenteral therapy is recommended with low-molecular weight heparin (LMWH) above unfractionated heparin (UH) infusion due to the rapid rise of therapeutic drug levels and decreased risk of heparin-induced thrombocytopenia. Furthermore, a meta-analysis demonstrated improved outcomes in PE patients initially treated with LMWH compared to UH, including a reduction in thrombotic complications, an increased safety profile for major hemorrhage, and lower risk of mortality [43]. Heparin infusions should be considered if there is concern for impending hemodynamic compromise and consideration for imminent endovascular intervention.

When stabilized and appropriate for discharge, direct oral anticoagulant (DOAC) therapy is frequently utilized due to ease of use. The safety and non-inferiority to vitamin K antagonists (VKA) of the direct oral anticoagulant (DOAC) agents is well established for PE treatment and incorporated in current practice guidelines [44–46]. In review of the major DOAC trials for thromboembolism, despite frequent DOAC utilization for treatment of intermediate-risk PE, the Hokusai-VTE investigators were the only group to specifically review the use of edoxaban in patients with right-ventricular dysfunction [47]. There was a reduction in VTE recurrence for patients with RV dysfunction treated with edoxaban compared to warfarin [47]. Important considerations for DOAC use include renal or hepatic function, as these agents are not well studied in patients with end-stage renal disease and should be avoided in patients with underlying hepatic dysfunction beyond Child–Pugh Class A. Patient history of bariatric surgery, potential medication interactions, patient weight, and financial feasibility should also be considered prior to prescription of DOAC therapy for first-line management of intermediate-risk PE, as these components can lead to subtherapeutic drug levels or non-compliance. Recent guidelines by the International Society on Thrombosis and Haemostasis support the use of apixaban and rivaroxaban for patients with a BMI > 35 or body weight > 120 kg; however, data are limited to support use in patients at weight extremes (BMI > 50 or body weight > 150 kg). The use of dabigatran or edoxaban in patients with a BMI > 35 or body weight > 120 kg has not been sufficiently studied and is not recommended [48]. For patients with unprovoked PE, antiphospholipid syndrome (APS) should be considered prior to dismissal on DOAC therapy, as patients with APS are known to have higher risk for DOAC failure. Additional serologic evaluation for inherited thrombophilias is not required prior to DOAC use in most patients. DOACs have also shown their effectiveness in cancer-associated PE and should be considered first-line in this population where traditionally LMWH has been used preferentially [49].

In patients with clinical contraindications or financial barriers to the use of DOAC therapies, anticoagulation with VKA is recommended. When used, monitoring for VKA therapy should be completed using international normalized ratio (INR) values with an anticipated range of 2.0–3.0. When VKA therapy is initiated, patients with acute VTE require bridging with LMWH until a therapeutic INR level can be achieved and for a minimum of 5 days. It is advised to treat with LMWH if the INR is below two during the first month after the event. A typical treatment course with therapeutic anticoagulation after intermediate-risk pulmonary embolism ranges from 3–6 months. Patients with unprovoked PE or patients with cancer-associated venous VTE should be strongly considered for extended VTE prophylaxis depending on the clinical scenario.

5. Escalation of Care Therapies

5.1. Role of Thrombolytic Therapy

In patients with concerning features for impending hemodynamic compromise, anticoagulation alone may not be a sufficient strategy to prevent clinical decline. The "Fibrinolysis for Patients with Intermediate-Risk Pulmonary Embolism" (PEITHO trial) was completed in 2014 to evaluate the use of tenecteplase (ranging from 30 to 50 mg) plus anticoagulation compared to placebo plus anticoagulation in a double-blind control study. Primary outcomes for this study included death or hemodynamic collapse within 7 days of enrollment, with a safety endpoint of major bleeding or stroke [50]. Although hemodynamic collapse in patients treated with tenecteplase plus heparin occurred less frequently when compared to the placebo group (2.6% vs. 5.6%, OR 0.44), this did not provide a net benefit at 30 days due to the increased risk of extracranial bleeding (6.3% vs. 1.2%) and hemorrhagic stroke in the tenecteplase group [50].

Due to concern for increased bleeding risk, the "Moderate Pulmonary Embolism Treated with Thrombolysis" (MOPETT trial) was conducted using low-dose tissue plasminogen activator (tPA; 0.5 mg/kg with maximum dose of 50 mg). The primary endpoints for this study were pulmonary hypertension, defined as a PASP of $\geq$40 mm Hg on echocardiogram, and a composite of pulmonary hypertension and recurrent PE after 28 months of follow-up. Pulmonary hypertension was noted in 16% of the low-dose thrombolytic group compared to 57% of the control group. Hospital duration was shorter for patients receiving low-dose thrombolytics (2.2 days vs. 4.9 days). A significant difference for death or PE recurrence was not appreciated in this study cohort. Therefore, low-dose thrombolytics are postulated to be safe; however, this has not yet been shown to alter other clinical outcomes [51]. It should be noted that this trial did include a small sample size. Conversely, a retrospective study comparing half-dose atleplase (50 mg) to full-dose (100 mg) suggested similar mortality rates and major bleeding events [52]. In summary, further large trials are needed to better ascertain the role of low-dose lytic therapy in this population.

Long-term outcome data for patients with intermediate-high-risk PE and thrombolytic therapy are limited. In 2017, the PEITHO group published long-term data in a subgroup with a median follow-up time of 37.8 months after systemic thrombolytic therapy. Survival was similar between the systemic thrombolysis and placebo groups (20.3% vs. 18.0%, respectively). Functional limitations and persistent dyspnea were similar between the two groups as well, approximately 33% in both arms. There was not a significant difference between echocardiographic findings for pulmonary hypertension or persistent RV dysfunction at follow-up [53]. To summarize, there was no significant difference for mortality, functional outcomes, or echocardiographic metrics to suggest long-term improvement for patients with intermediate-risk PE receiving thrombolytics.

In summary, while systemic thrombolytic therapy has shown reductions in pulmonary arterial pressures and reduced hospitalization length, no current evidence signals further mortality benefit in patients with intermediate-risk PE. However, these trials are not completely reflective of our current understanding of intermediate-high-risk PE nor are reflective of current recommended treatment strategies [54]. For example, the MOPETT trial enrolled patients with metrics consistent with symptomatic PE; however, evidence of RV dysfunction by imaging or cardiac biomarkers was not necessary for study enrollment [51]. Even in the PEITHO trial, RV dysfunction was defined by either echocardiographic or CT parameters, with a right-to-left ventricular end-diastolic diameter of >0.9 or right-to-left ventricular diameter ratio of >0.9 on CT. As mentioned earlier, these are not ideal metrics to define RV dysfunction. This highlights the need for further investigation into the role of systemic thrombolytics and the need to refine the definition of RV dysfunction for patients included in these trials. Furthermore, while prior studies of thrombolytic agents in intermediate-risk PE provided conflicting results, a recent meta-analysis completed in 2023 suggests that there may be further short-term benefits, though the evidence is overall weak [54]. With the rapid evolution of PE management, many prior reviews of thrombolytics included studies with antiquated agents or substandard doses. When only studies with current thrombolytic agents and standard dosing were included, a meta-analysis by Mathew et al. found that patients receiving systemic thrombolytics compared to anticoagulation alone had a decreased need for vasopressor support (RR 0.27, 95% CI 0.11–0.64) and rescue thrombolysis (RR 0.25, 95% CI 0.14–0.45). This occurred at the expense of increased intracranial hemorrhage and did not yield a significant in-hospital mortality difference between patients receiving thrombolytics versus those managed with anticoagulation alone [54].

5.2. Catheter-Based Strategies

The benefit of catheter-based therapies in high-risk PE is becoming well established; however, impacts on outcomes in intermediate-risk PE remain unclear [55]. Current invasive management strategies for intermediate-risk PE include mechanical thrombectomy and catheter-directed thrombolytic (CDT) systems, including ultrasound-facilitated systems (US CDT), which appeared on the market in the past decade. Mechanical thrombectomy devices available for clot retrieval include the Inari Medical (Irvine, CA, USA) FlowTriever, the Penumbra (Alameda, CA, USA) Indigo Aspiration Thrombectomy System, and the Angiodynamics (Latham, NY, USA) AngioVasc/AlphaVac. Potential benefits to mechanical thrombectomy include a measurable hemodynamic response while patients are in the interventional suite, reduced bleeding risk comparative to systemic lytic therapy in the short term, significantly shorter length of hospital stay, potential deferral of intensive care unit admission, and more rapid improvement in RV hemodynamic parameters compared to anticoagulation [56–58]. However, drawbacks include the risk for vascular or cardiac injury as well as a prolonged procedural time, depending on the nature of the thrombus being extracted. On retrospective review, compared to systemic thrombolytic therapy, patients undergoing catheter-directed thrombolytic therapy carry similar risk for major bleeding (RR 0.52: 95% CI 0.37–1.76) but lower risk for in-hospital mortality (RR 0.52, 95% CI 0.40–0.68) as well as intracranial hemorrhage (RR 0.66, 95% CI 0.47–0.94) [59]. However, these data are limited based on the retrospective nature of this study and by the lack of further classification based on PE risk.

Catheter-based thrombolytic strategies include EKOS (Boston Scientific, Marlborough, MA, USA), Bashir endovascular catheter (Thrombolex, New Britain, PA, USA), or the use of standard infusion catheters. Benefits to CDT include shorter procedural time; however, patients are generally admitted to the intensive care unit and response to treatment requires a minimum of several hours, along with the risk of patient discomfort due to necessary prolonged supine positioning. Patients with active bleeding, head trauma, or cerebral infarction in the preceding 3 months or known intracranial tumors/aneurysms have contraindications for these strategies. Relative contraindications include trauma or surgery within the preceding 10 days, uncontrolled hypertension (systolic BP > 180 mm Hg or diastolic > 110 mm Hg), or gastrointestinal bleeding within the preceding three months [60].

Notable studies for catheter-directed thrombolysis and mechanical thrombectomy in intermediate-risk PE are summarized in Table 3. Importantly, while randomized controlled trials examining the use of endovascular interventions exist, all the existing device trials include only a small subset of patients, which makes extrapolation difficult. Furthermore, most PE device studies for intermediate-risk PE examine only metrics of RV improvement, typically quantified by the RV/LV ratio, modified Miller score (a score for radiographic extent of thrombus), or PASP alone. The recently published REAL-PE trial, a retrospective study, signals that major bleeding occurs more frequently with mechanical thrombectomy when compared to ultrasound-directed CDT, including higher rates of intracranial hemorrhage. While these results provide insight into the bleeding risk and safety of endovascular strategies, the findings are somewhat counterintuitive. This is likely due to the retrospective trial design and confounding bias in patient selection for mechanical thrombectomy [61].

Table 3. Summary of device-related trials for treatment of intermediate-risk pulmonary embolism.

Trial	Device	Study Design/Aims	Outcomes	Limitations
Ultrasound-facilitated catheter-directed thrombolysis (US CDT)				
ULTIMA [56] (2013)	EkoSonic MACH4e Endovascular System	Randomized controlled trial. N = 59 patients. Aims: USAT + AC versus AC alone in the reversal of RV dilatation in *intermediate-risk* PE patients.	USAT + AC was superior to AC alone in reversing RV dilatation at 24 h. No increase in bleeding complications between the two arms.	Small study population size. Limited follow-up to 24 h reviewing ECHO metrics alone; no comparison for clinical outcomes.
SEATTLE II [57] (2015)	EkoSonic Endovascular System	Prospective, single-arm, multicenter study using US CDT and low-dose fibrinolytic therapy. N = 150 patients with proximal PE (included massive and submassive PE). Aims: change in RV/LV ratio and PA systolic pressure from baseline at 48 + 6 h after procedure. Safety outcome of major bleeding within 72 h and recurrent PE, all-cause mortality, and procedural complications.	Mean RV/LV diameter decreased (1.55 at baseline to 1.13 at 48 h). Mean PASP decreased (51.4 mm Hg at baseline to 37.5 mm Hg) at the end of procedure. Safety: 17 major bleeding events within 30 days of the procedure observed in 15 patients (10%).	Lack of comparator group for full-dose systemic fibrinolysis, half-dose systemic fibrinolysis, or anticoagulation alone. Excluded patients with stroke/TIA within 12 months, patients with INR > 3.0, or serum creatinine > 2.0. Limited follow-up to 30 days post-procedure. Limited follow-up to 24 h reviewing ECHO metrics alone; no comparison for clinical outcomes.
OPTALYSE PE [62] (2018)	EkoSonic Endovascular System	Intermediate-risk PE patients, randomized to one of four groups of varying timeframes and concentrations of tPA infusion. N = 101. Aim: reduction in RV:LV ratio by CTA and embolic burden by modified Miller score on CTPA at 48 h.	Improvement in RV:LV ratio and modified Miller score was observed in all groups. Four patients experienced MBE, two being intracranial hemorrhage.	Small study population size. Unclear if improvement in CTPA metrics translate into short or long-term clinical benefits or adverse outcomes.

Table 3. *Cont.*

Trial	Device	Study Design/Aims	Outcomes	Limitations
HI-PEITHO [63] (2022)	EKOS™ Endovascular System	Multi-center, prospective, randomized controlled trial for acute intermediate high-risk PE. Aim: EKOS + AC vs. AC alone for composite outcome of PE-related death, circulatory collapse, or non-fatal recurrence of PE.	Ongoing trial.	
Pharmacomechanical catheter-directed thrombolysis trials				
RESCUE [64] (2022)	Thrombolex-Bashir catheters	Multi-center, prospective trial. N = 109 patients. Aim: change in CTPA RV:LV ratio at 48 h and safety endpoint of serious adverse events in acute intermediate-risk PE.	RV/LV diameter ratio decreased by 0.56 (33.3%) and PA obstruction by refined modified Miller index was reduced (35.9%). Very low rate of adverse events or major bleeding (0.92%).	Small study population size. Lack of short-term or long-term clinical benefits or adverse outcomes data.
FLARE [65] (2019)	Inari FlowTriever catheters	Multi-center trial including symptomatic patients with RV/LV ratios > 0.9. N = 106 patients. Aim: Reduction in RV/LV ratio. Primary composite safety of device-related death, major bleeding, treatment related clinical decline, cardiac injury, or pulmonary vascular injury within 48 h.	RV/LV ratio was reduced by 0.38 at 48 h. Fourteen patients (13.2%) experienced serious adverse events at 30 days, with four (3.8%) occurring within 48 h of index procedure.	Small study population size. Lack of short-term or long-term clinical benefits or adverse outcomes data.
FLASH [66] (2022)	Inari FlowTriever catheters	Prospective, multi-center registry of high-risk or intermediate-risk PE. N = Goal of 250. Aim: composite endpoint for major adverse events including major bleeding, device-related bleeding, or death at 48 h.	Ongoing trial.	
PEERLESS [67] (2023)	Inari FlowTriever catheters	Prospective, multi-center, randomized controlled trial for intermediate or high-risk PE. N = goal of 550. Aims: composite endpoint for all-cause mortality, ICH, MBE, clinical deterioration, or ICU admission.	Ongoing trial.	

Table 3. Cont.

Trial	Device	Study Design/Aims	Outcomes	Limitations
FLAME [68] (2023)	Inari FlowTriever catheters	Prospective, multi-center, non-randomized controlled trial for high-risk PE. N = 115 patients. Aims: composite of all-cause mortality, bailout to alternate thrombus retrieval strategy, MBE, or clinical decline.	Lower in-hospital adverse outcomes (17.0%) versus historical data (32.0%). Reduction in high-risk PE mortality compared to historical data.	Limited study population size. Unclear definitions of historical and context comparison groups.
EXTRACT PE [69] (2021)	Penumbra Indigo aspiration system	Prospective, single-arm, multi-center study with symptomatic acute PE ≤ 14 days, SBP ≥ 90 mm Hg, and RV/LV ratio > 0.9. N = 119 patients. Aims: safety and efficacy by RV/LV ratio reduction at 48 h for patients with submassive PE.	Mean RV/LV ratio reduction from baseline was 0.43 at 48 h post-procedure. Two (1.7%) of patients experienced a major adverse event. Rates were low for cardiac or pulmonary vascular injury, MBE, or device related death at 48 h.	Small study population size. Lack of short-term (beyond 48 h) or long-term clinical benefits or adverse outcomes data.

Anticoagulation (AC), blood pressure (BP), brain natriuretic peptide (BNP), computed tomography (CT), computed tomography pulmonary angiogram (CTPA), echocardiogram (ECHO), heart rate (HR), intracranial hemorrhage (ICH), intensive care unit (ICU), major bleeding event (MBE), pulmonary embolism (PE), Pulmonary Embolism Severity Index (PESI), systolic blood pressure (SBP), tricuspid annular plane systolic excursion (TAPSE), right ventricle (RV), ultrasound-assisted catheter-directed thrombolysis (USAT), ultrasound-facilitated catheter-directed thrombolysis (US CDT).

To date, there remains a paucity of evidence to assess whether these acute hemodynamic changes improve clinical outcomes for patients, particularly as they pertain to the development of chronic thromboembolic pulmonary hypertension (CTEPH) or quality of life. It is also unclear whether there is a subset in the intermediate-risk PE population who may benefit from catheter-based therapies over others. For example, when analyzing patients with intermediate-high-risk PE, retrospective data suggest a mortality and bleeding benefit. Furthermore, an analysis of the National Inpatient Sample of cancer patients with intermediate or high-risk PE also suggested improved mortality, although higher bleeding [70]. Further data are urgently needed to prospectively analyze catheter-based therapies, particularly in the intermediate-high-risk PE population and its subsets.

6. Ongoing Trials for Intermediate-Risk Pulmonary Embolism

Current ongoing clinical trials include the Higher-Risk Pulmonary Embolism Thrombolysis (HI-PEITHO) study, which is currently enrolling patients with intermediate-high-risk PE with increased risk of death or hemodynamic compromise. This study aims to compare composite clinical outcomes at 7 days for patients receiving ultrasound-facilitated catheter-directed thrombolytic therapy with anticoagulation versus anticoagulation alone. Additional aims of the study include comparison of patients' functional status, quality of life indicators, and health-care utilization in the subsequent 30 days, 6 months, and 12 months after index PE [63].

The PE-TRACT study is another new multi-center randomized controlled trial investigating the use of catheter-directed thrombolytic (CDT) therapy in addition to standard anticoagulation compared to anticoagulation alone in patients with intermediate-risk PE. The anticipated enrollment will include 500 patients with an anticipated 6-year follow-up. The goal of this study is to examine routine use of CDT in patients with intermediate-risk

PE and could also provide new insight into the natural history of patients with intermediate PE [71].

Ongoing device trials include the FLASH and PEERLESS trials, examining the use of Inari FlowTriever systems in both intermediate and high-risk PE, respectively. The FlowTriever All-Comer Registry for Patient Safety and Hemodynamics (FLASH) study aims to compare safety outcomes at 48 h for patients undergoing thrombectomy with the Inari Flowtriever system compared to patients receiving conservative therapy with anticoagulation alone. Interim analysis of the initial 250 patients enrolled demonstrated a small number of major adverse events (1.2%) in the Inari group, which all resolved without sequelae. Intraprocedural hemodynamic improvements were also reported, with an average reduction of mean pulmonary artery pressure of 7.1 mmHg with patient-reported symptomatic improvement [66]. The PEERLESS trial, also utilizing the Inari FlowTriever system, is an ongoing randomized controlled study comparing intermediate-high-risk PE patients treated with mechanical thrombectomy (FlowTriever System) versus catheter-directed thrombolysis [67]. In May 2023, the Inari Medical group additionally announced its intention to start the PEERLESS II trial. As an expansion of the PEERLESS trial, PEERLESS II is another randomized controlled trial aiming to compare outcomes of patients with intermediate-risk PE treated with the FlowTriever system compared to those treated with anticoagulation alone [72]. A summary of prior and ongoing device trials is summarized in Table 3.

7. The Importance of Multidisciplinary Teams: The Pert

Given the high complexity, mortality risk, and evolving nature of available therapies for patients with intermediate-risk PE, a multidisciplinary team approach is crucial. Since 2012, Pulmonary Embolism Response Teams (PERTs) have become common at many institutions to streamline rapid assessment along with prompt implementation of EOC therapies for patients with intermediate or high-risk PE. Given the heterogeneity of hospitals, PERTs vary in composition between institutions, but generally consist of multidisciplinary teams including pulmonary critical care, cardiology, vascular medicine, interventional radiology, and interventional cardiology [1]. In the sentinel paper from Massachusetts General Hospital, the implementation of the PERT was rapidly adopted nationwide. Systemic anticoagulation was the primary treatment modality at the time of publication in 2016 [1,73]. However, since publication, catheter-directed therapies have rapidly developed and become accessible, strengthening the necessity for PERTs to assist in the nuanced decision-making for this population. Recent reviews of PERTs have found a decrease in ICU length of stay, reduced bleeding rates, decreased utilization of IVC filter placement, and short time-to-therapeutic anticoagulation when compared to historical controls [1,74–76]. It has been hypothesized that PERTs may reduce PE-related mortality; however, results are conflicting [1,74,76]. This may be in part due to the observational nature of some studies (pre- and post-PERT) which do not account for changing guidelines and therapies occurring simultaneously [1,74]. It is important to note that the expansion of PERTs across the nation has flourished. Although this expansion has facilitated interventional procedures, it is also important to recognize that the primary role of the PERT team should also be to carefully assess each patient and de-escalate management where bleeding risk predominates. There is additional benefit in a careful comprehensive assessment to exclude pre-existing pathologies which can confound the clinical presentation. A recommended outline for approaching a patient with intermediate-risk PE is summarized in Figure 2.

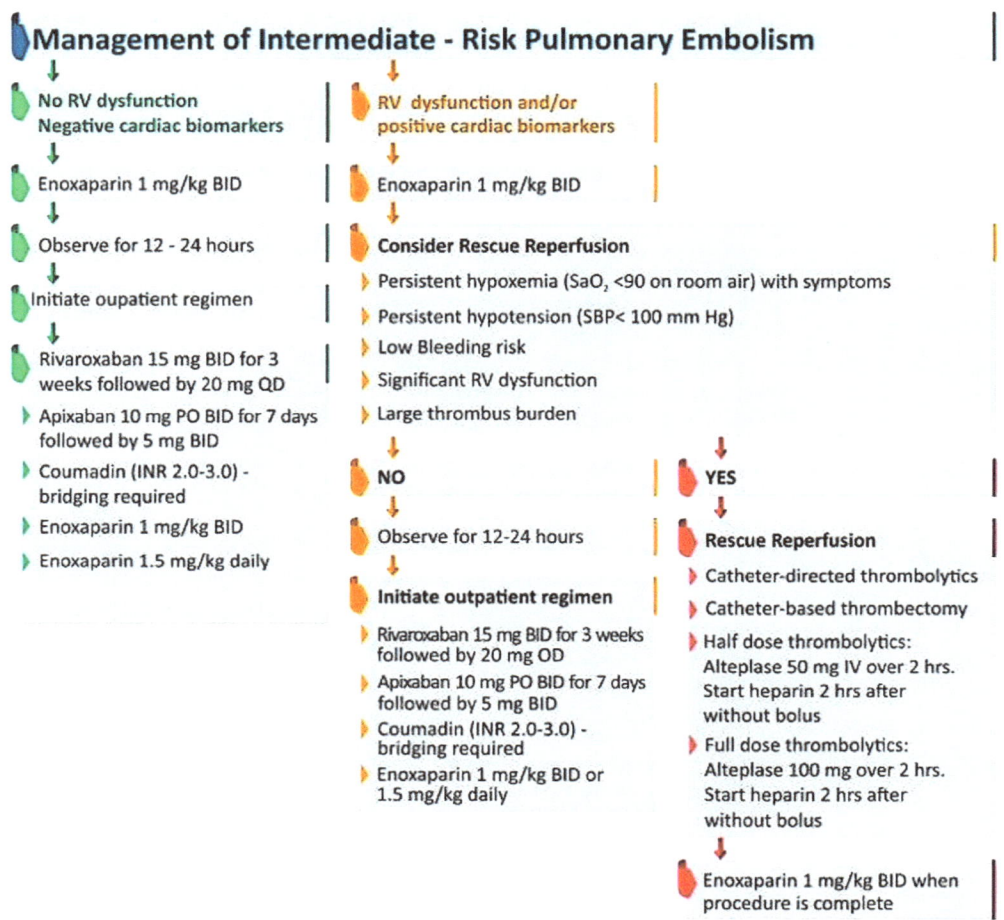

Figure 2. Decision–making in management of intermediate–risk pulmonary embolism.

8. Conclusions

The current understanding of intermediate-risk, previously submassive, PE is ever-evolving. We have reviewed the current definition of intermediate-risk PE, including caveats, with preference towards the current ESC guidelines as a framework to evaluate patients and have discussed the role of cardiac biomarkers and imaging findings to support diagnosis. Previous metrics for RV dysfunction may not be as clear, reproducible, or predictive in defining intermediate-risk PE. Further studies examining echocardiographic and CT parameters are needed. Anticoagulation remains the cornerstone of therapy. While the role of catheter-directed therapies with thrombolysis and mechanical thrombectomy have recently gained attention, their specific role in individualized care and influence on patient outcomes requires further longitudinal study. Lastly, decision-making for patients with intermediate-risk PE can be nuanced, and the use of multidisciplinary PERTs is recommended to direct patient care.

Funding: This research received no external funding.

Conflicts of Interest: The authors declare no conflict of interest.

References

1. Porres-Aguilar, M.; Rosovsky, R.P.; Rivera-Lebron, B.N.; Kaatz, S.; Mukherjee, D.; Anaya-Ayala, J.E.; Jimenez, D.; Jerjes-Sánchez, C. Pulmonary Embolism Response Teams: Changing the Paradigm in the Care for Acute Pulmonary Embolism. *J. Thromb. Haemost.* **2022**, *20*, 2457–2464. [CrossRef] [PubMed]
2. Keller, K.; Hobohm, L.; Ebner, M.; Kresoja, K.-P.; Münzel, T.; Konstantinides, S.V.; Lankeit, M. Trends in Thrombolytic Treatment and Outcomes of Acute Pulmonary Embolism in Germany. *Eur. Heart J.* **2020**, *41*, 522–529. [CrossRef] [PubMed]
3. Lehnert, P.; Lange, T.; Møller, C.H.; Olsen, P.S.; Carlsen, J. Acute Pulmonary Embolism in a National Danish Cohort: Increasing Incidence and Decreasing Mortality. *Thromb. Haemost.* **2018**, *118*, 539–546. [CrossRef] [PubMed]
4. 2019 ESC Guidelines for the Diagnosis and Management of Acute Pulmonary Embolism Developed in Collaboration with the European Respiratory Society (ERS) | European Heart Journal | Oxford Academic. Available online: https://academic.oup.com/eurheartj/article/41/4/543/5556136?login=true (accessed on 24 July 2023).
5. Piazza, G. Advanced Management of Intermediate- and High-Risk Pulmonary Embolism: JACC Focus Seminar. *J. Am. Coll. Cardiol.* **2020**, *76*, 2117–2127. [CrossRef] [PubMed]
6. Wendelboe, A.M.; Raskob, G.E. Global Burden of Thrombosis: Epidemiologic Aspects. *Circ. Res.* **2016**, *118*, 1340–1347. [CrossRef] [PubMed]
7. Pulmonary Embolism in Patients with COVID-19. American College of Cardiology. Available online: https://www.acc.org/latest-in-cardiology/journal-scans/2021/07/09/14/31/http://www.acc.org/latest-in-cardiology/journal-scans/2021/07/09/14/31/pulmonary-embolism-in-patients (accessed on 25 July 2023).
8. Katsoularis, I.; Fonseca-Rodríguez, O.; Farrington, P.; Jerndal, H.; Lundevaller, E.H.; Sund, M.; Lindmark, K.; Connolly, A.-M.F. Risks of Deep Vein Thrombosis, Pulmonary Embolism, and Bleeding after COVID-19: Nationwide Self-Controlled Cases Series and Matched Cohort Study. *BMJ* **2022**, *377*, e069590. [CrossRef]
9. Jaff, M.R.; McMurtry, M.S.; Archer, S.L.; Cushman, M.; Goldenberg, N.; Goldhaber, S.Z.; Jenkins, J.S.; Kline, J.A.; Michaels, A.D.; Thistlethwaite, P.; et al. Management of Massive and Submassive Pulmonary Embolism, Iliofemoral Deep Vein Thrombosis, and Chronic Thromboembolic Pulmonary Hypertension. *Circulation* **2011**, *123*, 1788–1830. [CrossRef]
10. Jiménez, D.; Yusen, R.D.; Otero, R.; Uresandi, F.; Nauffal, D.; Laserna, E.; Conget, F.; Oribe, M.; Cabezudo, M.A.; Díaz, G. Prognostic Models for Selecting Patients with Acute Pulmonary Embolism for Initial Outpatient Therapy. *Chest* **2007**, *132*, 24–30. [CrossRef]
11. Frémont, B.; Pacouret, G.; Jacobi, D.; Puglisi, R.; Charbonnier, B.; de Labriolle, A. Prognostic Value of Echocardiographic Right/Left Ventricular End-Diastolic Diameter Ratio in Patients with Acute Pulmonary Embolism: Results from a Monocenter Registry of 1,416 Patients. *Chest* **2008**, *133*, 358–362. [CrossRef]
12. Post, F.; Mertens, D.; Sinning, C.; Peetz, D.; Münzel, T. Decision for Aggressive Therapy in Acute Pulmonary Embolism: Implication of Elevated Troponin T. *Clin. Res. Cardiol.* **2009**, *98*, 401–408. [CrossRef]
13. Scridon, T.; Scridon, C.; Skali, H.; Alvarez, A.; Goldhaber, S.Z.; Solomon, S.D. Prognostic Significance of Troponin Elevation and Right Ventricular Enlargement in Acute Pulmonary Embolism. *Am. J. Cardiol.* **2005**, *96*, 303–305. [CrossRef] [PubMed]
14. Bova, C.; Pesavento, R.; Marchiori, A.; Palla, A.; Enea, I.; Pengo, V.; Visonà, A.; Noto, A.; Prandoni, P. Risk Stratification and Outcomes in Hemodynamically Stable Patients with Acute Pulmonary Embolism: A Prospective, Multicentre, Cohort Study with Three Months of Follow-Up. *J. Thromb. Haemost.* **2009**, *7*, 938–944. [CrossRef] [PubMed]
15. Kline, J.A.; Hernandez-Nino, J.; Rose, G.A.; Norton, H.J.; Camargo, C.A.J. Surrogate Markers for Adverse Outcomes in Normotensive Patients with Pulmonary Embolism. *Crit. Care Med.* **2006**, *34*, 2773. [CrossRef] [PubMed]
16. Secemsky, E.; Chang, Y.; Jain, C.C.; Beckman, J.A.; Giri, J.; Jaff, M.R.; Rosenfield, K.; Rosovsky, R.; Kabrhel, C.; Weinberg, I. Contemporary Management and Outcomes of Patients with Massive and Submassive Pulmonary Embolism. *Am. J. Med.* **2018**, *131*, 1506–1514. [CrossRef] [PubMed]
17. Lankeit, M.; Friesen, D.; Aschoff, J.; Dellas, C.; Hasenfuß, G.; Katus, H.; Konstantinides, S.; Giannitsis, E. Highly Sensitive Troponin T Assay in Normotensive Patients with Acute Pulmonary Embolism. *Eur. Heart J.* **2010**, *31*, 1836–1844. [CrossRef] [PubMed]
18. Giri, J.; Sista, A.K.; Weinberg, I.; Kearon, C.; Kumbhani, D.J.; Desai, N.D.; Piazza, G.; Gladwin, M.T.; Chatterjee, S.; Kobayashi, T.; et al. Interventional Therapies for Acute Pulmonary Embolism: Current Status and Principles for the Development of Novel Evidence: A Scientific Statement from the American Heart Association. *Circulation* **2019**, *140*, e774–e801. [CrossRef]
19. Aujesky, D.; Obrosky, D.S.; Stone, R.A.; Auble, T.E.; Perrier, A.; Cornuz, J.; Roy, P.-M.; Fine, M.J. Derivation and Validation of a Prognostic Model for Pulmonary Embolism. *Am. J. Respir. Crit. Care Med.* **2005**, *172*, 1041–1046. [CrossRef]
20. Jiménez, D.; Aujesky, D.; Moores, L.; Gómez, V.; Lobo, J.L.; Uresandi, F.; Otero, R.; Monreal, M.; Muriel, A.; Yusen, R.D.; et al. Simplification of the Pulmonary Embolism Severity Index for Prognostication in Patients with Acute Symptomatic Pulmonary Embolism. *Arch. Intern. Med.* **2010**, *170*, 1383–1389. [CrossRef]

21. Yamashita, Y.; Morimoto, T.; Amano, H.; Takase, T.; Hiramori, S.; Kim, K.; Oi, M.; Akao, M.; Kobayashi, Y.; Toyofuku, M.; et al. Validation of Simplified PESI Score for Identification of Low-Risk Patients with Pulmonary Embolism: From the COMMAND VTE Registry. *Eur. Heart J. Acute Cardiovasc. Care* **2020**, *9*, 262–270. [CrossRef]
22. Stevens, S.M.; Woller, S.C.; Kreuziger, L.B.; Bounameaux, H.; Doerschug, K.; Geersing, G.-J.; Huisman, M.V.; Kearon, C.; King, C.S.; Knighton, A.J.; et al. Antithrombotic Therapy for VTE Disease: Second Update of the CHEST Guideline and Expert Panel Report. *CHEST* **2021**, *160*, e545–e608. [CrossRef]
23. Bajaj, A.; Saleeb, M.; Rathor, P.; Sehgal, V.; Kabak, B.; Hosur, S. Prognostic Value of Troponins in Acute Nonmassive Pulmonary Embolism: A Meta-Analysis. *Heart Lung* **2015**, *44*, 327–334. [CrossRef] [PubMed]
24. Becattini, C.; Vedovati, M.C.; Agnelli, G. Prognostic Value of Troponins in Acute Pulmonary Embolism: A Meta-Analysis. *Circulation* **2007**, *116*, 427–433. [CrossRef] [PubMed]
25. Bikdeli, B.; Muriel, A.; Rodríguez, C.; González, S.; Briceño, W.; Mehdipoor, G.; Piazza, G.; Ballaz, A.; Lippi, G.; Yusen, R.D.; et al. High-Sensitivity vs Conventional Troponin Cutoffs for Risk Stratification in Patients With Acute Pulmonary Embolism. *JAMA Cardiol.* **2023**. [CrossRef] [PubMed]
26. Klok, F.A.; Mos, I.C.M.; Huisman, M.V. Brain-Type Natriuretic Peptide Levels in the Prediction of Adverse Outcome in Patients with Pulmonary Embolism: A Systematic Review and Meta-Analysis. *Am. J. Respir. Crit. Care Med.* **2008**, *178*, 425–430. [CrossRef] [PubMed]
27. Wu, J.; Gillam, L.; Solomon, S.; Bulwer, B. Echocardiography. In *Braunwald's Heart Disease: A Textbook of Cardiovascular Medicine*; Elsevier Inc.: Amsterdam, The Netherlands, 2022; pp. 196–267.
28. Dabbouseh, N.M.; Patel, J.J.; Bergl, P.A. Role of Echocardiography in Managing Acute Pulmonary Embolism. *Heart* **2019**, *105*, 1785–1792. [CrossRef]
29. Brailovsky, Y.; Lakhter, V.; Weinberg, I.; Porcaro, K.; Haines, J.; Morris, S.; Masic, D.; Mancl, E.; Bashir, R.; Alkhouli, M.; et al. Right Ventricular Outflow Doppler Predicts Low Cardiac Index in Intermediate Risk Pulmonary Embolism. *Clin. Appl. Thromb. Off. J. Int. Acad. Clin. Appl. Thromb.* **2019**, *25*, 1076029619886062. [CrossRef]
30. Cho, J.H.; Kutti Sridharan, G.; Kim, S.H.; Kaw, R.; Abburi, T.; Irfan, A.; Kocheril, A.G. Right Ventricular Dysfunction as an Echocardiographic Prognostic Factor in Hemodynamically Stable Patients with Acute Pulmonary Embolism: A Meta-Analysis. *BMC Cardiovasc. Disord.* **2014**, *14*, 64. [CrossRef]
31. Kurnicka, K.; Lichodziejewska, B.; Goliszek, S.; Dzikowska-Diduch, O.; Zdończyk, O.; Kozłowska, M.; Kostrubiec, M.; Ciurzyński, M.; Palczewski, P.; Grudzka, K.; et al. Echocardiographic Pattern of Acute Pulmonary Embolism: Analysis of 511 Consecutive Patients. *J. Am. Soc. Echocardiogr. Off. Publ. Am. Soc. Echocardiogr.* **2016**, *29*, 907–913. [CrossRef]
32. Hendriks, S.V.; Klok, F.A.; den Exter, P.L.; Eijsvogel, M.; Faber, L.M.; Hofstee, H.M.A.; Iglesias del Sol, A.; Kroft, L.J.M.; Mairuhu, A.T.A.; Huisman, M.V. Right Ventricle–to–Left Ventricle Diameter Ratio Measurement Seems to Have No Role in Low-Risk Patients with Pulmonary Embolism Treated at Home Triaged by Hestia Criteria. *Am. J. Respir. Crit. Care Med.* **2020**, *202*, 138–141. [CrossRef]
33. Contractor, S.; Maldjian, P.D.; Sharma, V.K.; Gor, D.M. Role of Helical CT in Detecting Right Ventricular Dysfunction Secondary to Acute Pulmonary Embolism. *J. Comput. Assist. Tomogr.* **2002**, *26*, 587. [CrossRef]
34. Lyhne, M.D.; Schultz, J.G.; MacMahon, P.J.; Haddad, F.; Kalra, M.; Tso, D.M.-K.; Muzikansky, A.; Lev, M.H.; Kabrhel, C. Septal Bowing and Pulmonary Artery Diameter on Computed Tomography Pulmonary Angiography Are Associated with Short-Term Outcomes in Patients with Acute Pulmonary Embolism. *Emerg. Radiol.* **2019**, *26*, 623–630. [CrossRef] [PubMed]
35. Becattini, C.; Agnelli, G.; Germini, F.; Vedovati, M.C. Computed Tomography to Assess Risk of Death in Acute Pulmonary Embolism: A Meta-Analysis. *Eur. Respir. J.* **2014**, *43*, 1678–1690. [CrossRef] [PubMed]
36. Yuriditsky, E.; Mitchell, O.J.L.; Sista, A.K.; Xia, Y.; Sibley, R.A.; Zhong, J.; Moore, W.H.; Amoroso, N.E.; Goldenberg, R.M.; Smith, D.E.; et al. Right Ventricular Stroke Distance Predicts Death and Clinical Deterioration in Patients with Pulmonary Embolism. *Thromb. Res.* **2020**, *195*, 29–34. [CrossRef]
37. Moceri, P.; Duchateau, N.; Sartre, B.; Baudouy, D.; Squara, F.; Sermesant, M.; Ferrari, E. Value of 3D Right Ventricular Function over 2D Assessment in Acute Pulmonary Embolism. *Echocardiography* **2021**, *38*, 1694–1701. [CrossRef] [PubMed]
38. Ammari, Z.; Al-Sarie, M.; Ea, A.; Sangera, R.; George, J.C.; Varghese, V.; Brewster, P.S.; Xie, Y.; Chen, T.; Sun, Z.; et al. Predictors of Reduced Cardiac Index in Patients with Acute Submassive Pulmonary Embolism. *Catheter. Cardiovasc. Interv.* **2021**, *97*, 292–298. [CrossRef] [PubMed]
39. He, Q.; Lin, Y.; Zhu, Y.; Gao, L.; Ji, M.; Zhang, L.; Xie, M.; Li, Y. Clinical Usefulness of Right Ventricle–Pulmonary Artery Coupling in Cardiovascular Disease. *J. Clin. Med.* **2023**, *12*, 2526. [CrossRef]
40. Hsu, S. Coupling Right Ventricular–Pulmonary Arterial Research to the Pulmonary Hypertension Patient Bedside. *Circ. Heart Fail.* **2019**, *12*, e005715. [CrossRef]
41. Ünlü, S.; Voigt, J.-U. Right Ventriculo-Arterial Coupling Assessed by Right Ventricular Strain Is a Superior Predictor of Clinical Outcome in Patients with Pulmonary Arterial Hypertension. *Eur. Heart J. Cardiovasc. Imaging* **2023**, *24*, e53. [CrossRef]
42. Barritt, D.W.; Jordan, S.C. Anticoagulant drugs in the treatment of pulmonary embolism: A controlled trial. *Lancet* **1960**, *275*, 1309–1312. [CrossRef]
43. Erkens, P.M.; Prins, M.H. Fixed Dose Subcutaneous Low Molecular Weight Heparins versus Adjusted Dose Unfractionated Heparin for Venous Thromboembolism. *Cochrane Database Syst. Rev.* **2010**, CD001100. [CrossRef]

44. Agnelli, G.; Becattini, C.; Bauersachs, R.; Brenner, B.; Campanini, M.; Cohen, A.; Connors, J.M.; Fontanella, A.; Gussoni, G.; Huisman, M.V.; et al. Apixaban versus Dalteparin for the Treatment of Acute Venous Thromboembolism in Patients with Cancer: The Caravaggio Study. *Thromb. Haemost.* **2018**, *118*, 1668–1678. [CrossRef] [PubMed]
45. EINSTEIN–PE Investigators. Oral Rivaroxaban for the Treatment of Symptomatic Pulmonary Embolism. *N. Engl. J. Med.* **2012**, *366*, 1287–1297. [CrossRef] [PubMed]
46. Agnelli, G.; Becattini, C.; Meyer, G.; Muñoz, A.; Huisman, M.V.; Connors, J.M.; Cohen, A.; Bauersachs, R.; Brenner, B.; Torbicki, A.; et al. Apixaban for the Treatment of Venous Thromboembolism Associated with Cancer. *N. Engl. J. Med.* **2020**, *382*, 1599–1607. [CrossRef] [PubMed]
47. The Hokusai-VTE Investigators. Edoxaban versus Warfarin for the Treatment of Symptomatic Venous Thromboembolism. *N. Engl. J. Med.* **2013**, *369*, 1406–1415. [CrossRef] [PubMed]
48. Martin, K.A.; Beyer-Westendorf, J.; Davidson, B.L.; Huisman, M.V.; Sandset, P.M.; Moll, S. Use of Direct Oral Anticoagulants in Patients with Obesity for Treatment and Prevention of Venous Thromboembolism: Updated Communication from the ISTH SSC Subcommittee on Control of Anticoagulation. *J. Thromb. Haemost.* **2021**, *19*, 1874–1882. [CrossRef]
49. Riaz, I.B.; Fuentes, H.; Deng, Y.; Naqvi, S.A.A.; Yao, X.; Sangaralingham, L.R.; Houghton, D.E.; Padrnos, L.J.; Shamoun, F.E.; Wysokinski, W.E.; et al. Comparative Effectiveness of Anticoagulants in Patients with Cancer-Associated Thrombosis. *JAMA Netw. Open* **2023**, *6*, e2325283. [CrossRef]
50. Meyer, G.; Vicaut, E.; Danays, T.; Agnelli, G.; Becattini, C.; Beyer-Westendorf, J.; Bluhmki, E.; Bouvaist, H.; Brenner, B.; Couturaud, F.; et al. Fibrinolysis for Patients with Intermediate-Risk Pulmonary Embolism. *N. Engl. J. Med.* **2014**, *370*, 1402–1411. [CrossRef]
51. Sharifi, M.; Bay, C.; Skrocki, L.; Rahimi, F.; Mehdipour, M. Moderate Pulmonary Embolism Treated with Thrombolysis (from the "MOPETT" Trial). *Am. J. Cardiol.* **2013**, *111*, 273–277. [CrossRef]
52. Kiser, T.H.; Burnham, E.L.; Clark, B.; Ho, P.M.; Allen, R.R.; Moss, M.; Vandivier, R.W. Half-Dose Versus Full-Dose Alteplase for Treatment of Pulmonary Embolism. *Crit. Care Med.* **2018**, *46*, 1617–1625. [CrossRef]
53. Konstantinides, S.V.; Vicaut, E.; Danays, T.; Becattini, C.; Bertoletti, L.; Beyer, W.J.; Bouvaist, H.; Couturaud, F.; Dellas, C.; Duerschmied, D.; et al. Impact of Thrombolytic Therapy on the Long-Term Outcome of Intermediate-Risk Pulmonary Embolism. *J. Am. Coll. Cardiol.* **2017**, *69*, 1536–1544. [CrossRef]
54. Mathew, D.; Seelam, S.; Bumrah, K.; Sherif, A.; Shrestha, U. Systemic Thrombolysis with Newer Thrombolytics vs Anticoagulation in Acute Intermediate Risk Pulmonary Embolism: A Systematic Review and Meta-Analysis. *BMC Cardiovasc. Disord.* **2023**, *23*, 482. [CrossRef] [PubMed]
55. Outcomes in High-Risk Pulmonary Embolism Patients Undergoing FlowTriever Mechanical Thrombectomy or Other Contemporary Therapies: Results from the FLAME Study | Circulation: Cardiovascular Interventions. Available online: https://www.ahajournals.org/doi/10.1161/CIRCINTERVENTIONS.123.013406 (accessed on 26 November 2023).
56. Kucher, N.; Boekstegers, P.; Müller, O.J.; Kupatt, C.; Beyer-Westendorf, J.; Heitzer, T.; Tebbe, U.; Horstkotte, J.; Müller, R.; Blessing, E.; et al. Randomized, Controlled Trial of Ultrasound-Assisted Catheter-Directed Thrombolysis for Acute Intermediate-Risk Pulmonary Embolism. *Circulation* **2014**, *129*, 479–486. [CrossRef] [PubMed]
57. Piazza, G.; Hohlfelder, B.; Jaff, M.R.; Ouriel, K.; Engelhardt, T.C.; Sterling, K.M.; Jones, N.J.; Gurley, J.C.; Bhatheja, R.; Kennedy, R.J.; et al. A Prospective, Single-Arm, Multicenter Trial of Ultrasound-Facilitated, Catheter-Directed, Low-Dose Fibrinolysis for Acute Massive and Submassive Pulmonary Embolism: The SEATTLE II Study. *JACC Cardiovasc. Interv.* **2015**, *8*, 1382–1392. [CrossRef] [PubMed]
58. Balanescu, D.V.; Tawney, A.M.; McNally, V.; Goldstein, J.A.; Bowers, T.R. C-37 | Outcomes of Escalation of Care Versus Standard Anticoagulation for Intermediate-High Risk Pulmonary Embolism: An Experienced PERT Approach. *J. Soc. Cardiovasc. Angiogr. Interv.* **2023**, *2*, 100825. [CrossRef]
59. Pasha, A.K.; Siddiqui, M.U.; Siddiqui, M.D.; Ahmed, A.; Abdullah, A.; Riaz, I.; Murad, M.H.; Bjarnason, H.; Wysokinski, W.E.; McBane, R.D. Catheter Directed Compared to Systemically Delivered Thrombolysis for Pulmonary Embolism: A Systematic Review and Meta-Analysis. *J. Thromb. Thrombolysis* **2022**, *53*, 454–466. [CrossRef] [PubMed]
60. Kohi, M.P.; Kohlbrenner, R.; Kolli, K.P.; Lehrman, E.; Taylor, A.G.; Fidelman, N. Catheter Directed Interventions for Acute Deep Vein Thrombosis. *Cardiovasc. Diagn. Ther.* **2016**, *6*, 599–611. [CrossRef]
61. Monteleone, P.; Ahern, R.; Banerjee, S.; Desai, K.R.; Kadian-Dodov, D.; Webber, E.; Omidvar, S.; Troy, P.; Parikh, S.A. Modern Treatment of Pulmonary Embolism (USCDT Versus MT): Results from a Real-World, Big Data Analysis (REAL-PE). *J. Soc. Cardiovasc. Angiogr. Interv.* **2023**, 101192. [CrossRef]
62. Tapson, V.F.; Sterling, K.; Jones, N.; Elder, M.; Tripathy, U.; Brower, J.; Maholic, R.L.; Ross, C.B.; Natarajan, K.; Fong, P.; et al. A Randomized Trial of the Optimum Duration of Acoustic Pulse Thrombolysis Procedure in Acute Intermediate-Risk Pulmonary Embolism: The OPTALYSE PE Trial. *JACC Cardiovasc. Interv.* **2018**, *11*, 1401–1410. [CrossRef]
63. Klok, F.A.; Piazza, G.; Sharp, A.S.P.; Ní Ainle, F.; Jaff, M.R.; Chauhan, N.; Patel, B.; Barco, S.; Goldhaber, S.Z.; Kucher, N.; et al. Ultrasound-Facilitated, Catheter-Directed Thrombolysis vs Anticoagulation Alone for Acute Intermediate-High-Risk Pulmonary Embolism: Rationale and Design of the HI-PEITHO Study. *Am. Heart J.* **2022**, *251*, 43–53. [CrossRef]
64. Bashir, R.; Foster, M.; Iskander, A.; Darki, A.; Jaber, W.; Rali, P.M.; Lakhter, V.; Gandhi, R.; Klein, A.; Bhatheja, R.; et al. Pharmacomechanical Catheter-Directed Thrombolysis with the Bashir Endovascular Catheter for Acute Pulmonary Embolism. *JACC Cardiovasc. Interv.* **2022**, *15*, 2427–2436. [CrossRef]

65. Tu, T.; Toma, C.; Tapson, V.F.; Adams, C.; Jaber, W.A.; Silver, M.; Khandhar, S.; Amin, R.; Weinberg, M.; Engelhardt, T.; et al. A Prospective, Single-Arm, Multicenter Trial of Catheter-Directed Mechanical Thrombectomy for Intermediate-Risk Acute Pulmonary Embolism: The FLARE Study. *JACC Cardiovasc. Interv.* **2019**, *12*, 859–869. [CrossRef] [PubMed]
66. Toma, C.; Bunte, M.C.; Cho, K.H.; Jaber, W.A.; Chambers, J.; Stegman, B.; Gondi, S.; Leung, D.A.; Savin, M.; Khandhar, S.; et al. Percutaneous Mechanical Thrombectomy in a Real-World Pulmonary Embolism Population: Interim Results of the FLASH Registry. *Catheter. Cardiovasc. Interv.* **2022**, *99*, 1345–1355. [CrossRef] [PubMed]
67. Inari Medical. The PEERLESS Study; Clinical Trial Registration NCT05111613; Clinicaltrials.gov. 2023. Available online: https://clinicaltrials.gov/study/NCT05111613 (accessed on 15 September 2023).
68. FLAME 2023—US | Inari Medical. Available online: https://www.inarimedical.com/flame/ (accessed on 17 September 2023).
69. Sista, A.K.; Horowitz, J.M.; Tapson, V.F.; Rosenberg, M.; Elder, M.D.; Schiro, B.J.; Dohad, S.; Amoroso, N.E.; Dexter, D.J.; Loh, C.T.; et al. Indigo Aspiration System for Treatment of Pulmonary Embolism. *JACC Cardiovasc. Interv.* **2021**, *14*, 319–329. [CrossRef] [PubMed]
70. Leiva, O.; Yuriditsky, E.; Postelnicu, R.; Yang, E.H.; Mukherjee, V.; Greco, A.; Horowitz, J.; Alviar, C.; Bangalore, S. Catheter-Based Therapy for Intermediate or High-Risk Pulmonary Embolism Is Associated with Lower in-Hospital Mortality in Patients with Cancer: Insights from the National Inpatient Sample. *Catheter. Cardiovasc. Interv. Off. J. Soc. Card. Angiogr. Interv.* **2023**, 1–11. [CrossRef] [PubMed]
71. NYU Langone Health. *Pulmonary Embolism-Thrombus Removal with Catheter-Directed Therapy*; Clinical Trial Registration NCT05591118; clinicaltrials.gov; 2023. Available online: https://clinicaltrials.gov/study/NCT05591118 (accessed on 31 December 2022).
72. Inari Medical Announces PEERLESS II, a Randomized Controlled Trial Evaluating Clinical Outcomes of the FlowTriever®System vs. Anticoagulation in Pulmonary Embolism Patients | Inari Medical, Inc. Available online: https://ir.inarimedical.com/news-releases/news-release-details/inari-medical-announces-peerless-ii-randomized-controlled-trial/ (accessed on 1 October 2023).
73. Kabrhel, C.; Rosovsky, R.; Channick, R.; Jaff, M.R.; Weinberg, I.; Sundt, T.; Dudzinski, D.M.; Rodriguez-Lopez, J.; Parry, B.A.; Harshbarger, S.; et al. A Multidisciplinary Pulmonary Embolism Response Team: Initial 30-Month Experience with a Novel Approach to Delivery of Care to Patients with Submassive and Massive Pulmonary Embolism. *CHEST* **2016**, *150*, 384–393. [CrossRef]
74. Wright, C.; Goldenberg, I.; Schleede, S.; McNitt, S.; Gosev, I.; Elbadawi, A.; Pietropaoli, A.; Barrus, B.; Chen, Y.L.; Mazzillo, J.; et al. Effect of a Multidisciplinary Pulmonary Embolism Response Team on Patient Mortality. *Am. J. Cardiol.* **2021**, *161*, 102–107. [CrossRef]
75. Chaudhury, P.; Gadre, S.K.; Schneider, E.; Renapurkar, R.D.; Gomes, M.; Haddadin, I.; Heresi, G.A.; Tong, M.Z.; Bartholomew, J.R. Impact of Multidisciplinary Pulmonary Embolism Response Team Availability on Management and Outcomes. *Am. J. Cardiol.* **2019**, *124*, 1465–1469. [CrossRef]
76. Carroll, B.J.; Beyer, S.E.; Mehegan, T.; Dicks, A.; Pribish, A.; Locke, A.; Godishala, A.; Soriano, K.; Kanduri, J.; Sack, K.; et al. Changes in Care for Acute Pulmonary Embolism Through a Multidisciplinary Pulmonary Embolism Response Team. *Am. J. Med.* **2020**, *133*, 1313–1321. [CrossRef]

Disclaimer/Publisher's Note: The statements, opinions and data contained in all publications are solely those of the individual author(s) and contributor(s) and not of MDPI and/or the editor(s). MDPI and/or the editor(s) disclaim responsibility for any injury to people or property resulting from any ideas, methods, instructions or products referred to in the content.

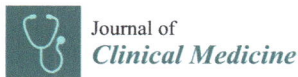

Review

Choice and Duration of Anticoagulation for Venous Thromboembolism

Aroosa Malik [1], Nghi B. Ha [2] and Geoffrey D. Barnes [1,*]

[1] Department of Internal Medicine, Division of Cardiovascular Medicine, Frankel Cardiovascular Center, University of Michigan, Ann Arbor, MI 48109, USA
[2] Pharmacy Innovations & Partnerships, University of Michigan, Ann Arbor, MI 48108, USA; nghih@med.umich.edu
* Correspondence: gbarnes@umich.edu

Abstract: Venous thromboembolism (VTE) is a prevalent medical condition with high morbidity, mortality, and associated costs. Anticoagulation remains the main treatment for VTE, though the decision on when, how, and for how long to administer anticoagulants is increasingly complex. This review highlights the different phases of VTE management, with special circumstances for consideration such as antiphospholipid syndrome, coronary artery disease, cancer-associated thrombus, COVID-19, and future anticoagulation options. Anticoagulation management will continue to be a complex decision, applying evidence-based medicine to individual patients with the hope of maximizing effectiveness while minimizing risks.

Keywords: venous thromboembolism; pulmonary embolism; deep vein thrombosis; anticoagulation; cardio-vascular disease

1. Introduction

Venous thromboembolism (VTE) is defined as a blood clot in the venous system, occurring as a deep vein thrombosis (DVT) or pulmonary embolism (PE). The annual incidence of VTE in the United States is estimated to be around 1–2 per 1000 people, or 300,000–600,000 cases. However, the incidence is noted to differ by age, with VTE occurring in 1 per 100 people aged ≥ 80 years old. The estimated total annual healthcare cost for VTE ranges from USD 2–10 billion. The disease process carries high morbidity and mortality, with 10–30% of patients having a 30-day mortality. Additionally, 20–25% of PE cases present with sudden death [1]. Around 60,000–100,000 deaths occur annually from VTE. A third of the people who have a VTE event will have a reoccurrence within 10 years, while a third of the patients with DVT will develop post-thrombotic syndrome [1,2]. This highlights the high burden of VTE on the healthcare system and the importance of its management, including preventing recurrence.

Traditionally, most VTE events are characterized according to the presence or absence of provoking risk factors. Provoked events can be further characterized as a transient risk factor vs. persistent risk factor, while for unprovoked events, they have no provoking factor, either transient or persistent [3] (Table 1).

Venous thromboembolism management continues to be an evolving field with considerations in choice and durations for anticoagulation. This review will outline VTE management decisions, focusing on various anticoagulation options, treatment length, and special considerations.

Table 1. Examples of VTE provoking risk factors.

Major Transient Risk Factors	Minor Transient Risk Factors	Persistent Risk Factors
-Cesarean section. -Confined to hospital bed for 3 days. -Surgery with general anesthesia for >30 min.	-Confined to bed out of hospital for 3 days. -Hospitalization < 3 days. -Leg injury. -Pregnancy. -Estrogen therapy. -Acute infectious illness (e.g., COVID-19) without hospitalization.	-Active cancer. -Inflammatory bowel disease. -Obesity. -Chronic inflammatory condition. -Advanced age. -Previous venous thromboembolism. -Genetic/acquired thrombophilia (APS, protein C&S deficiency, etc.).

2. Overview of Anticoagulation

Anticoagulation is the bedrock of VTE management, given its proven role in preventing VTE occurrence and recurrence. For nearly all patients with a proximal DVT or acute PE, anticoagulation is recommended as first-line therapy. The treatment for VTE is typically divided into three phases: the initiation phase, the treatment phase (primary treatment), and the extended phase (secondary prevention) (Figure 1). The goal of the initiation phase is to slow down any active thrombus formation, helping to prevent new thrombus from forming while allowing the body's natural thrombolytic process to proceed and restore/maintain venous blood flow. This can be achieved through either oral anticoagulation, with apixaban or rivaroxaban, or through parental medication (e.g., unfractionated heparin, low-molecular-weight heparin). For the treatment phase, all patients are recommended to receive 3–6 months of treatment with anticoagulation. This is the time when patients are at the highest risk of recurrence as an acute thrombus is being converted to fibrin [4]. Given their overall improved safety profile (especially lower rates of intracranial hemorrhage) and ease of administration, anticoagulation with apixaban, dabigatran, edoxaban, or rivaroxaban is recommended over vitamin K antagonist (VKA) for the treatment phase [5] (Table 2). For patients with a continued risk of VTE they will continue anticoagulation in the extended phase. In this phase, the risk vs. benefit of full-dose anticoagulation vs. reduced-dose anticoagulation vs. no anticoagulation will need to be considered depending on the patient's risk factors (Figure 1).

Apart from anticoagulation route selection, it is also important to decide where management should take place. For patients with a DVT, if there is rapid availability of ultrasound and ease of communication, then outpatient management is usually preferred. Exceptions would be for patients with a high risk of limb loss (e.g., phlegmasia cerula dolens) or an inability to reliably obtain anticoagulant medications in a timely manner and clinic follow-up. Most PEs are first evaluated in the emergency department where they are risk stratified for the risk of deterioration. Patients at low risk for complications should be offered an outpatient management strategy if there is appropriate availability of testing, medications, and clinical follow-up. A study has estimated that 20% or more of acute PE cases in the emergency department may be good candidates for outpatient treatment [6]. The remaining cases typically require a hospital stay.

An exception to routine anticoagulation for VTE treatment is in patients with distal DVT. Distal DVTs affect the deep veins, with the most proximal component being distal to the popliteal vein. The ninth edition of the CHEST guideline recommends serial ultrasound in 1–2 weeks without anticoagulation if the thrombus does not extend proximally. However, if there is extension into proximal veins, anticoagulation is strongly recommended [5]. Additionally, cases with distal DVT anticoagulation may be appropriate for patients with significant symptoms or a high risk of extension (e.g., underlying malignancy).

Another exception for routine anticoagulation treatment is in patients with isolated subsegmental PE without proximal DVT. In these patients, the risk of recurrence needs to be considered. In patients with a low risk of recurrent VTE, clinical surveillance can be considered, while for patients with a high risk of recurrent VTE, anticoagulation is recommended. These are both classified as weak recommendations by the most recent CHEST guidelines [5].

The third important exception is in patients with active bleeding, for whom anticoagulation should be avoided. It is also reasonable to consider avoiding anticoagulation for patients at very high risk of bleeding. The patient's risk vs. benefit of anticoagulation needs to be considered in the setting of VTE management and bleeding, with continued re-assessment. If anticoagulation is not being pursued, then the role of an IVC filter should be reviewed.

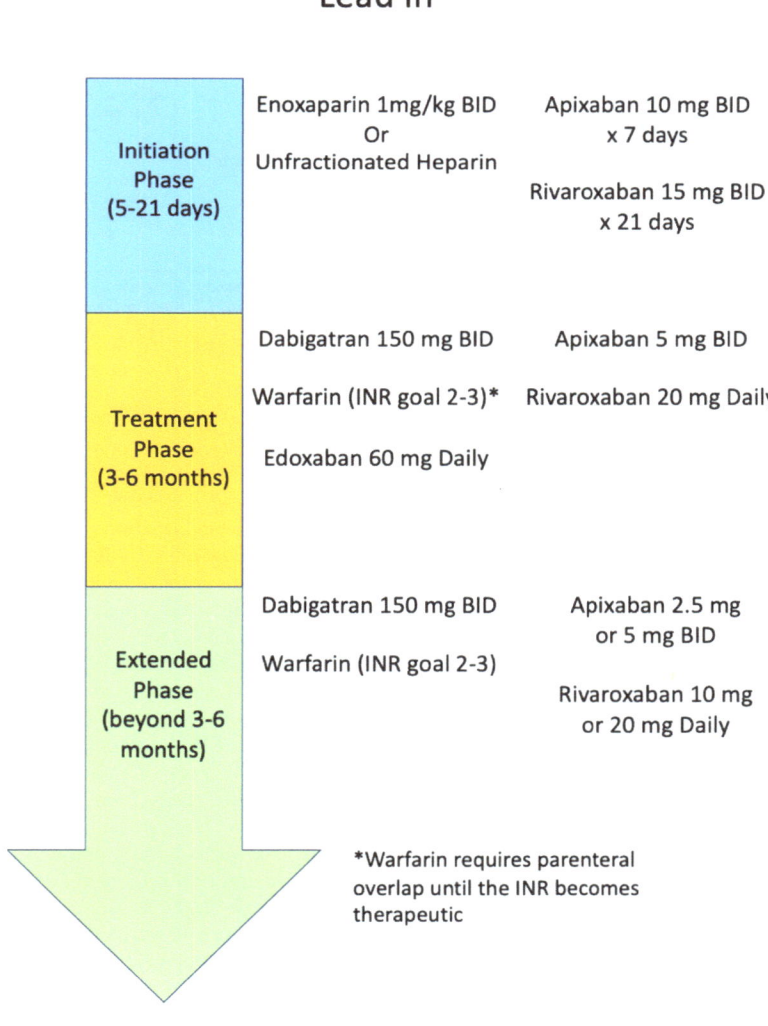

Figure 1. Choice and duration of anticoagulation for VTE.

Table 2. Oral anticoagulation for VTE.

Generic Name	Mechanism of Action	Dose and Regimen	Consideration of Renal Function	Consideration of Drug Interactions	Other Considerations
Apixaban	Factor Xa Inhibitor	10 mg BID × 7 days, followed by 5 mg BID	Not studied in patients with SCr ≥ 2.5 mg/dL or CrCl <25 mL/min	Reducing dose by 50% in patients taking strong dual *inhibitors* of p-glycoprotein and CYP 3A4. Avoiding in patients taking dual *inducers* of CYP 34A and p-glycoprotein.	N/a
Dabigatran	Direct Thrombin Inhibitor	150 mg BID after 5–10 days of parenteral anticoagulation lead in	Avoid in CrCl ≤ 30 mL/min	If CrCl ≤ 50 mL/min, patients taking p-glycoprotein *inhibitors* should avoid dabigatran. Patients taking p-glycoprotein *inducers* should avoid dabigatran.	N/a
Edoxaban	Factor Xa Inhibitor	60 mg daily after 5–10 days of parenteral anticoagulation lead in	Renally dose to 30 mg daily for CrCl 15–50 mL/min. Avoid in CrCl <15 mL/min	Reduce dose to 30 mg daily for patients taking p-glycoprotein *inhibitors*. Avoid using with p-glycoprotein *inducers*.	Reduce dose to 30 mg daily for body weight ≤ 60 kg.
Rivaroxaban	Factor Xa Inhibitor	15 mg twice a day for 21 days, then 20 mg daily	Avoid in CrCl ≤ 15 mL/min	In patients taking moderate dual *inhibitors* of CYP 3A4 and p-glycoprotein with CrCl ≤ 80 mL/min, use cautiously. Avoid use in patients taking strong dual *inhibitors* or *inducers* of CYP 3A4 and p-glycoprotein.	Administer with food.
Warfarin	Vitamin K Antagonist	Adjusted to target INR 2–3 Require parenteral anticoagulation overlap at initiation	None	Consider reducing starting dose to 2.5 mg for patients with drug–drug interactions expected to increase exposure to warfarin.	Consider reducing starting dose to 2.5 mg for patients with multiple comorbidities, advanced age, and advanced end-organ dysfunction.

BID = twice daily; CrCl = creatinine clearance as calculated by the Cockcroft–Gault equation with actual body weight; INR = international normalized ratio; N/a = not applicable; SCr = serum creatinine.

3. Phases of Management of VTE

3.1. Initiation Phase

During the initiation phase, the goal is to stop the growth of the thrombus and prevent embolism of the thrombus with anticoagulation. This can occur over 5 to 21 days, depending on the anticoagulation chosen. Traditionally, unfractionated heparin, or low-molecular-weight heparin, was the anticoagulant of choice. Now, apixaban and rivaroxaban are oral options that can be used for the initiation phase. Typically, if patients are hospitalized in the acute setting for VTE, they are initially started on a parenteral heparin agent and then transitioned to oral options prior to hospital discharge. For parenteral heparin agents, low-molecular-weight heparin (e.g., enoxaparin) is preferred over unfractionated heparin given the lower risk of HIT, subcutaneous administration, ease of dosing, and most importantly, a predictable anticoagulation level without requiring routine monitoring [4]. When this transition occurs before the completion of a typical initiation phase (e.g., a full 7 days for apixaban or 21 days of rivaroxaban), then the higher total daily dose of these oral medications is given to complete that initiation phase duration. Some clinicians will transition to the treatment phase dosing of oral anticoagulants if at least 5 days of parenteral heparin have been given, even if this strategy was not tested in the phase 3 randomized trials or included in the package label dosing recommendations.

For patients in the outpatient setting, direct oral anticoagulants (DOACs) with apixaban and rivaroxaban are effective oral-only options for patients who do not want parenteral lead in therapy (Figure 1). No single DOAC is recommended over another by most major society guidelines [5,7,8]. Apixaban and rivaroxaban are appropriate for use in patients with obesity with a BMI > 40 kg/m^2 or a weight >120 kg. Cost should be considered for DOAC therapy, which can be a barrier for patients. However, there are assistance programs available from drug manufacturers that can substantially reduce the out-of-pocket cost for many patients. Discussion with pharmacists and/or social workers is often helpful to connect patients with appropriate resources for DOAC coverage.

3.2. Treatment Phase

The treatment phase can last between 3 and 6 months, depending on the thrombus burden, symptoms, and patient clinical scenario. The American Society of Hematology recommends that this treatment phase last only 3–6 months rather than a more extended duration of 12 months [7]. DOACs are now the mainstay treatment in this phase. However, vitamin K antagonists (VKAs) are an acceptable alternative for most patients and may be preferred in selected patient groups (see below).

For patients using apixaban or rivaroxaban as an oral-only strategy during the initiation phase, these DOACs are typically continued into the treatment phase, but with a dose reduction (Figure 1). Dabigatran and edoxaban, on the other hand, are initiated in the treatment phase after a 5–10-day run-in period (initiation phase) with a parenteral anticoagulant. VKA with warfarin continues to be a well-studied anticoagulation option, though it can be difficult, requiring frequent lab work and a higher risk of bleeding. Warfarin needs to be monitored through the international normalized ratio (INR) with a goal of INR 2–3. There can be higher variability amongst patients for warfarin dosing given patient-specific factors such as diet, genetics, or other medications. Pharmacy costs of warfarin can be lower than DOACs for many patients, but the cost of INR laboratory testing or home testing must also be factored into the overall cost estimates. Most patients are started on warfarin 5 mg daily, with frequent INR testing at least weekly to help determine the warfarin dosing regimen. The mechanism of action plus special considerations for oral anticoagulation are outlined in Table 2. Overall, the treatment of choice for anticoagulation should be patient-specific, with shared decision-making between the patient and provider.

3.3. Extended Phase

Extended phase, or anticoagulation beyond the treatment phase of 3–6 months, is considered for certain patient populations depending on the patients' risk of recurrent VTE versus the risk of bleeding with continued treatment. Patient preference as well as risk scores (e.g., HERDOO2 Rule, Vienna Prediction Model, or DASH Prediction Score) [9–11] can assist with the decision-making process for extended-phase anticoagulation. In patients with a low risk of VTE recurrence who had a transiently provoked VTE (Table 1), anticoagulation beyond 3–6 months of the treatment phase is usually not necessary. Generally, for patients with unprovoked VTE, extended-phase treatment should be considered. Both DOACs and warfarin are viable options for extended-phase anticoagulation. For patients continuing on warfarin for VTE prevention, an INR goal of 2–3 is recommended. Dabigatran, apixaban, and rivaroxaban are all potential options for continued anticoagulation for secondary VTE prevention. These three DOACs have been compared to placebo in studies demonstrating superiority in preventing VTE recurrence without significant rates of major bleeding [12–15].

However, only apixaban and rivaroxaban have demonstrated both efficacy and safety in lower doses than their initial treatment phase doses for recurrent VTE prevention. In AMPLIFY-EXTEND, apixaban 5 mg BID was compared to apixaban 2.5 mg BID and placebo, demonstrating similar rates of recurrent VTE in both apixaban groups and superiority to the placebo group [14]. Patients who had a symptomatic DVT or PE and received treatment for 6–12 months without a recurrent VTE episode were included in the study. The EINSTEIN-CHOICE trial studied rivaroxaban 20 mg daily with rivaroxaban 10 mg daily and aspirin 100 mg daily. Both rivaroxaban groups had similar rates of recurrent VTE and a reduced rate of VTE compared to the aspirin group, while having no significant difference in the rate of major bleeding [15]. Patients who had an objectively confirmed, symptomatic proximal DVT or PE, anticoagulation for 6–12 months, and no interruption in anticoagulation 7 days prior to enrollment were included in the study. Given these studies, lower-dose DOACs compared to standard therapy should be considered for continued anticoagulation in the prevention of recurrent VTE. Once again, this decision is patient-specific, weighing the risk vs. benefit of full vs. reduced DOAC dosing.

The guidelines recommend that patients with recurrent VTE and/or patients with a history of strong thrombophilia be offered extended-phase anticoagulation therapy [5,7]. This recommendation is based on the higher risk of VTE recurrence, which outweighs the risk of bleeding with extended anticoagulation therapy.

4. Special Considerations

Special circumstances need to be considered when deciding on management for VTE. Briefly, below, we will review VTE management in cancer-associated thrombosis (CAT), antiphospholipid syndrome (APS), coronary artery disease (CAD), and COVID-19.

4.1. Cancer-Associated Thrombosis Treatment

Cancer is among the most common risk factors for VTE, with approximately 20% of all VTE cases occurring in patients with cancer. In these patients, more than 50% of VTE cases occur within 3 months of the cancer diagnosis. Both the American College of Chest Physicians (ACCP) and ASH have guideline recommendations specifically on the management of CAT. ACCP guidelines recommend DOAC over other anticoagulation for acute VTE in the cancer setting [5], while for ASH, both DOACs (apixaban or rivaroxaban) or low-molecular-weight heparin (LMWH) are recommended. The SELECT-D study examined rivaroxaban vs. dalteparin monotherapy and found that the DOAC group at 6 months had significantly fewer recurrent VTE episodes but higher rates of bleeding [16]. The ADAM VTE and Caravaggio studies both looked at apixaban vs. dalteparin, noting a lower risk of recurrent VTE, while the Caravaggio study found no difference in the major bleeding risk [17,18]. For short-term treatment (3–6 months), DOAC is recommended over LMWH. In patients with active cancer and VTE, long-term anticoagulation is recommended for secondary prophylaxis, which can be achieved through DOAC or LMWH. In patients with cancer and recurrent VTE on anticoagulation, an inferior vena cava filter is not recommended [19]. These recommendations should be considered when treating VTE in patients with cancer-associated thrombosis. It is worth noting that special considerations should be made for gastrointestinal or genitourinary malignancies, as in these select populations, DOACs have demonstrated higher rates of bleeding [20]. Additionally, there should be close communication with the patient's oncologist given drug–drug interactions with DOACs and cancer therapies. DOAC uptake is dependent on the P-glycoprotein system, while metabolism is dependent on the cytochrome P450 system. DOACs should be avoided when co-administered with cancer therapies that are strong P-glycoprotein or CYP3A4 inducers or inhibitors [21].

4.2. Thrombophilia and Antiphospholipid Syndrome Treatment

Warfarin and other VKAs have been the mainstream treatment for thrombotic antiphospholipid syndrome (APS). However, given the increased use of DOACs for other conditions, the use of DOACs for APS remains controversial. While DOACs are far more convenient for patients and are associated with lower rates of bleeding than VKA, it is unclear if they are as effective as VKA in patients with APS. Khairani et al. conducted a systematic review and meta-analysis of RCTs comparing DOACs vs. VKA for the treatment of VTE in patients with APS. Four open-labeled RCTs were included, as summarized in Table 3 [22–26]. The study found that DOACs, compared to VKA, have an increased risk of arterial thrombosis but a similar risk of subsequent VTE or major bleeding. Overall, the findings did not support the routine use of DOACs for patients with thrombotic APS [22]. Additionally, all major societal guidelines recommend the use of VKA over DOACs for APS [5,7,8]. However, there may still be select cases where DOAC therapy is appropriate for a patient with APS, especially if that strongly aligns with the patient's values/preferences and they are well informed of the current outcome data. In particular, patients with only one or two positive antibodies, patients who have previously tolerated VKA therapy, and/or patients who express a strong preference for VKA therapy over DOAC may be appropriate for VKA therapy. However, it is important for clinicians to engage in a shared decision–discussion with the patient before selecting DOAC over VKA therapy.

Table 3. Randomized trials of oral anticoagulation for antiphospholipid syndrome patients with venous thromboembolism.

Clinical Trial (Ref. #)	Included Patients	N	Trial Design	Length of Follow-Up	Treatment Groups	Primary Efficacy Outcomes	Efficacy Outcomes	Major Bleeding Outcomes
RAPS [23]	Patients with APS who were taking warfarin for previous VTE	116	Open-label RCT	210 days	Continue warfarin vs. rivaroxaban 20 mg daily	Percentage change in endogenous thrombin potential at day 42, with non-inferiority set at less than 20% difference from warfarin	ETP (nmol/L per min): Rivaroxaban 1086 vs. warfarin 548 Treatment effect (ratio): 2.0 (1.7–2.4)	Rivaroxaban: 0 Warfarin: 0
TRAPS [24]	Patients with APS (triple positivity) with history of thrombus	120	Open-label RCT	569 days (mean)	Rivaroxaban 20 mg or 15 mg daily (dependent on creatine clearance) vs. warfarin	Cumulative incidence of thromboembolic events, major bleeding, and vascular death	Rivaroxaban: 19% Warfarin: 3% HR: 6.7 (1.5–30.5)	Rivaroxaban: 7% Warfarin: 3% HR: 2.5 (0.5–13.6)
Ordi-Ros et al. [25]	Patients with APS (positive result on aPL testing on 2 occasions at least 3 months apart) with history of thrombus	190	Open-label RCT	36 months	Rivaroxaban 20 mg or 15 mg daily (dependent on creatine clearance) vs. warfarin	Proportion of patients with new thrombotic event	Rivaroxaban: 11.6% Warfarin: 6.3% HR: 1.94 (0.72–5.24)	Rivaroxaban: 6.3% Warfarin: 7.4% HR: 0.88 (0.3–2.63)
ASTRO-APS [26]	Patients with thrombotic antiphospholipid syndrome on anticoagulation for secondary prevention	48	Open-label RCT	12 months	Apixaban 2.5 mg BID then increased to 5 mg BID (after 25 patient was randomized) vs. warfarin	Thrombosis and vascular death	Apixaban: 6 thrombotic events Warfarin: no thrombotic events	Apixaban: 0 Warfarin: 1 event

APS = antiphospholipid syndrome; BID = twice daily; ETP = endogenous thrombin potential; HR = hazard ratio; RCT = randomized control trial; VTE = venous thromboembolism.

Patients with other thrombophilias can be safely treated with DOAC therapy. In a meta-analysis of randomized trials, patients with thrombophilia had similar rates of recurrent VTE and bleeding when treated with DOAC as a VKA therapy [27]. However, care must be taken when ordering and interpreting thrombophilia laboratory tests while being treated with DOAC therapy, as many anticoagulants can interfere with thrombophilia testing processes [28].

4.3. Concurrent Coronary Artery Disease and Venous Thromboembolism

The optimal antithrombotic regimen can be difficult to determine for patients with both CAD and VTE. Historically, patients have been treated with triple therapy, including two antiplatelet agents (low-dose aspirin and P2Y12 inhibitors) and anticoagulation. However, this triple therapy combination increases the risk of bleeding up to 3-fold compared to oral anticoagulation alone [29]. Studies examining the risk of bleeding on oral anticoagulation have demonstrated lower rates of bleeding in patients with VTE as compared to those with AF, likely due to their younger age and fewer comorbidities. However, several key factors are critical to consider when a patient on anticoagulation for VTE undergoes percutaneous coronary intervention (PCI). These include the planned duration of anticoagulation, the urgency of PCI, and how best to combine anticoagulation with anti-platelet therapy to decrease bleeding risk.

The American College of Cardiology (ACC) has developed clinical pathways to assist with anticoagulation and antiplatelet therapy. The first key distinction to make is the duration of anticoagulation and if it will be indefinite therapy, as discussed prior. Next, the reason for PCI (stable ischemic heart disease vs. acute coronary syndrome (ACS)) divides the pathways in length and choice of antiplatelet therapy. (Figure 2). Finally, all patients should be started on proton pump inhibitors or H2 blockers to decrease the risk of bleeding when they are using multiple antithrombotic agents concurrently [30]. The use of DOAC is preferred over warfarin while on antiplatelet therapy, given the lower risk of major, intracranial, or fatal bleeding with DOAC therapy. However, special considerations (e.g., the use of warfarin for APS) must be taken into account for individual patients [30].

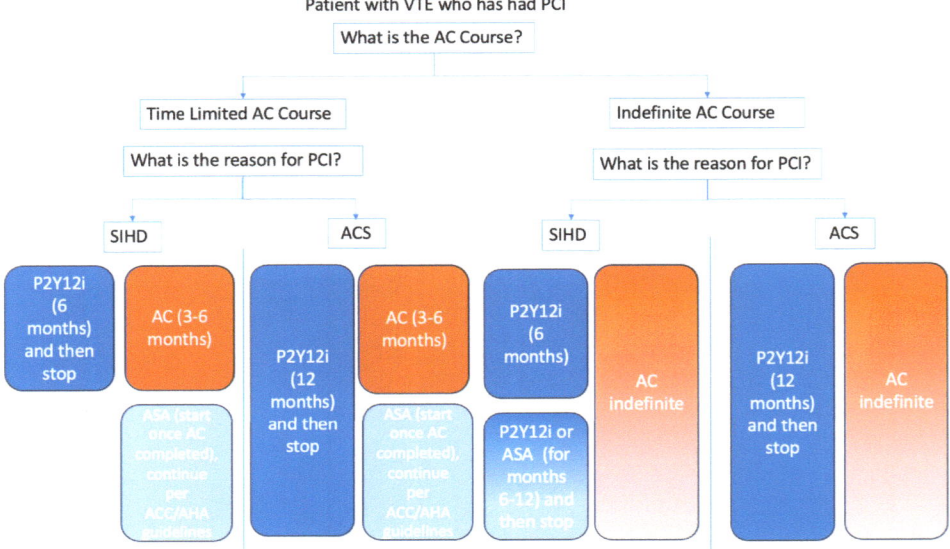

AC=anticoagulation; ACS=acute coronary syndrome; ASA= baby aspirin; P2Y12i=P2Y12 inhibitor; PCI=percutaneous coronary intervention; SIHD=stable ischemic heart disease; VTE=venous thromboembolism

Figure 2. VTE and CAD antithrombotic therapy.

4.4. COVID-19 Infection

The COVID-19 infection creates a pro-inflammatory state that often increases a patient's risk for VTE, especially when the infection is severe enough to require hospitalization. For patients who develop VTE concurrently with a COVID-19 acute infection, standard anticoagulation therapy as outlined above is recommended. These patients are typically considered to have experienced a transient, reversibly provoked VTE, so a shorter course of 3–6 months of anticoagulation is most common [31].

The pro-inflammatory and thrombotic nature of COVID-19 has led to evolving recommendations regarding the use of anticoagulation for VTE thromboprophylaxis. The recommendations require a balance between thrombotic risk and bleeding risk, as well as the patient's overall risk of survival. In general, patients with COVID-19 can be categorized into one of three groups: ambulatory, hospitalized non-critically ill, and hospitalized critically ill. Based on the results of several randomized trials in patients who require oxygen but are not critically ill (i.e., not in intensive care), a therapeutic dose of heparin (preferentially LMWH) is recommended for patients with D-dimer above the upper limit of normal and without increased bleeding risk [31–35]. These patients should continue therapeutic-intensity thromboprophylaxis for 14 days or until discharge/escalation of care to an intensive care unit. All other hospitalized patients should receive standard VTE thromboprophylaxis with prophylactic doses of heparin. The use of DOACs for inpatient thromboprophylaxis is generally not recommended [35,36]. However, consideration can be made for the use of extended post-hospital thromboprophylaxis with low-dose rivaroxaban in select patients at high thromboembolic risk but low bleeding risk [37]. Finally, antiplatelet therapy to prevent COVID progression or death is not recommended based on the negative results of the ACTIV-4a and RECOVERY trials [32–38].

5. Future Anticoagulation Options

Anticoagulation management for VTE looks different today than twenty years ago. DOACs revolutionized VTE management with their increased ease of administration and lower risk of bleeding, but they are more limited in terms of clinical applications. There continue to be ongoing clinical trials examining new anticoagulation medications. Table 4 summarizes the current ongoing trials for VTE and Factor XI/XIa inhibitors [39–41]. These agents might allow for further reductions in the bleeding risk by uncoupling thrombosis and hemostasis. Furthermore, they may provide further advantages over DOACs by eliminating concerns about renal clearance and longer half-lives to address issues of medication compliance. However, their efficacy in preventing VTE or VTE recurrence remains to be proven in rigorous phase 3 randomized trials.

Table 4. Factor XI ongoing clinical trials for VTE.

Clinical Trial Reference (Status)	Drug	Mechanism of Action	N	Clinical Trial Summary	Results
ASTER NCT05171049 (Ongoing) [39]	Abelacimab	Binds and inhibits Factor XI and Factor XIa	1655	Phase III trial comparing the effect of abelacimab relative to apixaban on VTE recurrence and bleeding in patients with CAT	No results currently
MAGNOLIA NCT05171075 (Ongoing) [40]	Abelacimab	Binds and inhibits Factor XI and Factor XIa	1020	Phase III trial comparing the effect of abelacimab vs. dalteparin on VTE recurrence and bleeding in patients with gastrointestinal or genitourinary CAT	No results currently
NCT04465760 (Recruiting) [41]	Xisomab	Binds Factor XI and blocks activation by Factor XIIa	50	Phase II trial examining the efficacy of xisomab as measured by incidence of catheter associated thrombosis in individuals with a central venous catheter	No results currently

CAT = cancer-associated thrombosis; VTE = venous thromboembolism.

6. Final Thoughts

VTE is a highly prevalent condition associated with significant morbidity and mortality. While anticoagulation is the mainstream therapy for VTE, the decision on when, how, and for how long to administer anticoagulants is increasingly complex. By considering each individual patient's underlying thromboembolic and bleeding risk, clinicians can then apply evidence from both randomized and observational data to personalize anticoagulation therapy. Anticoagulation management will continue to evolve with new agents and new evidence that aim to maximize effectiveness and minimize risk.

Author Contributions: Writing—original draft preparation, writing—review and editing, visualization, A.M., N.B.H. and G.D.B. Supervision, G.D.B. All authors have read and agreed to the published version of the manuscript.

Funding: This research received no external funding.

Data Availability Statement: Not applicable.

Conflicts of Interest: GDB: Grant Funding—Boston Scientific; Consulting—Pfizer, Bristol-Myers Squibb, Janssen, Bayer, AstraZeneca, Sanofi, Anthos, Abbott Vascular, Boston Scientific; DSMB—Translational Sciences (Clinical Events Adjudication Committee); Board of Directors—Anticoagulation Forum. AM and NH—none.

References

1. Beckman, M.G.; Hooper, W.C.; Critchley, S.E.; Ortel, T.L. Venous thromboembolism: A public health concern. *Am. J. Prev. Med.* **2010**, *38* (Suppl. S4), S495–S501. [CrossRef]
2. CDC. Data and Statistics on Venous Thromboembolism. Available online: https://www.cdc.gov/ncbddd/dvt/data.html (accessed on 6 November 2023).
3. Kearon, C.; Ageno, W.; Cannegieter, S.C.; Cosmi, B.; Geersing, G.J.; Kyrle, P.A. Categorization of patients as having provoked or unprovoked venous thromboembolism: Guidance from the SSC of ISTH. *J. Thromb. Haemost.* **2016**, *14*, 1480–1483. [CrossRef] [PubMed]
4. Renner, E.; Barnes, G.D. Antithrombotic Management of Venous Thromboembolism: JACC Focus Seminar. *J. Am. Coll. Cardiol.* **2020**, *76*, 2142–2154. [CrossRef] [PubMed]
5. Stevens, S.M.; Woller, S.C.; Baumann Kreuziger, L.; Bounameaux, H.; Doerschug, K.; Geersing, G.-J.; Huisman, M.V.; Kearon, C.; King, C.S.; Knighton, A.J.; et al. Executive Summary: Antithrombotic Therapy for VTE Disease: Second Update of the CHEST Guideline and Expert Panel Report. *Chest* **2021**, *160*, 2247–2259. [CrossRef] [PubMed]
6. Vinson, D.R.; Ballard, D.W.; Huang, J.; Reed, M.E.; Lin, J.S.; Kene, M.V.; Sax, D.R.; Rauchwerger, A.S.; Wang, D.H.; McLachlan, D.I.; et al. MAPLE Investigators of the KP CREST Network. Outpatient Management of Emergency Department Patients with Acute Pulmonary Embolism: Variation, Patient Characteristics, and Outcomes. *Ann. Emerg. Med.* **2018**, *72*, 62–72.e3. [CrossRef] [PubMed]
7. Ortel, T.L.; Neuman, I.; Ageno, W.; Beyth, R.; Clark, N.P.; Cuker, A.; Hutten, B.A.; Jaff, M.R.; Manja, V.; Schulman, S.; et al. American Society of Hematology 2020 guidelines for management of venous thromboembolism: Treatment of deep vein thrombosis and pulmonary embolism. *Blood Adv.* **2020**, *4*, 4693–4738. [CrossRef] [PubMed]
8. Konstantinides, S.V.; Meyer, G.; Becattini, C.; Bueno, H.; Geersing, G.J.; Harjola, V.P.; Huisman, M.V.; Humbert, M.; Jennings, C.S.; Jiménez, D.; et al. 2019 ESC Guidelines for the diagnosis and management of acute pulmonary embolism developed in collaboration with the European Respiratory Society (ERS): The Task Force for the diagnosis and management of acute pulmonary embolism of the European Society of Cardiology (ESC). *Eur. Heart J.* **2020**, *41*, 543–603. [PubMed]
9. Eichinger, S.; Heinze, G.; Jandeck, L.M.; Kyrle, P.A. Risk assessment of recurrence in patients with unprovoked deep vein thrombosis or pulmonary embolism: The Vienna prediction model. *Circulation* **2010**, *121*, 1630–1636. [CrossRef]
10. Rodger, M.A.; Kahn, S.R.; Wells, P.S.; Anderson, D.A.; Chagnon, I.; Le Gal, G.; Solymoss, S.; Crowther, M.; Perrier, A.; White, R.; et al. Identifying unprovoked thromboembolism patients at low risk for recurrence who can discontinue anticoagulant therapy. *CMAJ* **2008**, *179*, 417–426. [CrossRef]
11. Tosetto, A.; Iorio, A.; Marcucci, M.; Baglin, T.; Cushman, M.; Eichinger, S.; Palareti, G.; Poli, D.; Tait, R.C.; Douketis, J. Predicting disease recurrence in patients with previous unprovoked venous thromboembolism: A proposed prediction score (DASH). *J. Thromb. Haemost.* **2012**, *10*, 1019–1025. [CrossRef]
12. Bauersachs, R.; Berkowitz, S.D.; Brenner, B.; Buller, H.R.; Decousus, H.; Gallus, A.S.; Lensing, A.W.; Misselwitz, F.; Prins, M.H.; Raskob, G.E.; et al. Oral rivaroxaban for symptomatic venous thromboembolism. *N. Engl. J. Med.* **2010**, *363*, 2499–2510. [PubMed]
13. Schulman, S.; Kearon, C.; Kakkar, A.K.; Schellong, S.; Eriksson, H.; Baanstra, D.; Kvamme, A.M.; Friedman, J.; Mismetti, P.; Goldhaber, S.Z. Extended use of dabigatran, warfarin, or placebo in venous thromboembolism. *N. Engl. J. Med.* **2013**, *368*, 709–718. [CrossRef] [PubMed]
14. Agnelli, G.; Buller, H.R.; Cohen, A.; Curto, M.; Gallus, A.S.; Johnson, M.; Porcari, A.; Raskob, G.E.; Weitz, J.I. Apixaban for extended treatment of venous thromboembolism. *N. Engl. J. Med.* **2013**, *368*, 699–708. [CrossRef] [PubMed]
15. Weitz, J.I.; Lensing, A.W.A.; Prins, M.H.; Bauersachs, R.; Beyer-Westendorf, J.; Bounameaux, H.; Brighton, T.A.; Cohen, A.T.; Davidson, B.L.; Decousus, H.; et al. Rivaroxaban or aspirin for extended treatment of venous thromboembolism. *N. Engl. J. Med.* **2017**, *376*, 1211–1222. [CrossRef] [PubMed]
16. Young, A.M.; Marshall, A.; Thirlwall, J.; Chapman, O.; Lokare, A.; Hill, C.; Hale, D.; Dunn, J.A.; Lyman, G.H.; Hutchinson, C.; et al. Comparison of an oral factor Xa inhibitor with low molecular weight heparin in patients with cancer with venous thromboembolism: Results of a randomized trial (SELECT-D). *J. Clin. Oncol.* **2018**, *36*, 2017–2023. [CrossRef] [PubMed]
17. McBane, R., 2nd; Wysokinski, W.E.; Le-Rademacher, J.G.; Zemla, T.; Ashrani, A.; Tafur, A.; Perepu, U.; Anderson, D.; Gundabolu, K.; Kuzma, C.; et al. Apixaban and dalteparin inactive malignancy-associated venous thromboembolism: The ADAM VTE trial. *J. Thromb. Haemost.* **2020**, *18*, 411–421. [CrossRef] [PubMed]
18. Agnelli, G.; Becattini, C.; Meyer, G.; Muñoz, A.; Huisman, M.V.; Connors, J.M.; Cohen, A.; Bauersachs, R.; Brenner, B.; Torbicki, A.; et al. Apixaban for the treatment of venous thromboembolism associated with cancer. *N. Engl. J. Med.* **2020**, *382*, 1599–1607. [CrossRef]
19. Lyman, G.H.; Carrier, M.; Ay, C.; Di Nisio, M.; Hicks, L.K.; Khorana, A.A.; Leavitt, A.D.; Lee, A.Y.; Macbeth, F.; Morgan, R.L.; et al. American Society of Hematology 2021 guidelines for management of venous thromboembolism: Prevention and treatment in patients with cancer. *Blood Adv.* **2021**, *5*, 927–974. [CrossRef]
20. Li, A.; Garcia, D.A.; Lyman, G.H.; Carrier, M. Direct oral anticoagulant (DOAC) versus low-molecular weight heparin (LMWH) for treatment of cancer associated thrombosis (CAT): A systematic review and meta-analysis. *Thromb. Res.* **2019**, *173*, 158–163. [CrossRef]
21. Mosarla, R.C.; Vaduganathan, M.; Qamar, A.; Moslehi, J.; Piazza, G.; Giugliano, R.P. Anticoagulation Strategies in Patients With Cancer: JACC Review Topic of the Week. *J. Am. Coll. Cardiol.* **2019**, *73*, 1336–1349. [CrossRef]

22. Khairani, C.D.; Bejjani, A.; Piazza, G.; Jimenez, D.; Monreal, M.; Chatterjee, S.; Pengo, V.; Woller, S.C.; Cortes-Hernandez, J.; Connors, J.M.; et al. Direct Oral Anticoagulants vs Vitamin K Antagonists in Patients With Antiphospholipid Syndromes: Meta-Analysis of Randomized Trials. *J. Am. Coll. Cardiol.* **2023**, *81*, 16–30. [CrossRef] [PubMed]
23. Cohen, H.; Hunt, B.J.; Efthymiou, M.; Arachchillage, D.R.J.; Mackie, I.J.; Clawson, S.; Sylvestre, Y.; Machin, S.J.; Bertolaccini, M.L.; Ruiz-Castellano, M.; et al. Rivaroxaban versus warfarin to treat patients with thrombotic antiphospholipid syndrome, with or without systemic lupus erythematosus (RAPS): A randomised, controlled, open-label, phase 2/3, non-inferiority trial. *Lancet Haematol.* **2016**, *3*, e426–e436. [CrossRef] [PubMed]
24. Pengo, V.; Denas, G.; Zoppellaro, G.; Jose, S.P.; Hoxha, A.; Ruffatti, A.; Andreoli, L.; Tincani, A.; Cenci, C.; Prisco, D.; et al. Rivaroxaban vs warfarin in high-risk patients with antiphospholipid syndrome. *Blood* **2018**, *132*, 1365–1371. [CrossRef] [PubMed]
25. Ordi-Ros, J.; Saez-Comet, L.; Perez-Conesa, M.; Vidal, X.; Riera-Mestre, A.; Castro-Salomó, A.; Cuquet-Pedragosa, J.; Ortiz-Santamaria, V.; Mauri-Plana, M.; Solé, C.; et al. Rivaroxaban versus vitamin K antagonist in antiphospholipid syndrome: A randomized noninferiority trial. *Ann. Intern. Med.* **2019**, *171*, 685–694. [CrossRef]
26. Woller, S.C.; Stevens, S.M.; Kaplan, D.; Wang, T.F.; Branch, D.W.; Groat, D.; Wilson, E.L.; Armbruster, B.; Aston, V.T.; Lloyd, J.F.; et al. Apixaban compared with warfarin to prevent thrombosis in thrombotic antiphospholipid syndrome: A randomized trial. *Blood Adv.* **2022**, *6*, 1661–1670. [CrossRef]
27. Elsebaie, M.A.T.; van Es, N.; Langston, A.; Büller, H.R.; Gaddh, M. Direct oral anticoagulants in patients with venous thromboembolism and thrombophilia: A systematic review and meta-analysis. *J. Thromb. Haemost.* **2019**, *17*, 1538–7933.
28. Kovacs, M.R.; Lazo-Langner, A.; Louzada, M.L.; Kovacs, M.J. Thrombophilia testing in patients receiving rivaroxaban or apixaban for the treatment of venous thromboembolism. *Thromb. Res.* **2020**, *195*, 231–232. [CrossRef] [PubMed]
29. Hansen, M.L.; Sorensen, R.; Clausen, M.T.; Fog-Petersen, M.L.; Raunsø, J.; Gadsbøll, N.; Gislason, G.H.; Folke, F.; Andersen, S.S.; Schramm, T.K.; et al. Risk of bleeding with single, dual, or triple therapy with warfarin, aspirin, and clopidogrel in patients with atrial fibrillation. *Arch. Intern. Med.* **2010**, *170*, 1433–1441. [CrossRef]
30. Kumbhani, D.J.; Cannon, C.P.; Beavers, C.J.; Bhatt, D.L.; Cuker, A.; Gluckman, T.J.; Marine, J.E.; Mehran, R.; Messe, S.R.; Patel, N.S.; et al. 2020 ACC Expert Consensus Decision Pathway for Anticoagulant and Antiplatelet Therapy in Patients With Atrial Fibrillation or Venous Thromboembolism Undergoing Percutaneous Coronary Intervention or With Atherosclerotic Cardiovascular Disease: A Report of the American College of Cardiology Solution Set Oversight Committee. *J. Am. Coll. Cardiol.* **2021**, *77*, 629–658.
31. NIH. Antithrombotic Therapy in Patients with COVID-19. Available online: https://www.covid19treatmentguidelines.nih.gov/therapies/antithrombotic-therapy (accessed on 26 November 2023).
32. ATTACC, ACTIV-4a, and REMAP-CAP Investigators. Therapeutic anticoagulation with heparin in noncritically ill patients with COVID-19. *N. Engl. J. Med.* **2021**, *385*, 790–802. [CrossRef]
33. Sholzberg, M.; Tang, G.H.; Rahhal, H.; AlHamzah, M.; Kreuziger, L.B.; Áinle, F.N.; Alomran, F.; Alayed, K.; Alsheef, M.; AlSumait, F.; et al. Effectiveness of therapeutic heparin versus prophylactic heparin on death, mechanical ventilation, or intensive care unit admission in moderately ill patients with COVID-19 admitted to hospital: RAPID randomised clinical trial. *BMJ* **2021**, *375*, n2400. [CrossRef] [PubMed]
34. Spyropoulos, A.C.; Goldin, M.; Giannis, D.; Diab, W.; Wang, J.; Khanijo, S.; Mignatti, A.; Gianos, E.; Cohen, M.; Sharifova, G.; et al. Efficacy and safety of therapeutic-dose heparin vs standard prophylactic or intermediate-dose heparins for thromboprophylaxis in high-risk hospitalized patients with COVID-19: The HEP-COVID randomized clinical trial. *JAMA Intern. Med.* **2021**, *181*, 1612–1620. [CrossRef]
35. Stone, G.W.; Farkouh, M.E.; Lala, A.; Tinuoye, E.; Dressler, O.; Moreno, P.R.; Palacios, I.F.; Goodman, S.G.; Esper, R.B.; Abizaid, A.; et al. Randomized trial of anticoagulation strategies for noncritically ill patients hospitalized with COVID-19. *J. Am. Coll. Cardiol.* **2023**, *81*, 1747–1762. [CrossRef]
36. Lopes, R.D.; de Barros, E.S.P.G.M.; Furtado, R.H.M.; Macedo, A.V.S.; Bronhara, B.; Damiani, L.P.; Barbosa, L.M.; de Aveiro Morata, J.; Ramacciotti, E.; de Aquino Martins, P.; et al. Therapeutic versus prophylactic anticoagulation for patients admitted to hospital with COVID-19 and elevated D-dimer concentration (ACTION): An open-label, multicentre, randomised, controlled trial. *Lancet* **2021**, *397*, 2253–2263. [CrossRef]
37. Ramacciotti, E.; Agati, L.B.; Calderaro, D.; Aguiar, V.C.R.; Spyropoulos, A.C.; de Oliveira, C.C.C.; dos Santos, J.L.; Volpiani, G.G.; Sobreira, M.L.; Joviliano, E.E.; et al. Rivaroxaban versus no anticoagulation for post-discharge thromboprophylaxis after hospitalisation for COVID-19 (MICHELLE): An open-label, multicentre, randomised, controlled trial. *Lancet* **2022**, *399*, 50–59. [CrossRef]
38. RECOVERY Collaborative Group. Aspirin in patients admitted to hospital with COVID-19 (RECOVERY): A randomised, controlled, open-label, platform trial. *Lancet* **2022**, *399*, 143–151. [CrossRef]
39. A Study Comparing Abelacimab to Apixaban in the Treatment of Cancer-associated VTE (ASTER). Available online: https://www.clinicaltrials.gov/study/NCT05171049 (accessed on 26 November 2023).

40. A Study Comparing Abelacimab to Dalteparin in the Treatment of Gastrointestinal/Genitourinary Cancer and Associated VTE (MAGNOLIA). Available online: https://www.clinicaltrials.gov/study/NCT05171075 (accessed on 26 November 2023).
41. Xisomab 3G3 for the Prevention of Catheter-Associated Thrombosis in Patients with Cancer Receiving Chemotherapy. Available online: https://clinicaltrials.gov/study/NCT04465760 (accessed on 26 November 2023).

Disclaimer/Publisher's Note: The statements, opinions and data contained in all publications are solely those of the individual author(s) and contributor(s) and not of MDPI and/or the editor(s). MDPI and/or the editor(s) disclaim responsibility for any injury to people or property resulting from any ideas, methods, instructions or products referred to in the content.

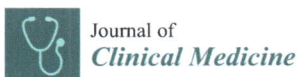 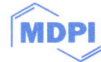

Review

The Role of IVC Filters in the Management of Acute Pulmonary Embolism

Samer Asmar [1,*], George Michael [2], Vincent Gallo [2] and Mitchell D. Weinberg [1]

1. Division of Cardiology, Department of Internal Medicine, Staten Island University Hospital, Staten Island, NY 10305, USA; mweinberg4@northwell.edu
2. Division of Vascular & Interventional Radiology, Department of Radiology, Staten Island University Hospital—Northwell Health, Staten Island, NY 10305, USA; gmichael@northwell.edu (G.M.); vgallo2@northwell.edu (V.G.)
* Correspondence: sasmar1@northwell.edu; Tel.: +1-(718)-226-9000

Abstract: Venous thromboembolism (VTE), comprising deep venous thrombosis (DVT) and pulmonary embolism (PE), is a prevalent cardiovascular condition, ranking third globally after myocardial infarction and stroke. The risk of VTE rises with age, posing a growing concern in aging populations. Acute PE, with its high morbidity and mortality, emphasizes the need for early diagnosis and intervention. This review explores prognostic factors for acute PE, categorizing it into low-risk, intermediate-risk, and high-risk based on hemodynamic stability and right ventricular strain. Timely classification is crucial for triage and treatment decisions. In the contemporary landscape, low-risk PE patients are often treated with Direct Oral Anticoagulants (DOACS) and rapidly discharged for outpatient follow-up. Intermediate- and high-risk patients may require advanced therapies, such as systemic thrombolysis, catheter-directed thrombolysis, mechanical thrombectomy, and IVC filter placement. The latter, particularly IVC filters, has witnessed increased usage, with evolving types like retrievable and convertible filters. However, concerns arise regarding complications and the need for timely retrieval. This review delves into the role of IVC filters in acute PE management, addressing their indications, types, complications, and retrieval considerations. The ongoing debate surrounding IVC filter use, especially in patients with less conventional indications, reflects the need for further research and data. Despite complications, recent studies suggest that clinically significant issues are rare, sparking discussions on the appropriate and safe utilization of IVC filters in select PE cases. The review concludes by highlighting current trends, gaps in knowledge, and potential avenues for advancing the role of IVC filters in future acute PE management.

Keywords: pulmonary embolism; IVC filter; high-risk PE; intermediate-risk PE

Citation: Asmar, S.; Michael, G.; Gallo, V.; Weinberg, M.D. The Role of IVC Filters in the Management of Acute Pulmonary Embolism. *J. Clin. Med.* **2024**, *13*, 1494. https://doi.org/10.3390/jcm13051494

Academic Editor: Brett Carroll

Received: 18 January 2024
Revised: 21 February 2024
Accepted: 4 March 2024
Published: 5 March 2024

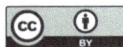

Copyright: © 2024 by the authors. Licensee MDPI, Basel, Switzerland. This article is an open access article distributed under the terms and conditions of the Creative Commons Attribution (CC BY) license (https://creativecommons.org/licenses/by/4.0/).

1. Introduction

Venous thromboembolism (VTE), including deep venous thrombosis (DVT) and pulmonary embolism (PE), ranks as the third most common cardiovascular ailment after myocardial infarction and stroke [1]. The risk of VTE doubles with each decade beyond age 40 and is thus becoming increasingly important in countries with aging populations [2]. Acute PE carries a high morbidity and mortality and, as such, necessitates an emphasis on early diagnosis and treatment [3]. A variety of rapidly expanding clinical, serologic, and imaging-based factors help prognostication of patients with acute PE [4]. PE can be categorized into low-risk, intermediate-risk (or sub-massive), and high-risk based on hemodynamic stability and the presence of right ventricular strain. Hemodynamically unstable patients are identified by a systolic blood pressure (SBP) below 90 mmHg, a drop in SBP of 40 mmHg or more from baseline, or the need for inotropes or vasopressors. Among hemodynamically stable patients, PE is considered low-risk if there is no evidence of right heart strain, and intermediate-risk in the presence of right heart strain identified through imaging, cardiac biomarker, and/or echocardiographic changes. PE is classified as high-risk when there is hemodynamic instability [5]. Appropriately categorizing a patient with PE as high-risk, intermediate-risk, or low-risk at the time of their presentation is uniquely impactful for early triage and treatment decisions.

In the modern era, low-risk patients are typically treated with Direct Oral Anticoagulants (DOACS) and, in appropriate settings, rapidly discharged for outpatient follow-up. Intermediate- and high-risk PE patients require parenteral anticoagulation and are considered for more advanced therapies in appropriate clinical scenarios, specifically those patients with high-risk PE and those intermediate-risk PE patients with certain high-risk features [6]. Such therapies include systemic thrombolysis, catheter-directed thrombolysis, mechanical thrombectomy, surgical thrombectomy, ECMO (extracorporeal membrane oxygenation), and inferior vena cava (IVC) filter placement. The data around the appropriate use of such therapies are still being generated via a plethora of ongoing trials, making this topic of advanced therapies for PE a topic of interest worldwide. Somewhat less glamorous but still important is the role of IVC interrupting devices in patients with PE. While IVC filters do not directly address acute VTE, they aim to prevent acute larger PE when the source of embolism originates in the venous system distal to the filter implantation site. However, smaller clots can still flow through the larger spaces of the filtering structure and is an acceptable trade-off between the filter catching all clots while maintaining IVC patency. This introduces an important distinction that should be made regarding filter implantation in patients with acute PE and confirmed DVT and in those whose imaging did not show the presence of thrombi in proximal or distal veins. Although the process is straightforward, it entails transporting the patient to the catheterization laboratory, puncturing a major vein (jugular, femoral, or arm vein), temporary immobilization of the patient, fluoroscopy, applying pressure to the vascular access site post-procedure, and, occasionally, readmission to remove the filter. It should be acknowledged that the procedure presents both organizational and economic challenges and may subject the patient to additional discomfort and anxiety. Indications for IVC filter placement in acute PE may be grouped into classic, well-accepted indications for use, and "extended", less uniformly accepted indications. IVC filter use truly hinges on risk assessment and Eized considerations, especially when the indication for placement is less well-accepted [7]. Classic indications include patients with documented acute PE possessing absolute contraindications to anticoagulation or patients with high-risk PE considered to be at risk of death despite anticoagulation, or patients with VTE and a complication of anticoagulation. Far more controversial is the use of IVC filters in patients who have medical comorbidities that are thought to limit their cardiopulmonary reserve [8,9], a decision based on the concern that another PE in such a patient could be fatal, and thus, IVC filter placement is indicated in the absence of a conventional indication.

IVC filters provide protection from life-threatening PE in the early period, but over time long-term risks and filter complications increase. Over the time-period of an IVC filter, an initial favorable risk/benefit ratio changes to be less benefit and more risk at which point the filter should be removed [10,11]. The Society of Interventional Radiology (SIR) has established defined complications and acceptable thresholds for IVC filters. Supplementary Table S1 summarizes the most reported complications by clinicians, and Supplementary Figure S1 shows radiographic images of such complications. This has prompted considerable focus within the vascular and interventional radiology communities on prompt removal of retrievable filters within weeks to months, a window that varies by retrievable filter type. In early generation retrievable IVC filters, some devices had recommendations about the window of opportunity for removal, but current generation devices and even many early generation IVC filters can now be safely removed with interventional radiology techniques [12,13]. Importantly, Johnson et al.'s findings from The Predicting the Safety and Effectiveness of IVC Filters (PRESERVE) trial showed that while IVC filter complications do occur, those that are clinically significant are rare with currently available filters [14]. While both appropriate and inappropriate IVC filter use are associated with risk, a role remains for IVC filter use in select patients with PE. Selecting such patients, however, is limited by the paucity of high-quality data in the field. This review aims to explore the available data on IVC filters in acute PE management, discuss current trends impacting decision-making, and highlight opportunities for advancements that may potentially enhance the role of IVC filters in the future management of acute PE.

2. Historical Overview and Currently Available IVC Filters

From a historic perspective, surgery was used to place clips around the IVC or sutures to segment the IVC before IVC filters were applied by Lazar Greenfield. This filter was placed using either a cutdown of the jugular or femoral vein and used a 24 Fr sheath. Interventional radiologists adopted the technique using percutaneous access (Dr. Dorfman, Brown University) [7]. Since then, IVC filter delivery systems have been greatly reduced in size making insertion much easier, and the use of IVC filters in the United States has steadily increased since the introduction of the Greenfield filter in 1972 [7]. In 2003, the FDA approved modifications to three permanent filters, enabling percutaneous retrieval [7]. Currently, IVC filters are categorized as permanent or optional, with the latter including temporary, retrievable, and convertible types. Retrievable IVC filters are sometimes referred to as temporary filters, even though they are FDA-cleared for both permanent and temporary placement, while temporary filters are specifically designed to be implanted only on a temporary basis and cannot be used permanently. Temporary filters are designed for short-term use and are suspended by catheters or wires. Convertible filters may be transformed into stents when IVC filtration is no longer needed. Retrievable filters possess tethering hooks for anchoring, like many permanent devices, but also possess a hook for later retrieval [10,11]. The filters used in the PRESERVE trial were ALN (ALN ± hook), Argon (Option Elite), B. Braun (LP, VenaTech Convertible), CR Bard (Denali), Cook (Gunther Tulip), Cordis (OptEase, TrapEase), and Philips Volcano (Crux) [14]. Figure 1 depicts some of the different types of IVC filters.

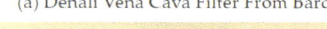

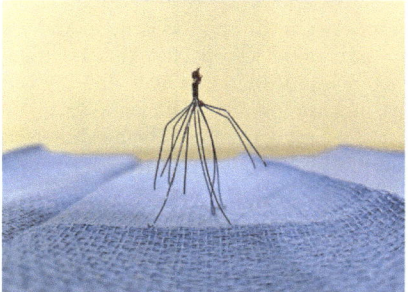 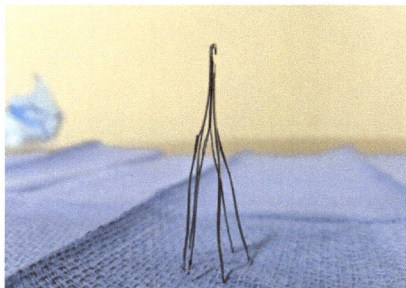

Figure 1. Different types of IVC filters available.

3. The Evolution in the Role of IVC Filters in the Management of Acute PE: The Two Eras

Our understanding of IVC filter use is best perceived upon the timeline of advancing PE therapeutics. Our initial understanding of the use of IVC filters in acute PE, until approximately 2010, was driven by a few data sets of limited size established when PE therapeutics were effectively simple. The introduction of PE multi-disciplinary care teams and the rapid advances in PE catheter-based technologies together drove a more aggressive strategy toward treating both high-risk and intermediate-risk PE. Systemic lysis at varying doses, catheter-based intervention, surgical thrombectomy, and ECMO use have all become more common as clinical understanding and related therapeutic strategies have evolved [10]. Data sets generated during this latter period are, of course, different than those generated in years prior to these advances. Thus, we will examine IVC filter data generated in these two very different eras: the early PE era and the current era.

3.1. The Early Era of PE Care: Marked by Registries, Trials, and In-Hospital Data

3.1.1. Registries Demonstrate Limited PE Therapies during the Early Era

The landmark PE trial of the early era was The International Cooperative Pulmonary Embolism Registry (ICOPER). ICOPER was a large-scale, multicenter, prospective registry dedicated to the study of acute PE conducted in the mid-1990s and enrolled 2454 patients with acute PE across 52 institutions in North America and Europe. The study concluded that PE continues to be a significant clinical challenge with a high mortality rate (12 to 14% 90-day mortality) and provided valuable insights for the planning of future trials involving high-risk PE patients [15]. The Emergency Medicine Pulmonary Embolism in the Real-World Registry (EMPEROR) was a registry comprising consecutive emergency department (ED) outpatients diagnosed with acute PE over a 26-month period from 2006 to 2008 across 22 hospitals in the United States. 1880 patients with confirmed acute PE were enrolled, and the study concluded that these patients have high functional status and 1% mortality. It also highlighted that the management of acute PE patients in the ED with anticoagulation is poorly standardized and encouraged more research to improve outcomes in these patients [16]. Results from the EMPEROR registry and ICOPER also provided important information on IVC filter use. In the ICOPER, none of the 11 (10.1%) patients who received an IVC filter developed recurrent PE within 90 days, and 10 (90.9%) survived at least 90 days. They showed that IVC filters were associated with a reduction in 90-day mortality (hazard ratio, 0.12; 95% CI, 0.02 to 0.85) [14]. In EMPEROR, 9 out of 58 patients with massive PE (defined as SBP < 90 mm Hg) received IVC filters, and 273 out of 1817 patients with non-massive PE (defined as SBP $\geq$ 90 mm Hg) received IVC filters. Unfortunately, no sub-analysis was performed to look at whether the use of IVC filters improves mortality or not [16]. Reports from both the EMPEROR registry and ICOPER indicated low rates of systemic thrombolysis administration in patients with high-risk PE. In ICOPER, 33 patients (30.5%) underwent thrombolysis, 1 (0.9%) underwent catheter-directed therapy, and 3 (2.7%) had surgical embolectomy [14]. In EMPEROR, 7 patients (12.1%) underwent thrombolysis, none underwent catheter-directed therapy, and 2 (3.4%) had surgical embolectomy [16]. This therapeutic style is in stark contrast to a recent analysis which demonstrated that over 70% of patients with high-risk PE received advanced therapies, including systemic thrombolysis, which was the most common but still less than half, and a variety of other advanced therapies including catheter-directed thrombolysis and surgical embolectomy [17].

3.1.2. The Trials

Randomized controlled trials (RCT) evaluating IVC filter use from the early era are few and limited by sample size. Perhaps the most important was the Prévention du Risque d'Embolie Pulmonaire par Interruption Cave II (PREPIC II) investigation. In the PREPIC II RCT, 200 stable patients with PE, along with DVT or superficial venous thrombosis and at least one additional high-risk criterion, received a retrievable IVC filter along with anticoagulation, while 199 patients received anticoagulation alone. Results at three and six months post-filter-insertion revealed comparable rates of recurrent PE, fatal PE, and all-cause mortality in those who received an IVC filter compared with those who did not [18]. The PREPIC II was limited in terms of assessment of utility for IVC filters in patients receiving anticoagulation; it helped further solidify the general approach to avoid filters in patients that can receive anticoagulation but did not help in understanding appropriateness in patients with a contraindication to anticoagulation, the group where filters are most commonly utilized. Other limitations included the exclusion of unstable patients and the absence of subgroup analysis given the small sample size. The PRESERVE trial is a large-scale, multi-specialty, nonrandomized prospective clinical study at 54 sites in the United States that enrolled 1429 participants who received IVC filters between 2015 and 2019. Patients were evaluated at baseline and followed up, even if the filter was removed, to determine the safety and effectiveness of vena cava filters. The PRESERVE trial by Johnson et al. affirmed the safety of IVC filters but faced challenges in claiming effectiveness. Limitations included the absence of a control group, inclusion of patients with anticoagulation history, and a lack of routine imaging for recurrent VTE assessment. The study's design impedes a direct comparison between IVC filter placement and medical management, hindering a clear assertion of the intervention's effectiveness [14,19]. Bikdeli et al. conducted a systematic review and meta-analysis that included six RCT and five prospective observational studies to further evaluate the safety and efficacy of IVC filters versus none in 4204 patients at risk of PE. They concluded that IVC filters reduced the risk of subsequent PE (odds ratio, 0.50; 95% CI, 0.33 to 0.75), increased the risk for DVT (odds ratio, 1.70; 95% CI, 1.17 to 2.48), and had no significant effect on neither PE-related mortality (odds ratio, 0.51; 95% CI, 0.25 to 1.05) nor overall mortality (odds ratio, 0.91; 95% CI, 0.70 to 1.19). However, on post hoc analysis of three studies whose patients had contraindications to anticoagulation and recurrent PE despite adequate anticoagulation, the nonsignificant reduction in PE-related mortality reached statistical significance (odds ratio, 0.47; 95% CI, 0.21 to 1.04) [1]. This study subgroup is most reflective of current guideline-recommended indications guiding IVC filter placement. Important limitations disclosed by the authors included the lack of a control procedure which may potentially bias the results of the individual studies and thereby contribute to pooled estimates, a likely underestimation of the rates of IVC-filter-related complications, and the exclusion of all retrospective studies.

3.1.3. In-Hospital Data

Registry data from the early era suggested the opposite, that IVC filters might be useful in patients with acute PE and certain high-risk features. Stein et al. conducted an analysis of the 1979 to 1999 National Hospital Discharge Survey (NHDS) database and revealed a consistent linear increase in the percentage of acute PE patients who underwent IVC filter insertion over a 21-year observation period [20]. This increase in the utilization of IVC filters in the management of acute PE provided a rich data set to potentially answer questions regarding the clinical utility of IVC filters in acute PE. Stein et al., in a review article, assessed the utility of IVC filters in stable patients with acute PE [21]. Results suggested that a variety of patient subsets, such as those undergoing pulmonary embolectomy, receiving thrombolytic therapy, experiencing recurrent PE while on treatment, hospitalized with solid malignant tumors (particularly if aged > 60 years), hospitalized with chronic obstructive pulmonary disease (COPD) (especially if aged > 50 years), and affected by PE when elderly (aged > 80 years), all exhibited reduced mortality with the addition of an IVC filter [21].

3.2. The Second Era: Marked by Novel Changes

The second era is marked by a set of clinical and device-related advances in the care of patients with acute PE. These advances in interventional tools, PE risk stratification, lytic dosing strategy, IVC filter technology, and shock management have reinvigorated the diagnosis and treatment of high- and intermediate-risk PE and prompted a reevaluation of IVC filter usage in PE patients. Another major change in PE was the development of safer and more reliable retrievable IVC filters. Before this, a patient with VTE had a permanent device inserted which may indwell for decades. While the development of the filters perhaps lowered the threshold to apply them in VTE, the difficulty is identifying the subset(s) of patient who will benefit the most from IVC filtration (Figure 2).

Secemsky et al. analyzed 630 patients with high- and intermediate-risk PE and found that advanced therapies were independently associated with 61% reduction in mortality despite major bleeding events. Of these patients, 37.9% received advanced therapy distributed as follows: IVC filter (20.7%), systemic thrombolysis (4.7%), catheter-directed thrombolysis (13.9%), endovascular suction embolectomy (0.9%), surgical embolectomy (4.4%), or ECMO (2.1%) [22]. Advanced therapies are increasingly being looked at and utilized, and further investigation is needed to determine their optimal use.

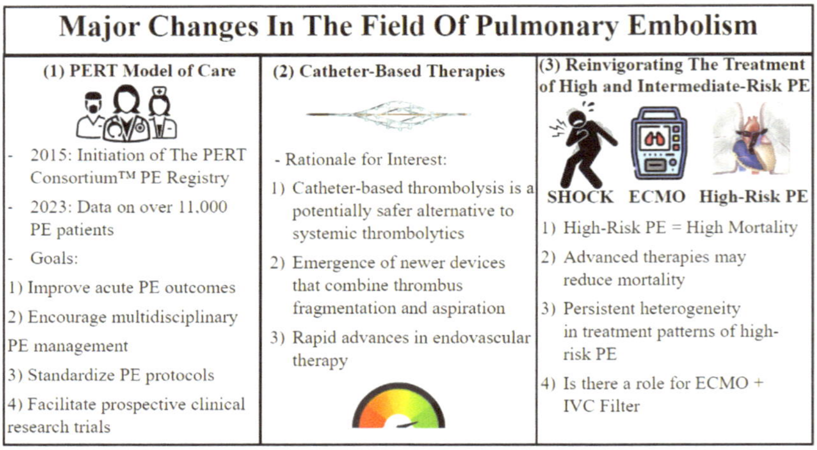

Major Changes In The Field Of Pulmonary Embolism		
(1) PERT Model of Care	**(2) Catheter-Based Therapies**	**(3) Reinvigorating The Treatment of High and Intermediate-Risk PE**
- 2015: Initiation of The PERT Consortium™ PE Registry - 2023: Data on over 11,000 PE patients - Goals: 1) Improve acute PE outcomes 2) Encourage multidisciplinary PE management 3) Standardize PE protocols 4) Facilitate prospective clinical research trials	- Rationale for Interest: 1) Catheter-based thrombolysis is a potentially safer alternative to systemic thrombolytics 2) Emergence of newer devices that combine thrombus fragmentation and aspiration 3) Rapid advances in endovascular therapy	SHOCK ECMO High-Risk PE 1) High-Risk PE = High Mortality 2) Advanced therapies may reduce mortality 3) Persistent heterogeneity in treatment patterns of high-risk PE 4) Is there a role for ECMO + IVC Filter

Figure 2. Major changes in the field of pulmonary embolism.

4. PERT and Other Societal Interest in IVC-Related Research

The PE Response Team (PERT) Consortium™ PE Registry is a contemporary multicenter registry designed to adapt to the evolving healthcare landscape, emphasizing a value-based system that prioritizes measurable aspects of quality, cost, and patient experience. This registry established and promoted the multidisciplinary PERT model of care delivery. Early publications from the PERT Consortium™ PE Registry included studies on PE mortality risk scores, risk stratification, and management practices among PE experts [10,23]. Variability in practice patterns was observed among participating centers, with advanced therapy implementation ranging from 16% to 46%, and 30-day mortality varying from 9% to 44% [10]. The diverse practices observed in the studies emphasize the urgency of establishing guidelines that promote optimal care, reduce variability, and improve overall quality in the management of acute PE. Driven by the PERT consortium, a renewed focus and societal interest on PE-related research occurred, and novel studies emerged discussing the role of IVC filters in acute PE. The American College of Chest Physicians, the American Heart Association, and the SIR have published guidelines for IVC filter insertion. The guidelines from the American College of Chest Physicians were perhaps the most conservative when it comes to insertion of IVC filters. The Eastern Association for the Surgery of Trauma also has guidelines for IVC filter placement in trauma patients [9]. However, the multiplicity of groups and varying recommendations makes it confusing for many as to when and who should get IVC filters.

5. Exploring the Role of IVC Filters in Diverse Patient Populations with Acute PE

5.1. High-Risk and Intermediate-Risk PE

No randomized controlled trials have been conducted to assess the efficacy of thrombolytic therapy, pulmonary embolectomy, or IVC filters in patients experiencing high-risk PE, characterized by shock or the need for ventilator support. Among intermediate-risk PERT-assessed patients in the registry, 32% received catheter-directed therapies, and 7% had an IVC filter placed. For high-risk patients, 37% underwent catheter-directed therapies, 25% received tissue plasminogen activator, 12% had an IVC filter implanted, and 14% were placed on ECMO [10]. These findings derived from the PERT consortium guided the design of observational studies to address the indications of IVC filters in the management of acute PE. Important inclusion/exclusion criteria include the patient's hemodynamic status (stable or unstable) at the time of acute PE and whether advanced therapies (systemic thrombolysis, catheter-directed thrombolysis, endovascular suction embolectomy, surgical embolectomy, or ECMO) were used. Elderly patients and patients with recurrent PE are unique populations with separate indications for IVC filter placement. The subsequent discussion provides a review of the studies supporting the use of IVC filters in different patients with acute PE. Despite the absence of such trials, numerous investigations have explored these treatments based on retrospective cohort studies utilizing administrative data from large government and commercial databases.

5.1.1. Patients Receiving Thrombolytic Therapy

A variety of non-randomized analyses have suggested that IVC filters may improve mortality when used in intermediate- and high-risk PE patients receiving lytic therapy. To ascertain the role of IVC filters in acute PE management, Stein et al., using administrative data from large government and commercial databases, demonstrated that outcomes of thrombolytic therapy were significantly enhanced when IVC filters were incorporated. Specifically, IVC filters demonstrated a reduction in in-hospital all-cause mortality not only when used alongside anticoagulants alone (mortality IVC filter 32% vs. mortality no IVC filter 51%, $p < 0.0001$) or in pulmonary embolectomy (mortality IVC filter 24% vs. mortality no IVC filter 58%, $p < 0.0001$), but also in conjunction with thrombolytic therapy (mortality IVC filter 8% vs. mortality no IVC filter 18%, $p < 0.0001$) across all age groups in individuals with high-risk PE. The effectiveness of IVC filters in reducing mortality was particularly notable when inserted on the day of admission or the following day, during the period when the patient is most fragile. This suggests that the optimal treatment for patients with high-risk PE involves the combination of thrombolytic therapy and IVC filter insertion in the early stage when the patient is actively unstable. The authors conclude that this combined treatment approach is recommended for all high-risk PE patients, regardless of age [24]. In a single-center prospective study, Secemsky et al. evaluated outcomes in acute PE patients and noted that mortality was highest during the index hospitalization for high-risk PE patients, a risk that dissipated at the time of discharge. However, in the patients with intermediate-risk PE, the mortality risk persisted beyond the time of discharge [22]. Notably, advanced therapies, including IVC filters, were commonly used in this population and demonstrated an independent association with lower mortality (hazard ratio, 0.39, 95% CI, 0.20 to 0.76; $p < 0.01$), a finding consistent with other studies [22,25]. A subsequent analysis by Stein et al. reinforced the importance of early IVC filter insertion and demonstrated that in-hospital all-cause mortality appeared to be reduced with IVC filter placement (mortality IVC filter 19.4% vs. mortality no IVC filter 40.8%, $p < 0.0001$) only when the filter was inserted on the first (mortality IVC filter 21.4% vs. mortality no IVC filter 40.8%, $p = 0.017$) or second day of admission (mortality IVC filter 14.8% vs. mortality no IVC filter 29.2%, $p = 0.023$). This outcome benefit was independent of thrombolytic therapy administration [26]. Interestingly, a separate study demonstrated that advanced age should not be a limiting factor when considering an IVC filter in high-risk patients with PE [27]. Combining these more recent studies with the results of NIS database analyses from the early era makes for a convincing argument for IVC filter placement in high-risk and intermediate-risk PE patients.

5.1.2. Patients Receiving Pulmonary Embolectomy

The American College of Chest Physicians recommends surgical pulmonary embolectomy in cases where patients have contraindications to thrombolytic therapy, have experienced failed thrombolysis or catheter-assisted embolectomy, or are in a state of shock that is likely to lead to death before the effects of thrombolysis can take place, provided that surgical expertise and resources are available [28]. Notably, three retrospective cohort studies, spanning different time periods and utilizing various databases such as the Nationwide Inpatient Sample (NIS) (1999–2008) (mortality IVC filter 25% vs. mortality no IVC filter 58%, $p < 0.0001$), the Premier Healthcare Database (2010–2014) (mortality IVC filter 5.9% vs. mortality no IVC filter 44%, $p = 0.01$), and the NIS (2009–2014) (mortality IVC filter 18.1% vs. mortality no IVC filter 50.1%, $p < 0.0001$), demonstrated a lower mortality associated with the use of IVC filters in high-risk PE patients who underwent pulmonary embolectomy [29–31].

Stein et al. conducted a retrospective analysis using data from the 2010–2014 Premier Healthcare Database to evaluate the impact of IVC filters on mortality in patients with high-risk PE and those who underwent pulmonary embolectomy [30]. Their findings indicated that patients with high-risk PE who received an IVC filter exhibited lower in-hospital all-cause mortality (mortality IVC filter 23% vs. mortality no IVC filter 45%, $p < 0.0001$) and lower 3-month all-cause mortality (mortality IVC filter 25% vs. mortality no IVC filter 45%, $p < 0.0001$) compared to those without an IVC filter. This reduction in mortality was observed in patients receiving thrombolytic therapy, undergoing pulmonary embolectomy, and those receiving neither. Moreover, mortality attributable to PE at both in-hospital and 3-month intervals was also lower in patients who received an IVC filter in each subgroup [30].

5.1.3. Patients Receiving ECMO or Surgical Thrombectomy

Patients with high- and intermediate-risk PE may be excellent candidates for veno-arterial (VA)-ECMO and some potential indications for ECMO include patients with absolute contraindications to thrombolysis, persistent instability despite thrombolysis (lytic failure), and the stabilization of a patient prior to intubation. Future potential roles in the management of high- and intermediate-risk PE patients may include its role as a temporizing bridging therapy until anticoagulation efficacy, controlled thrombolysis, or definitive interventional therapy is performed [32]. Liu et al. performed a 2018–2021 single-center retrospective review of a prospectively maintained registry and included nine patients with high- and intermediate-risk PE who underwent VA-ECMO for initial hemodynamic stabilization, with or without percutaneous mechanical thrombectomy. Only two of the nine patients (22.2%) received IVC filters. They concluded that an ECMO-first strategy in these patients was safe and efficacious. Specifically, they consider VA-ECMO as a feasible option for initial stabilization, serving as a bridge to therapy, particularly in cases where surgery is not feasible for high-risk PE. To date, obtaining high-level evidence is challenging due to the rarity of situations requiring VA-ECMO in acute PE and the restricted availability of ECMO to specialized centers [33]. In recent years, surgical thrombectomy, once considered risky and generally ineffective, has experienced a resurgence. The current mortality rate for the procedure is approximately 10%, deemed acceptable in specific high-risk cases. Potential indications for surgical thrombectomy include high-risk PE in patients with absolute contraindications to thrombolysis or cases of thrombolytic failure. Currently, there is no high-level evidence comparing surgical thrombectomy to interventional radiology clot extraction but advances in catheter embolectomy, such as the Inari Flowtriever system, may offer superior outcomes in many cases, but further study is needed [34]. Informal discussions between many interventional radiology groups in the San Diego area, where utilization of these suction thrombectomy devices is increasingly being utilized, suggests improved patient hemodynamics, successful outcomes, and faster hospital discharges. However, the ideal patients who are the best candidates for such, more aggressive, therapies remain a topic of debate. While it is difficult to give a strong recommendation to place an IVC filter in patients on ECMO, case reports suggest placing one in high-risk PE patients with idiopathic hypercoagulability and residual thrombus despite thrombolytic therapy, regardless of the use of percutaneous mechanical thrombectomy. Implanting the IVC filter should be performed in tandem with ECMO decannulation to avoid potentially lethal complications [33,35].

5.2. Stable Acute PE

Stein et al. utilized the 2010–2014 Premier Healthcare Database to demonstrate that among stable patients with acute PE who underwent thrombolytic therapy, those who additionally received an IVC filter experienced lower in-hospital all-cause mortality (mortality IVC filter 5.2% vs. mortality no IVC filter 16.1%, $p < 0.0001$). This reduction in in-hospital mortality was observed across all age groups from 31 years and older for individuals who received an IVC filter in conjunction with thrombolytic therapy [36]. Results from the 2009–2014 NIS database showed similar benefits in stable acute PE patients who underwent pulmonary embolectomy and received IVC filters (mortality IVC filter 4.1% vs. mortality no IVC filter 27%, $p < 0.0001$), specifically if filters were inserted within the first 4 or 5 days following embolectomy [31]. The older literature derived from the 1999–2014 NIS database showed that there is no substantial evidence supporting a clinically meaningful reduction in mortality with IVC filters in stable patients, unless they are aged over 80 years [27]. Despite these positive outcomes, the studies highlighted a concerning trend; the proportion of unstable patients receiving IVC filters is decreasing, with the largest number of filters continuing to be inserted in stable patients with acute PE [26,37].

5.3. Elderly Patients with Acute PE

In an investigation focusing on elderly patients ($\geq$65 years old) with stable acute PE who did not receive thrombolytic therapy, a national cohort study of Medicare beneficiaries revealed that the use of IVC filters did not result in lower all-cause mortality at 30 days [38]. However, in a subsequent assessment by Stein et al., utilizing more recent data from the NIS, they concluded that in very elderly stable patients (aged >80 years) with a primary or secondary diagnosis of acute PE, with (mortality IVC filter 6.1% vs. mortality no IVC filter 10.5%, $p < 0.0001$) or without (mortality IVC filter 3.3% vs. mortality no IVC filter 6.3%, $p < 0.0001$) comorbid conditions, the use of IVC filters led to a reduction in mortality [27]. Furthermore, in another study by Stein et al., stable patients with PE and heart failure (HF) who were aged >80 years exhibited reduced in-hospital all-cause mortality (mortality IVC filter 4.1% vs. mortality no IVC filter 6.8%, $p = 0.0012$) when IVC filters were employed [39]. Another special population that may benefit from IVC filters in acute PE includes stable patients with PE and solid malignant tumors, specifically those older than 60 years. This subgroup demonstrated lower in-hospital all-cause mortality (mortality IVC filter 7.4% vs. mortality no IVC filter 11.2%, $p < 0.0001$) and lower 3-month mortality (mortality IVC filter 15.1% vs. mortality no IVC filter 17.4%, $p < 0.0001$) compared to those who did not receive an IVC filter [40].

5.4. Patients Experiencing Recurrent PE

In 2016, a cohort study involving patients from the Registro Informatizado de la Enfermedad Tromboembolica (RIETE registry) demonstrated a lower mortality (mortality IVC filter 2.1% vs. mortality no IVC filter 25.3%, $p = 0.02$) associated with the use of IVC filters in patients experiencing recurrent PE while on anticoagulant therapy [41]. Additionally, Stein et al. conducted a retrospective cohort study spanning six years, using administrative data from the Premier Healthcare Database. Their findings concluded that patients with PE who suffered a recurrent PE within the first three months after an index PE exhibited reduced mortality (mortality IVC filter 3.0% vs. mortality no IVC filter 39.3%, $p < 0.0001$) if they received an IVC filter at the time of recurrence. This reduction in mortality was observed in stable patients who did not receive thrombolytic therapy or undergo pulmonary embolectomy (mortality IVC filter 2.6% vs. mortality no IVC filter 42.6%, $p < 0.0001$). The study emphasized the importance of IVC filters in reducing mortality in stable patients with recurrent PE, underscoring the risk of death associated with early recurrences [42]. The high mortality rates reported in these studies suggest that patients with recurrent PE, despite therapeutic anticoagulation, are at the highest risk of mortality and IVC filters should be used in these cases.

6. Classic and Extended Indications for IVC Filters in Acute PE: Expert Panel Recommendations

Kaufman et al. conducted a systematic review and identified a total of 34 studies that provided the evidence base for the guidelines guiding IVC filter placement. The expert panel consisted of renowned experts across various medical, surgical, and interventional societies who agreed on the following recommendations with respect to acute PE [8,9]. However, they conclude that the efficacy of IVC filters in acute PE remains debatable, necessitating personalized assessments considering risks and benefits. Table 1 summarizes some of the recognized and potential advantages of IVC filter placement. Classic indications involve documented acute PE with absolute anticoagulation contraindications or a massive PE posing a risk of death despite anticoagulation. Despite the limited availability of robust evidence, the consensus among experts suggests that individuals facing acute PE along with contraindications to anticoagulation should generally be considered for IVC filter placement. Important factors influencing this decision encompass the patient's cardiopulmonary condition, hemodynamic response to PE, and the anticipated duration of contraindication to anticoagulation. In patients with massive PE, hemodynamic shock, and/or requiring ventilatory support, the panel deems that the potential benefits, including a likely reduction in in-hospital mortality from recurrent PE, justify the intervention in this specific and select patient population. The expert panel concluded that, in these cases, the benefits associated with IVC filter placement, including a reduction in short-term PE recurrence and potentially a decrease in mortality, outweigh the potential harms.

Table 1. Recognized and potential advantages of IVC filters.

Recognized Advantages of IVC Filters	Potential Advantages of IVC Filters
Prevent acute larger PE when the source of embolism originates in the venous system distal to the filter implantation site	Development of newer and safer IVC Filters may lead to more utilization with better outcomes
Classic Indications: A Role In: (1) Patients with documented acute PE possessing absolute contraindications to anticoagulation (2) Patients with high-risk PE considered to be at risk of death despite anticoagulation (3) Patients with VTE and a complication of anticoagulation	Extended Indications: A Role In: (1) Patients treated with thrombolysis or thrombectomy (2) Acute PE in individuals with limited cardiopulmonary reserve (3) Acute PE and undergoing ECMO (4) Acute PE in unstable conditions such as hemodynamic shock and requiring ventilatory support (5) Patients with acute PE and documented iliocaval DVT or large, free-floating proximal DVT
Role in recurrent PE despite therapeutic anticoagulation	Role in elderly patients with acute PE

Extended indications encompass cases treated with thrombolysis or thrombectomy and acute PE in individuals with limited cardiopulmonary reserve. In patients experiencing acute PE and undergoing advanced therapies, the expert panel issues a recommendation with limited strength for IVC filter placement, particularly in those with unstable conditions such as hemodynamic shock, requiring ventilatory support, and/or limited cardiopulmonary reserve. This recommendation is grounded in low-quality retrospective observational studies. The panel deems that the potential benefits, including a likely reduction in in-hospital mortality from recurrent PE, justify the intervention in this specific and select patient population. The panel also introduced the importance of making a distinction regarding IVC filter implantation in patients with acute PE regardless of advanced therapies and confirmed DVT to those whose imaging did not reveal the presence of thrombi in the proximal or distal veins. The panel deems those patients with acute PE and documented iliocaval DVT or large, free-floating proximal DVT as candidates for IVC filter placement satisfying extended indications.

7. Devising Novel IVC Filters and Retrieval Programs

Technological advance in the current era of PE care has not been limited to the treatment of PE in isolation. Currently, there are continuous efforts to improve IVC filter devices and design effective retrieval programs to improve outcomes in acute PE patients. These advances were built on Johnson et al.'s findings from the ongoing PRESERVE trial in which major IVC filter manufacturers are actively involved [14].

(A) Novel IVC Filter Advance

The PRESERVE trial showed low complications with currently available filters: strut perforation greater than 5 mm was demonstrated in 31 of 201 (15.4%) filters, of which only 3 (0.2%) were considered clinically significant, and filter-related perioperative adverse events occurred in 7 of 1421 (0.5%) patients. On follow-up, VTE (none of which were fatal) occurred in 93 patients (6.5%), including DVT (80 events in 74 patients [5.2%]), PE (23 events in 23 patients [1.6%]), and/or caval thrombotic occlusions (15 events in 15 patients [1.1%]), and no PE occurred in patients following prophylactic placement [14]. IVC filter advances involve enhanced comprehension of filter-associated complications and novel filter manufacturing. The development of convertible and bio-convertible filters like Sentry and VenaTech models eliminates the need for additional removal procedures and addresses potential complications associated with indwelling filters, providing temporary protection against PE before retraction of the filter arms and stent-like incorporation into its surrounding vasculature [43]. Clinical trials, such as the investigational device exemption multicenter trial with a convertible IVC filter, report favorable conversion rates and low adverse effects [44]. Additionally, the FDA-approved triple-lumen central venous catheter with a deployable IVC filter provides protection in critically ill patients and must be removed before discharge to avoid long-term complications [45]. As filter technology continues to develop, so will the determination of their indications, safety, and efficacy.

(B) Rigorous IVC Filter Retrieval Programs and Their Efficacy

The future direction of IVC filter utilization in managing PE emphasizes the importance of increasing retrieval rates and avoiding potential long-term complications. Timely retrieval of IVC filters is an important quality metric which multidisciplinary PERT aims to improve by reducing unnecessary filter use, streamlining outpatient follow-up, and expediting filter removal. The time window for safe retrieval varies by filter subtype. The FDA issued a safety communication in 2014 based on reports of adverse events associated with IVC filters and recommended that implanting physicians consider removing the filter as soon as blood clots are no longer a risk for the patient. After this report, many operators became more serious about IVC filter removals, and referrals for IVC filters declined from previous levels [7]. Johnson et al.'s findings from the PRESERVE trial affirm the safety of IVC filters in contemporary medical practice. IVC filters were removed from 632 of 640 (98.8%) patients who underwent attempted removal, 620 (96.8%) of which were removed at first attempt. Only one patient died during attempted filter retrieval [14]. Similarly, De Gregorio et al. conducted a study in the Spanish multicenter real-life registry (REFiVeC), reporting a 94.15% global retrieval rate after adjustment with no major complications [46]. Efforts at improving retrieval rates should focus on physician accountability, emphasizing that practitioners should only place IVC filters when strong indications exist and that they are also responsible for removing them when they are no longer indicated. This can be better accomplished with well-designed and enforced follow-up plans at the time of placement. Improved expertise in advanced retrieval techniques is also crucial, with an acceptable target retrieval success rate of 95%. Lastly, standardizing rigorous protocols to enhance the retrieval rates and provide high-quality care for patients can only succeed when a multidisciplinary team-based approach is followed.

8. Conclusions

The percutaneous image-guided insertion of an IVC filter represents a crucial therapeutic option in the management of specific patients with acute PE. However, the strength of recommendations in various clinical scenarios is limited by the lack of high-quality data, which is a persistent challenge in the field. The multiplicity of guidelines across various medical disciplines adds to confusion and uncertainty about appropriate use of IVC filters. While it is crucial to approach the inference of lower mortality with IVC filters cautiously, given the reliance on comparative effectiveness research using national observational data, the prospect of conducting an RCT in these specific subcategories of acute PE patients appears remote. The decision on whether patients are better served by the proactive insertion of an IVC filter based on retrospective cohort studies or by withholding IVC filters until an RCT can be conducted requires careful consideration.

Supplementary Materials: The following supporting information can be downloaded at: https://www.mdpi.com/article/10.3390/jcm13051494/s1, Table S1. IVC-Filter-Related Complications and Definitions; Figure S1. Radiographic Images of IVC-Filter-Related Complications.

Author Contributions: Conceptualization, S.A. and M.D.W.; methodology, S.A. and M.D.W.; software, G.M.; validation, S.A., M.D.W. and V.G.; formal analysis, G.M.; investigation, S.A.; resources, S.A.; data curation, S.A.; writing—original draft preparation, S.A.; writing—review and editing, S.A. and M.D.W.; visualization, G.M.; supervision, M.D.W. and V.G.; project administration, M.D.W.; funding acquisition, NA. All authors have read and agreed to the published version of the manuscript.

Funding: This research received no external funding.

Data Availability Statement: Not applicable.

Conflicts of Interest: There are no identifiable conflicts of interest to report. The authors have no financial or proprietary interest in the subject matter or materials discussed in the manuscript.

References

1. Bikdeli, B.; Chatterjee, S.; Desai, N.R.; Kirtane, A.J.; Desai, M.M.; Bracken, M.B.; Spencer, F.A.; Monreal, M.; Goldhaber, S.Z.; Krumholz, H.M. Inferior Vena Cava Filters to Prevent Pulmonary Embolism: Systematic Review and Meta-Analysis. *J. Am. Coll. Cardiol.* **2017**, *70*, 1587–1597. [CrossRef] [PubMed]
2. Raskob, G.E.; Angchaisuksiri, P.; Blanco, A.N.; Buller, H.; Gallus, A.; Hunt, B.J.; Hylek, E.M.; Kakkar, A.; Konstantinides, S.V.; Mccumber, M.; et al. Thrombosis: A major contributor to global disease burden. *Arterioscler. Thromb. Vasc. Biol.* **2014**, *34*, 2363–2371. [CrossRef] [PubMed]
3. Aujesky, D.; Obrosky, D.S.; Stone, R.A.; Auble, T.E.; Perrier, A.; Cornuz, J.; Roy, P.M.; Fine, M.J. A prediction rule to identify low-risk patients with pulmonary embolism. *Arch. Intern. Med.* **2006**, *166*, 169–175. [CrossRef] [PubMed]
4. Wood, K.E. Major pulmonary embolism: Review of a pathophysiologic approach to the golden hour of hemodynamically significant pulmonary embolism. *Chest* **2002**, *121*, 877–905. [CrossRef] [PubMed]
5. Balakrishna, M.A.; Reddi, V.; Belford, P.M.; Alvarez, M.; Jaber, W.A.; Zhao, D.X.; Vallabhajosyula, S. Intermediate-Risk Pulmonary Embolism: A Review of Contemporary Diagnosis, Risk Stratification and Management. *Medicina* **2022**, *58*, 1186. [CrossRef] [PubMed]
6. Tapson, V.F. Acute pulmonary embolism. *N. Engl. J. Med.* **2008**, *358*, 1037–1052. [CrossRef]
7. Muriel, A.; Jiménez, D.; Aujesky, D.; Bertoletti, L.; Decousus, H.; Laporte, S.; Mismetti, P.; Muñoz, F.J.; Yusen, R.; Monreal, M.; et al. Survival effects of inferior vena cava filter in patients with acute symptomatic venous thromboembolism and a significant bleeding risk. *J. Am. Coll. Cardiol.* **2014**, *63*, 1675–1683. [CrossRef]
8. Kaufman, J.A.; Barnes, G.D.; Chaer, R.A.; Cuschieri, J.; Eberhardt, R.T.; Johnson, M.S.; Kuo, W.T.; Murin, S.; Patel, S.; Rajasekhar, A.; et al. Society of Interventional Radiology Clinical Practice Guideline for Inferior Vena Cava Filters in the Treatment of Patients with Venous Thromboembolic Disease: Developed in collaboration with the American College of Cardiology, American College of Chest Physicians, American College of Surgeons Committee on Trauma, American Heart Association, Society for Vascular Surgery, and Society for Vascular Medicine. *J. Vasc. Interv. Radiol.* **2020**, *31*, 1529–1544.
9. DeYoung, E.; Minocha, J. Inferior Vena Cava Filters: Guidelines, Best Practice, and Expanding Indications. *Semin. Interv. Radiol.* **2016**, *33*, 65–70. [CrossRef]
10. Schultz, J.; Giordano, N.; Zheng, H.; Parry, B.A.; Barnes, G.D.; Heresi, G.A.; Jaber, W.; Wood, T.; Todoran, T.; Courtney, D.M.; et al. EXPRESS: A Multidisciplinary Pulmonary Embolism Response Team (PERT)—Experience from a national multicenter consortium. *Pulm Circ.* **2019**, *9*, 2045894018824563. [CrossRef]
11. Ortel, T.L.; Neumann, I.; Ageno, W.; Beyth, R.; Clark, N.P.; Cuker, A.; Hutten, B.A.; Jaff, M.R.; Manja, V.; Schulman, S.; et al. American Society of Hematology 2020 guidelines for management of venous thromboembolism: Treatment of deep vein thrombosis and pulmonary embolism. *Blood Adv.* **2020**, *4*, 4693–4738. [CrossRef]
12. Duffett, L.; Carrier, M. Inferior vena cava filters. *J. Thromb. Haemost.* **2017**, *15*, 3–12. [CrossRef]

13. Morales, J.P.; Li, X.; Irony, T.Z.; Ibrahim, N.G.; Moynahan, M.; Cavanaugh, K.J. Decision analysis of retrievable inferior vena cava filters in patients without pulmonary embolism. *J. Vasc. Surg. Venous Lymphat. Disord.* **2013**, *1*, 376–384. [CrossRef]
14. Johnson, M.S.; Spies, J.B.; Scott, K.T.; Kato, B.S.; Mu, X.; Rectenwald, J.E.; White, R.A.; Lewandowski, R.J.; Khaja, M.S.; Zuckerman, D.A.; et al. Predicting the Safety and Effectiveness of Inferior Vena Cava Filters (PRESERVE): Outcomes at 12 months. *J. Vasc. Surg. Venous Lymphat. Disord.* **2023**, *11*, 573–585. [CrossRef]
15. Goldhaber, S.Z.; Visani, L.; De Rosa, M. Acute pulmonary embolism: Clinical outcomes in the International Cooperative Pulmonary Embolism Registry (ICOPER). *Lancet* **1999**, *353*, 1386–1389. [CrossRef]
16. Pollack, C.V.; Schreiber, D.; Goldhaber, S.Z.; Slattery, D.; Fanikos, J.; O'Neil, B.J.; Thompson, J.R.; Hiestand, B.; Briese, B.A.; Pendleton, R.C.; et al. Clinical characteristics, management, and outcomes of patients diagnosed with acute pulmonary embolism in the emergency department: Initial report of EMPEROR (Multicenter Emergency Medicine Pulmonary Embolism in the Real World Registry). *J. Am. Coll. Cardiol.* **2011**, *57*, 700–706. [CrossRef]
17. Lin, B.W.; Schreiber, D.H.; Liu, G.; Briese, B.; Hiestand, B.; Slattery, D.; Kline, J.A.; Goldhaber, S.Z.; Pollack, C.V. Therapy and outcomes in massive pulmonary embolism from the Emergency Medicine Pulmonary Embolism in the Real World Registry. *Am. J. Emerg. Med.* **2012**, *30*, 1774–1781. [CrossRef] [PubMed]
18. Mismetti, P.; Laporte, S.; Pellerin, O.; Ennezat, P.V.; Couturaud, F.; Elias, A.; Falvo, N.; Meneveau, N.; Quere, I.; Roy, P.M.; et al. Effect of a retrievable inferior vena cava filter plus anticoagulation vs anticoagulation alone on risk of recurrent pulmonary embolism: A randomized clinical trial. *JAMA* **2015**, *313*, 1627–1635. [CrossRef]
19. Dawson, D.L. PRESERVE trial confirms low risk for most inferior vena cava filters, but benefit remains uncertain. *J. Vasc. Surg. Venous Lymphat. Disord.* **2023**, *11*, 586. [CrossRef] [PubMed]
20. Stein, P.D.; Kayali, F.; Olson, R.E. Twenty-one-year trends in the use of inferior vena cava filters. *Arch. Intern. Med.* **2004**, *164*, 1541–1545. [CrossRef] [PubMed]
21. Stein, P.D.; Matta, F.; Hughes, M.J. Usefulness of Inferior Vena Cava Filters in Stable Patients with Acute Pulmonary Embolism. *Am. J. Cardiol.* **2019**, *123*, 1874–1877. [CrossRef]
22. Secemsky, E.; Chang, Y.; Jain, C.C.; Beckman, J.A.; Giri, J.; Jaff, M.R.; Rosenfield, K.; Rosovsky, R.; Kabrhel, C.; Weinberg, I. Contemporary Management and Outcomes of Patients with Massive and Submassive Pulmonary Embolism. *Am. J. Med.* **2018**, *131*, 1506–1514. [CrossRef]
23. Kabrhel, C.; Rosovsky, R.; Channick, R.; Jaff, M.R.; Weinberg, I.; Sundt, T.; Dudzinski, D.M.; Rodriguez-Lopez, J.; Parry, B.A.; Harshbarger, S.; et al. A Multidisciplinary Pulmonary Embolism Response Team: Initial 30-Month Experience with a Novel Approach to Delivery of Care to Patients with Submassive and Massive Pulmonary Embolism. *Chest* **2016**, *150*, 384–393. [CrossRef] [PubMed]
24. Stein, P.D.; Dalen, J.E.; Matta, F.; Hughes, M.J. Optimal Therapy for Unstable Pulmonary Embolism. *Am. J. Med.* **2019**, *132*, 168–171. [CrossRef]
25. Kobayashi, T.; Pugliese, S.; Sethi, S.S.; Parikh, S.A.; Goldberg, J.; Alkhafan, F.; Vitarello, C.; Rosenfield, K.; Lookstein, R.; Keeling, B.; et al. Contemporary Management and Outcomes of Patients with High-Risk Pulmonary Embolism. *J. Am. Coll. Cardiol.* **2024**, *83*, 35–43. [CrossRef]
26. Stein, P.D.; Matta, F.; Lawrence, F.R.; Hughes, M.J. Importance of Early Insertion of Inferior Vena Cava Filters in Unstable Patients with Acute Pulmonary Embolism. *Am. J. Med.* **2018**, *131*, 1104–1109. [CrossRef]
27. Stein, P.D.; Matta, F.; Hughes, M.J. Inferior Vena Cava Filters in Elderly Patients with Stable Acute Pulmonary Embolism. *Am. J. Med.* **2017**, *130*, 356–364. [CrossRef] [PubMed]
28. Rousseau, H.; Del Giudice, C.; Sanchez, O.; Ferrari, E.; Sapoval, M.; Marek, P.; Delmas, C.; Zadro, C.; Revel-Mouroz, P. Endovascular therapies for pulmonary embolism. *Heliyon* **2021**, *7*, e06574. [CrossRef]
29. Stein, P.D.; Matta, F. Case fatality rate with pulmonary embolectomy for acute pulmonary embolism. *Am. J. Med.* **2012**, *125*, 471–477. [CrossRef]
30. Stein, P.D.; Matta, F.; Lawrence, F.R.; Hughes, M.J. Usefulness of Inferior Vena Cava Filters in Unstable Patients with Acute Pulmonary Embolism and Patients Who Underwent Pulmonary Embolectomy. *Am. J. Med.* **2018**, *121*, 495–500. [CrossRef]
31. Stein, P.D.; Matta, F.; Hughes, M.J. Effect on Mortality with Inferior Vena Cava Filters in Patients Undergoing Pulmonary Embolectomy. *Am. J. Med.* **2020**, *125*, 1276–1279. [CrossRef]
32. Davies, M.G.; Hart, J.P. Current status of ECMO for massive pulmonary embolism. *Front. Cardiovasc. Med.* **2023**, *10*, 1298686. [CrossRef]
33. Liu, Z.; Chen, J.; Xu, X.; Lan, F.; He, M.; Shao, C.; Xu, Y.; Han, P.; Chen, Y.; Zhu, Y.; et al. Extracorporeal Membrane Oxygenation-First Strategy for Acute Life-Threatening Pulmonary Embolism. *Front. Cardiovasc. Med.* **2022**, *9*, 875021. [CrossRef]
34. Farkas, J. Internet Book of Critical Care (IBCC). Available online: https://emcrit.org/ibcc/pe/#surgical_thrombectomy (accessed on 12 December 2023).
35. Sherk, W.M.; Khaja, M.S.; Jo, A.; Marko, X.; Williams, D.M. Bedside intravascular ultrasound-guided fibrin sheath balloon maceration and inferior vena cava filter placement during extracorporeal membranous oxygenation decannulation. *J. Vasc. Surg. Cases Innov. Tech.* **2020**, *6*, 56–58. [CrossRef]
36. Stein, P.D.; Matta, F.; Hughes, M.J. Inferior Vena Cava Filters in Stable Patients with Acute Pulmonary Embolism Who Receive Thrombolytic Therapy. *Am. J. Med.* **2018**, *131*, 97–99. [CrossRef]

37. Stein, P.D.; Matta, F.; Hughes, M.J. Effectiveness of Inferior Vena Cava Filters in Patients with Stable and Unstable Pulmonary Embolism and Trends in Their Use. *Am. J. Med.* **2020**, *133*, 323–330. [CrossRef]
38. Bikdeli, B.; Wang, Y.; Minges, K.E.; Desai, N.R.; Kim, N.; Desai, M.M.; Spertus, J.A.; Masoudi, F.A.; Nallamothu, B.K.; Goldhaber, S.Z.; et al. Vena Caval Filter Utilization and Outcomes in Pulmonary Embolism: Medicare Hospitalizations from 1999 to 2010. *J. Am. Coll. Cardiol.* **2016**, *67*, 1027–1035. [CrossRef]
39. Stein, P.D.; Matta, F.; Hughes, M.J. Inferior Vena Cava Filters in Stable Patients with Pulmonary Embolism and Heart Failure. *Am. J. Cardiol.* **2019**, *124*, 292–295. [CrossRef]
40. Stein, P.D.; Matta, F.; Lawrence, F.R.; Hughes, M.J. Inferior Vena Cava Filters in Patients with Acute Pulmonary Embolism and Cancer. *Am. J. Med.* **2018**, *131*, 442.e9–442.e12. [CrossRef]
41. Mellado, M.; Pijoan, J.I.; Jiménez, D.; Muriel, A.; Aujesky, D.; Bertoletti, L.; Decousus, H.; Barrios, D.; Clará, A.; Yusen, R.D.; et al. Outcomes Associated with Inferior Vena Cava Filters Among Patients with Thromboembolic Recurrence during Anticoagulant Therapy. *JACC Cardiovasc. Interv.* **2016**, *9*, 2440–2448. [CrossRef]
42. Stein, P.D.; Matta, F.; Lawrence, F.R.; Hughes, M.J. Inferior Vena Cava Filters in Patients with Recurrent Pulmonary Embolism. *Am. J. Med.* **2019**, *132*, 88–92. [CrossRef] [PubMed]
43. Bajda, J.; Park, A.N.; Raj, A.; Raj, R.; Gorantla, V.R. Inferior Vena Cava Filters and Complications: A Systematic Review. *Cureus* **2023**, *15*, e40038. [CrossRef] [PubMed]
44. Hohenwalter, E.J.; Stone, J.R.; O'Moore, P.V.; Smith, S.J.; Selby, J.B.; Lewandowski, R.J.; Samuels, S.; Kiproff, P.M.; Trost, D.W.; Madoff, D.C.; et al. Multicenter Trial of the VenaTech Convertible Vena Cava Filter. *J. Vasc. Interv. Radiol.* **2017**, *28*, 1353–1362. [CrossRef] [PubMed]
45. Covello, B.; Radvany, M. Back to the Basics: Inferior Vena Cava Filters. *Semin. Interv. Radiol.* **2022**, *39*, 226–233. [CrossRef]
46. De Gregorio, M.A.; Guirola, J.A.; Urbano, J.; Díaz-Lorenzo, I.; Muñoz, J.J.; Villacastin, E.; Lopez-Medina, A.; Figueredo, A.L.; Guerrero, J.; Sierre, S.; et al. Spanish multicenter real—Life registry of retrievable vena cava filters (REFiVeC). *CVIR Endovasc.* **2020**, *3*, 26. [CrossRef]

Disclaimer/Publisher's Note: The statements, opinions and data contained in all publications are solely those of the individual author(s) and contributor(s) and not of MDPI and/or the editor(s). MDPI and/or the editor(s) disclaim responsibility for any injury to people or property resulting from any ideas, methods, instructions or products referred to in the content.

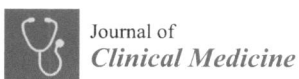

Review

Sequelae of Acute Pulmonary Embolism: From Post-Pulmonary Embolism Functional Impairment to Chronic Thromboembolic Disease

John H. Fountain [1,2], Tyler J. Peck [1,2,*,†] and David Furfaro [1,2,†]

1. Division of Pulmonary, Critical Care and Sleep Medicine, Beth Israel Deaconess Medical Center, Boston, MA 02215, USA; jfounta2@bidmc.harvard.edu (J.H.F.); dfurfaro@bidmc.harvard.edu (D.F.)
2. Harvard Medical School, Boston, MA 02115, USA
* Correspondence: tpeck2@bidmc.harvard.edu
† These authors contributed equally to this work.

Abstract: Among survivors of acute pulmonary embolism (PE), roughly half report persistent dyspnea, impaired functional status, and decreased quality of life. Post-pulmonary embolism syndrome (PPES) is a broad condition which has been increasingly recognized in recent years and may be due to post-pulmonary embolism functional impairment, chronic thromboembolic disease, or the most severe long-term complication of PE, chronic thromboembolic pulmonary hypertension. Despite guideline recommendations for appropriate follow-up for post-pulmonary embolism patients, PPES remains underrecognized and diagnostic testing underutilized. Patients with symptoms suggestive of PPES at follow-up should undergo a transthoracic echocardiogram to screen for the presence of pulmonary hypertension; additional testing, such as a ventilation/perfusion scan, right heart catheterization, and cardiopulmonary exercise testing may be indicated. The pathophysiology of post-pulmonary embolism syndrome is complex and heterogeneous. In chronic thromboembolic pulmonary hypertension, the pathophysiology reflects persistent pulmonary arterial thrombi and a progressive small vessel vasculopathy. In patients with chronic thromboembolic disease or chronic thromboembolic pulmonary hypertension, medical therapy, balloon pulmonary angioplasty, or pulmonary thromboendarterectomy should be considered, and in cases of chronic thromboembolic pulmonary hypertension, pulmonary thromboendarterectomy significantly improves mortality. In all causes of post-pulmonary embolism syndrome, rehabilitation is a safe treatment option that may improve quality of life.

Keywords: pulmonary embolism; pulmonary hypertension; CTED; CTEPH; post-pulmonary embolism syndrome; quality of life

Citation: Fountain, J.H.; Peck, T.J.; Furfaro, D. Sequelae of Acute Pulmonary Embolism: From Post-Pulmonary Embolism Functional Impairment to Chronic Thromboembolic Disease. *J. Clin. Med.* **2024**, *13*, 6510. https://doi.org/10.3390/jcm13216510

Academic Editor: Raimondo De Cristofaro

Received: 1 September 2024
Revised: 25 October 2024
Accepted: 28 October 2024
Published: 30 October 2024

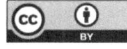

Copyright: © 2024 by the authors. Licensee MDPI, Basel, Switzerland. This article is an open access article distributed under the terms and conditions of the Creative Commons Attribution (CC BY) license (https://creativecommons.org/licenses/by/4.0/).

1. Introduction

Post-pulmonary embolism syndrome (PPES) is a broad and heterogeneous condition that has been increasingly recognized after acute pulmonary embolism (PE). Despite advances in the detection and management of acute PE, roughly half of patients report dyspnea, exercise intolerance, impaired functional status, or decreased quality of life at follow-up [1–4]. While complications of PE, such as recurrent venous thromboembolism (VTE) and anticoagulant-related bleeding, have been well-described, PPES remains underrecognized and undertreated.

2. Definition and Epidemiology

PPES is heterogeneous and is described as one of the following syndromes despite at least three months of anticoagulation after acute PE: post-PE functional impairment, chronic thromboembolic pulmonary disease (CTED), or chronic thromboembolic pulmonary hypertension (CTEPH) (Table 1) [1]. Post-PE functional impairment—defined as the presence of dyspnea, impaired exercise tolerance, or diminished functional status without an identified non-PE explanation, CTED, or CTEPH—represents the most common form of PPES.

Table 1. Definition, epidemiology, and diagnosis of the spectrum of post-pulmonary embolism syndrome (PPES).

Syndrome	Definition *	Epidemiology	Diagnostic Testing for Detection
Post-pulmonary embolism (PE) functional impairment	Dyspnea, impaired exercise tolerance, or diminished functional status after acute PE without an identified non-PE explanation, CTED, or CTEPH	Poorly reported, up to 56% of patients after acute PE have PPES [5]	6MWD, QoL questionnaire, CPET and rule out CTED or CTEPH
Chronic thromboembolic disease (CTED)	Persistent pulmonary vascular obstruction and functional limitation or symptoms without the presence of resting pulmonary hypertension	29–38% [6,7] of patients have residual perfusion defects after acute PE	Confirm persistent vascular obstruction: V/Q scan, CTPA, pulmonary angiography and rule out CTEPH with TTE and RHC
Chronic thromboembolic pulmonary hypertension (CTEPH)	Persistent pulmonary vascular obstruction and the presence of pre-capillary pulmonary hypertension on right heart catheterization	0.56% in all comers after PE [8]	Confirm persistent vascular obstruction: V/Q scan, CTPA, pulmonary angiography and RHC with mPA $\geq$ 20 mmHg, PCWP $\leq$ 15 mmHg and PVR $\geq$ 2 woods units [9]

* All diagnoses can only be made after 3 months of effective anticoagulation following acute PE. PPES = post-pulmonary embolism syndrome; PE = pulmonary embolism; CTED = chronic thromboembolic disease; CTEPH = chronic thromboembolic pulmonary hypertension; CPET = cardiopulmonary exercise test; V/Q = ventilation/perfusion; CTPA = computed tomography pulmonary angiogram; TTE = transthoracic echocardiogram; RHC = right heart catheterization; mPA = mean pulmonary artery pressure; PCWP = pulmonary capillary wedge pressure; PVR = pulmonary vascular resistance identified non-PE explanation; CTED or CTEPH—represents the most common form of PPES. Among patients with persistent pulmonary vascular obstruction on imaging, there are two groups of patients: those without pulmonary hypertension at rest but with functional limitation, who are described as having CTED, and those who meet criteria for CTEPH with pulmonary hypertension at rest (mean pulmonary arterial [PA] pressure $\geq$ 20 mmHg with pulmonary capillary wedge pressure $\leq$ 15 mmHg and pulmonary vascular resistance [PVR] $\geq$ 2 woods units [9]). CTEPH is the most severe long-term complication of PE.

The symptoms of PPES are non-specific and thus it remains under-recognized and diagnostic testing is under-utilized. In a retrospective cohort study of 21,297 patients with their first PE, PPES was present in 56.2% of patients at follow-up; however, only 42.8% of these patients had an appropriate diagnostic testing ordered [5]. While the high incidence of PPES after PE is replicated in multiple patient cohorts, the risk factors have not been fully elucidated and vary across the spectrum of PPES [1,3,4,10–12]. Cardiopulmonary comorbidities, age, higher BMI, and smoking are predictive of post-PE functional impairment [2]. Several risk factors for the development of CTEPH have been identified, which include prior VTE, malignancy, the presence of antiphospholipid antibodies, history of splenectomy, chronic inflammatory disease, ventriculoatrial shunts, and hypothyroidism [8,13,14].

While there has been great interest in therapies for acute PE to prevent decompensation and mortality, these treatments have yet to demonstrate prevention of PPES or CTEPH. Among 109 previously healthy patients with submassive PE treated with anticoagulation alone, the cornerstone of PE therapy, 41% had abnormal cardiopulmonary function at a 6 month follow up, characterized by an abnormal right ventricular size and/or function, an impaired 6-min walk distance, and/or a NYHA functional class > II [4]. Notably, in a long-term follow up of the PEITHO trial—which evaluated fibrinolysis for intermediate-risk PE—there was no difference in the proportion of patients who had CTEPH or post-PE impairment between the anticoagulation and tenecteplase treatment arms [15]. Further, to date, there is no evidence that mechanical thrombectomy or catheter-directed therapies reduce the risk of PPES.

Importantly, reported symptoms of PPES correlate well with objective findings of exercise performance. The ELOPE study evaluated patients after their first PE and performed quality of life (QoL) questionnaires, a 6-min walk test (6MWT), and a cardiopulmonary exercise test (CPET) at 1 and 12 months, as well as a ventilation/perfusion (V/Q) scan and computed tomography pulmonary angiography (CT-PA) at 6 and 12 months. Patients with a VO2 peak < 80% predicted had worse generic and PE-specific QoL scores, dyspnea scores, and 6-min walk distances (6MWD) [3]. While these relationships are well replicated, the significance of other findings, such as residual pulmonary vascular obstruction, remains less clear. In the ELOPE study, the mean obstruction index on CT-PA was similar between patients with reduced and normal VO2 peaks, suggesting that both initial and residual obstruction does not directly correlate to symptoms after PE [3]. In contrast, other studies have found that thrombus resolution is associated with improved NYHA functional class and thus the presence of residual obstruction may represent a risk factor for PPES [11].

The timely diagnosis of PPES is crucial, particularly to identify patients with CTEPH given its mortality if left untreated and the multiple available treatment modalities, including curative surgical options. The incidence of CTEPH has been estimated from 0.79–3.8% after PE, and a recent meta-analysis estimates its incidence to be 3.2% in survivors of PE and 0.56% in all-comers after PE [8,12,13,16–18]. Further making the diagnosis of PPES more challenging, up to 25% of patients with CTEPH have no known history of PE [19].

3. Pathophysiology

3.1. Post-PE Functional Impairment

Of the etiologies of PPES, post-PE functional impairment remains the least well understood. It is hypothesized to be due to deconditioning secondary to dyspnea from PE, persistent chest pain, or fear of complications or recurrence of PE [1]. Many survivors of PE report mental health conditions that contribute to functional impairment including depression, anxiety, and post-traumatic stress [20,21]. It remains a diagnosis of exclusion in symptomatic patients who have been confirmed not to have CTED or CTEPH. Further data, such as tissue pathology from biopsy or autopsy, may help elucidate its etiology.

3.2. CTED and CTEPH

Patients with CTED and CTEPH demonstrate residual obstruction in the pulmonary vasculature, though the fact that only some patients develop pulmonary hypertension indicates a complex physiologic pathway beyond just organization of chronic thrombus (Figure 1). Patients with PE are well known to be at high risk of recurrent VTE, with 10.1% of patients having recurrent VTE at 6 months and 40% at 10 years [22]. Further, patients with CTEPH demonstrate increased platelet activation and have higher rates of lupus anticoagulant, antiphospholipid antibodies, and factor V Leiden compared to patients with non-CTEPH pulmonary hypertension [23,24]. Additionally, fibrin resistance to plasmin-mediated lysis has been observed in CTEPH patients, suggesting a role of impaired fibrinolysis in the development of persistent luminal abnormalities following PE in this population [25]. As such, thorough evaluations for hypercoagulable disorders and recurrent VTE are essential in the evaluation of CTED and CTEPH.

Invasive hemodynamic and imaging studies have shown that >25% of the cumulative pulmonary arterial lumen must be obstructed in acute PE prior to the PA pressure rising, which suggests that vascular changes occur in areas beyond those with unresolved thrombus [2]. Histopathology from surgical specimens after PTE provide insight into these progressive vascular changes, and demonstrate small vessel arteriopathy [26], with findings historically characteristic of pulmonary arterial hypertension (PAH): plexogenic lesions, smooth muscle hypertrophy, and intimal proliferation and fibrosis [26,27]. Notably, these changes can be seen both in vessels distal to PE and those free of thrombus, and, compared to patients with PAH, they generally occur in larger caliber vessels in CTEPH and are more heterogeneous [27]. The presence of arteriopathy distal to obstructed vessels may be due to the development of bronchial-to-pulmonary vascular anastomoses, pulmonary arterial remodeling, and abnormal vascular reactivity with related endothelial cell dysfunction [24,27]. The cause of remodeling in non-obstructed vessels is not fully understood but may be related to high flow rates and higher-pressure circulation in these areas [28].

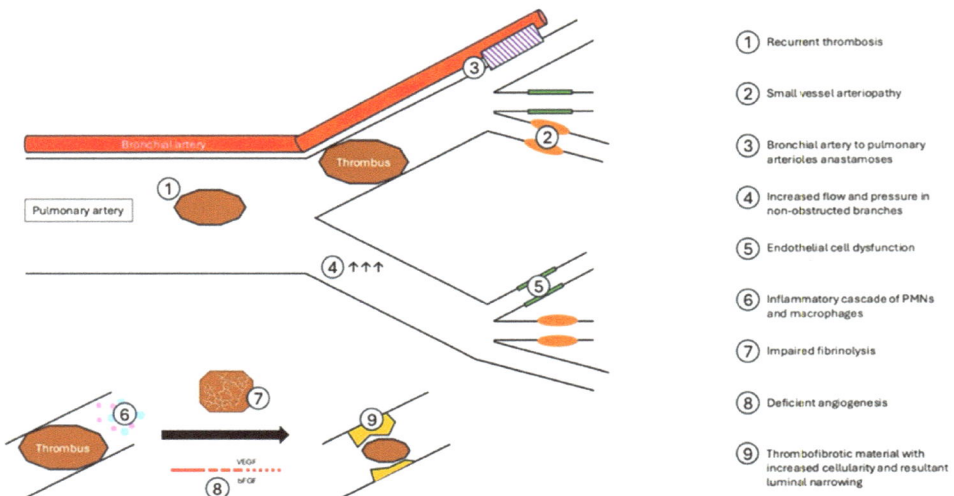

Figure 1. Pathophysiology of CTEPH.

After acute PE, there is a rapid inflammatory response consisting of inflammatory cells, cytokines, and chemokines [29]. In a rat model of PE, there was a significant increase in neutrophil and macrophage concentration within the vasa vasorum at 1 and 2 days after PE with increased intimal wall thickness at 4 days and increased cellularity through 14 days [29]. Impairments within the usual process of organization and degradation of thrombus, recanalization and remodeling of the vascular wall may lead to excessive remodeling [24]. Resultant CTEPH may also be secondary to deficient angiogenesis, in which abnormalities in neovascularization, mediated by vascular endothelial growth factor (VEGF) and basic fibroblast growth factor (bFGF), lead to impaired penetration of an occlusive thrombus and impaired recanalization [24].

4. Detection and Imaging Findings

The timely identification of PPES is paramount, particularly to identify CTEPH. Despite increases in the awareness of PPES, and particularly CTEPH, the median time from the development of symptoms to diagnosis was 14.1 months in a registry of 679 patients with CTEPH [19]. As a result, guidelines for the diagnosis and management of acute PE recommend transthoracic echocardiogram (TTE) at 3–6 months after PE if dyspnea or functional limitation persist despite anticoagulation [30]. Acknowledging the practical limitations of obtaining TTE in some settings, the InShape II trial evaluated an algorithm utilizing clinical characteristics, electrocardiogram, and biomarkers to identify patients who were unlikely to have CTEPH, and thus did not warrant TTE. Of 424 patients with acute PE, 81 (19%) were referred to TTE based on their algorithm, and only 1 out of 343 (0.29%) patients who were deemed low risk was subsequently found to have CTEPH [31]. This may represent a viable option for screening in resource-limited settings.

Patients with intermediate- or high-probability of pulmonary hypertension on TTE should undergo further diagnostic evaluation for persistent vascular obstruction in order to diagnose or exonerate CTEPH. V/Q scan is the first line imaging modality for diagnosing CTED and has a sensitivity of 96–97% and specificity of 90–95% [30]. While CT-PA remains an excellent test for the diagnosis of acute PE, it is not recommended in isolation for evaluation of CTEPH; among a cohort of patients with CTEPH who underwent both a V/Q scan and a CT-PA, the sensitivity of the V/Q scan was 98.9% compared to 65.9% for the CT-PA [32]. Nonetheless, imaging findings on the CT-PAs that are suggestive of CTEPH are helpful when present, and include the presence of persistent thrombus, eccentric wall-adherent thrombus, pulmonary arterial webs, abrupt tapering of the pulmonary arteries, bronchial artery collaterals, and a widening of the main pulmonary artery [33]. Other imaging modalities, such as single-photon emission computed tomography (SPECT) [34], dual-energy CT, and magnetic resonance (MR) pulmonary angiography, can also demonstrate perfusion defects and may play a role in CTEPH diagnosis in the future, especially given the increased resolution that these studies provide [35].

Cardiopulmonary exercise testing (CPET) remains a useful diagnostic tool for those with dyspnea after PE and may be diagnostic or highly suggestive of CTED or CTEPH based on characteristic physiologic abnormalities. Patients with post-PE functional impairment without CTED/CTEPH generally have a reduction in peak VO2, which supports deconditioning as its cause. In patients with CTED and CTEPH, however, CPET demonstrates an increase in ventilatory dead space proportion (VD/VT), which corresponds to areas of impaired perfusion due to persistent thrombus [36]. Held et al. evaluated the use of a 4- and 6-score parameter test using CPET in patients with CTEPH that had normal or unmeasurable right ventricular systolic pressure on a TTE [37]. Their 4-score parameter testing evaluated increases in the alveolar–arterial oxygen gradient, minute ventilation to carbon dioxide production (VE/VCO$_2$) slope, capillary to end-tidal carbon dioxide gradient (P[c-ET]CO$_2$), and end-tidal partial pressure of CO$_2$ at anaerobic threshold (PETCO$_2$ at AT), and was 83.3% sensitive and 92.2% specific for CTEPH [37].

Ultimately, right heart catheterization (RHC) is the gold standard for diagnosis of pulmonary hypertension and is required to definitively diagnose CTEPH. CTEPH is confirmed when patients have persistent perfusion abnormalities after effective anticoagulation and the presence of pre-capillary pulmonary hypertension on RHC. Pre-capillary pulmonary hypertension is defined as PA pressure $\geq$ 20 mmHg with pulmonary capillary wedge pressure $\leq$ 15 mmHg and PVR $\geq$ 2 woods units [9]. Concomitant pulmonary angiography is helpful to confirm vascular obstruction and determine whether patients are a candidate for surgical or interventional management. All patients with confirmed CTEPH should be tested for anti-phospholipid syndrome, and hypercoagulability work up in patients with PPES should otherwise be considered based on patient risk factors, clotting history, and family history.

5. Management

Guidelines recommend the referral of CTEPH patients to a CTEPH expert center once diagnosed for consideration of surgical/interventional treatment options, medical therapy, and multimodal therapy [9,38,39].

5.1. Anticoagulation

The backbone of therapy for patients with CTEPH is indefinite anticoagulation (Table 2). For patients with post-PE functional impairment and CTED without PH, the duration of anticoagulation should be determined based on guideline recommendations following acute PE and patient-level decision making; the nuances of anticoagulant choice and duration after PE are beyond the scope of this review [30,40,41]. For patients with CTEPH, vitamin K antagonists (i.e., warfarin) are the preferred anticoagulants based on retrospective data, suggesting that patients on direct oral anticoagulants have increased rates of recurrent VTE with similar bleeding rates [42,43]. As patients with prior VTE are at risk of recurrent thrombosis, they should be monitored for the presence of new thrombotic events at follow up.

Table 2. Treatments for post-pulmonary embolism syndrome (PPES).

Syndrome	Treatment
Post-pulmonary embolism (PE) functional impairment	Anticoagulation • Duration and agent per guidelines following acute PE and patient risk factors Pulmonary rehabilitation Treatment for concomitant mental health conditions common after PE (depression, anxiety, PTSD)
Chronic thromboembolic disease (CTED)	Anticoagulation • Duration and agent per guidelines following acute PE and patient risk factors • Consider longer duration or lifelong in presence of significant persistent perfusion defects Pulmonary rehabilitation Consider PTE • Small studies of use in patients with CTED Further studies needed
Chronic thromboembolic pulmonary hypertension (CTEPH)	Indefinite anticoagulation • Vitamin K antagonists preferred over DOACs Pulmonary rehabilitation PTE • Multidisciplinary discussion of candidacy for all patients • Gold standard treatment for patients with surgically amenable disease and appropriate risk/benefit profile BPA • For patients with inoperable CTEPH • For patients with persistent or recurrent CTEPH after PTE Pulmonary vasodilators • Riociguat • ERAs • Subcutaneous Treprostinil • Off-label use of other class of pulmonary vasodilators (PDE5i, prostacyclin analogs) • Consider combination therapy

PE = pulmonary embolism; PTSD = post-traumatic stress disorder; CTED = chronic thromboembolic disease; PTE = pulmonary thromboendarterectomy; DOAC = direct oral anticoagulant; CTEPH = chronic thromboembolic pulmonary hypertension; BPA = balloon pulmonary angioplasty; ERA = endothelin receptor antagonist; PDE5i = phosphodiesterase type 5 inhibitor.

5.2. Pulmonary Thromboendarterectomy

Pulmonary thromboendarterectomy (PTE) has become a well-established procedure that is performed on patients with CTED and CTEPH. The technique of PTE is well described in the literature and a few key points warrant mentioning. An effective PTE is by definition bilateral, and thus requires a midline sternotomy. A cardiopulmonary bypass and a brief circulatory arrest are necessary in contributing to the risk profile of the procedure. An endarterectomy is performed by dissection into the pulmonary vasculature as well as a removal of pathologically remodeled tissue in addition to organized thrombus; this is performed on the subsegmental branches [44,45].

All patients with CTEPH should have multidisciplinary evaluation for PTE, as it represents a potentially curative treatment. Surgical candidacy depends on the anatomy of the disease (proximal vs. distal), the severity of the pulmonary hypertension, the risk profile of the patient, and the experience level of the treating center [9,45]. Left untreated, CTEPH leads to progressive RV failure and death, and in one cohort, the untreated mortality at 3 years was 90% in patients with a mean PA pressure of >30 mm Hg [46]. To that end, multiple studies have evaluated the efficacy and safety of PTE for CTEPH. In a Canadian study of 401 patients who underwent PTE, the 30-day mortality was 2.8% and the 5-year survival rate was 80–91% depending on disease type [47]. These patients demonstrated a significant improvement in 6MWD, right ventricular systolic pressure, and PVR, and a significant reduction in NYHA functional class. Patients with severe pulmonary hypertension (based on PVR >1000 dynes/s/cm^{-5}) had a higher need for ECMO, and a longer duration of intubation, ICU, and hospital stay but had a similar 30-day mortality rate to patients with PVR < 1000 dynes/s/cm^{-5} and a 10-year survival of 84% [48]. Among >1500 patients treated at University of California San Diego, in-hospital mortality decreased temporally and with increased experience from 5.5% to 2.2%, and cumulative survival at 5 years was 92% [45]. Notably, this cohort included a large proportion of patients with distal disease indicating that with appropriate experience even distal chronic perfusion defects can be treated effectively and definitively with PTE [45]. Beyond survival, both echocardiographic and CPET parameters show improvement after PTE; sustained improvements in RV size, right ventricular systolic pressure, and TR at 1-year post-surgery [49] and improvements in peak VO2 and reduction in VE/VCO$_2$ slope over the first year after PTE [50] have been demonstrated.

Historically, PTE was indicated only for patients with CTEPH; however, recent data has supported its use in patients with CTED. A 2014 study performed PTE in patients with CTED with a concomitant IVC filter placement and demonstrated a reduction in mean PA pressure from 21 to 18 mm Hg, an increase in 6MWD from 372 to 421m, a reduction in PVR from 164 to 128 dynes/s/cm^{-5}, and an improvement in NYHA functional class [51]. All patients were alive at hospital discharge, though two died after discharge, resulting in a mortality of 5%. A 2018 study of 23 patients showed similar results and survival characteristics [52]. Of note, given the changes in the ERS/ESC diagnostic criteria for pulmonary hypertension, was that many of the patients in these studies would meet the criteria for CTEPH by the updated definition, so the utility of PTE in CTED requires further investigation.

5.3. Balloon Pulmonary Angioplasty

Balloon pulmonary angioplasty (BPA) is a treatment option for patients with inoperable CTEPH or persistent or recurrent pulmonary hypertension after PTE, and there have been multiple studies evaluating its safety and efficacy. BPA is performed endovascularly, primarily in the catheterization laboratory, with advancement of a catheter to chronic thromboembolic lesions and inflation of a balloon causing disruption to intimal caps, the dilation of fibrotic luminal obstructions, the compression of organized thrombotic material, and the stretching of the pulmonary vessels [53,54]. In a Japanese cohort of 308 patients, the average 6MWD increased from 318 to 429.7m with an improvement in the b-type natriuretic peptide (BNP) from 239.5 to 38.7 pg/mL, PVR from 853.7 to 288.1 dynes/s/cm^{-5}, and mean PA pressure from 43.2 to 22.5 mm Hg [55]. Average NYHA functional class improved from III to II. Mortality was 3.9% at follow up, with eight patients (2.6%) dying within 30 days of BPA. French [56], German [57], and American [58] registries demonstrate similar improvements in hemodynamics and 6MWD after BPA as well as low mortality in the peri-procedural period (2.2%, 1.8%, and 1.3%, respectively) with patients undergoing an average of 5.4, 4.8, and 2.7 sessions, respectively.

As clinicians may offer procedural therapy and/or medical therapy to patients with CTEPH, trials have sought to elucidate their efficacy and safety in head-to-head trials. Recently, the RACE trial evaluated 105 patients randomized to riociguat, an oral medication that both sensitizes soluble guanylate cyclase to nitric oxide and acts as a soluble guanylate cyclase agonist causing vasodilation of the pulmonary vasculature, or BPA. In patients who underwent BPA, there was an average reduction in PVR of 458.4 dynes/s/cm^{-5} compared to 200.8 in patients treated with riociguat [59]. There was no difference in 6MWD between the two groups; however, there were improvements in the borg dyspnea scale, WHO-FC, NT-proBNP, and mean PA pressure in patients who underwent BPA compared to treatment with riociguat [59]. Similar findings were noted in the MR BPA trial, which randomized patients to treatment with riociguat or BPA and demonstrated reduction in the mean PA pressure of 16.3 mm Hg in the BPA group and 9.3 mm Hg in the riociguat group at 12 months [60]. However, especially considering the frequent need for multiple sessions, the procedural risk of BPA warrants careful consideration. The most common complications across both cohorts were lung injury and hemoptysis [59,60], and unsurprisingly, an increase in BPA experience reduced the complication rate [56].

Given these, and other similar results, BPA is increasingly utilized for CTEPH, while acknowledging that PTE is the gold standard to pursue if feasible. The current ESC/ERS guidelines for the management of pulmonary hypertension recommend BPA as a class I indication for patients with residual PH after PTE or who are technically inoperable, with weaker recommendations to consider BPA for patients based on surgical risk profile alone [9].

5.4. Medical Therapy

Medical therapy remains a well-tolerated option for patients with CTEPH and has been evaluated in patients with residual pulmonary hypertension after PTE or BPA as well as in those with inoperable disease. The most well-studied medication for CTEPH is riociguat. In the CHEST-1 study and its subsequent follow up, CHEST-2, riociguat was shown to reduce PVR and increase 6MWD compared to a placebo, with similar rates of adverse events between the two groups [61,62].

Endothelin receptor antagonists have also been evaluated in CTEPH. The MERIT-1 trial demonstrated a reduction in PVR and increase in 6MWD with the use of macitentan compared to a placebo [63], while the BENEFIT trial demonstrated a reduction in PVR and an increase in 6MWD with the use of bosentan compared to a placebo [64].

For patients with severe disease and functional impairment, subcutaneous treprostinil has been studied in a randomized controlled trial of 105 patients and demonstrated improvement in 6MWD [65]. While other medical therapies for pulmonary hypertension are not specifically approved for CTEPH, such as phosphodiesterase type 5 inhibitors and other forms of prostacyclin analogs, registry data demonstrates that they are frequently used for monotherapy or combination therapy at the discretion of specialists [66,67].

5.5. Rehabilitation

Rehabilitation is a safe and low risk treatment option for all causes of PPES. Several studies have demonstrated the safety of rehabilitation after venous thromboembolism [68–71]; there were no deaths and few adverse events related to VTE in any patients in these studies. Notably, the majority of studies do not differentiate between patients with post-PE functional impairment, CTED, and CTEPH, making results difficult to generalize by disease process. Among 23 patients with PE (5 of whom had massive PE), a 3-month exercise program led to an improvement in peak VO2 by 3.9 mL/kg/min, the time to walk 400 m by 1.1 min, and an improvement in QoL questionnaires [69]. Patients enrolled in a 6-week pulmonary rehabilitation program after PE demonstrated an increase in 6MWD by 49.4 m, with 78% of patients reporting an improvement in their health status after rehabilitation [72]. In patients with PPES but without CTEPH, a study of 27 patients demonstrated an improvement in the QoL questionnaires and an improvement in post-VTE functional status with the use of a 12-week pulmonary rehabilitation program [73]. These results have been replicated for patients with confirmed CTEPH. In a study of 35 patients with inoperable or residual CTEPH, a 3-week in-hospital followed by 15-week out of hospital exercise program led to an improvement in 6MWD QoL questionnaires and peak oxygen consumption [74].

6. Conclusions

Post-pulmonary embolism syndrome is common, underdiagnosed, and warrants early consideration in patients with dyspnea, exercise intolerance, impaired functional status, or worse QoLs after PE. Evaluation with a TTE, a V/Q scan, and/or a CPET can identify patients who may benefit from treatment with medical, interventional, or rehabilitation-based therapy.

Author Contributions: Conceptualization, J.H.F., T.J.P. and D.F.; writing—original draft preparation, J.H.F.; writing—review and editing, J.H.F., T.J.P. and D.F.; visualization, D.F.; supervision, T.J.P. and D.F. All authors have read and agreed to the published version of the manuscript.

Funding: This research received no external funding.

Conflicts of Interest: The authors declare no conflicts of interest.

References

1. Luijten, D.; de Jong, C.M.M.; Ninaber, M.K.; Spruit, M.A.; Huisman, M.V.; Klok, F.A. Post-Pulmonary Embolism Syndrome and Functional Outcomes after Acute Pulmonary Embolism. *Semin. Thromb. Hemost.* **2023**, *49*, 848–860. [CrossRef] [PubMed]
2. Klok, F.A.; van der Hulle, T.; den Exter, P.L.; Lankeit, M.; Huisman, M.V.; Konstantinides, S. The Post-PE Syndrome: A New Concept for Chronic Complications of Pulmonary Embolism. *Blood Rev.* **2014**, *28*, 221–226. [CrossRef] [PubMed]
3. Kahn, S.R.; Hirsch, A.M.; Akaberi, A.; Hernandez, P.; Anderson, D.R.; Wells, P.S.; Rodger, M.A.; Solymoss, S.; Kovacs, M.J.; Rudski, L.; et al. Functional and Exercise Limitations After a First Episode of Pulmonary Embolism. *Chest* **2017**, *151*, 1058–1068. [CrossRef] [PubMed]
4. Stevinson, B.G.; Hernandez-Nino, J.; Rose, G.; Kline, J.A. Echocardiographic and Functional Cardiopulmonary Problems 6 Months after First-Time Pulmonary Embolism in Previously Healthy Patients. *Eur. Heart J.* **2007**, *28*, 2517–2524. [CrossRef]
5. Aggarwal, V.; Hyder, S.N.; Kamdar, N.; Zghouzi, M.; Visovatti, S.H.; Yin, Z.; Barnes, G.; Froehlich, J.; Moles, V.M.; Cascino, T.; et al. Symptoms Suggestive of Postpulmonary Embolism Syndrome and Utilization of Diagnostic Testing. *J. Soc. Cardiovasc. Angiogr. Interv.* **2023**, *2*, 101063. [CrossRef]
6. Chang, H.-Y.; Chang, W.-T.; Chen, P.-W.; Lin, C.-C.; Hsu, C.-H. Pulmonary Thromboembolism with Computed Tomography Defined Chronic Thrombus Is Associated with Higher Mortality. *Pulm. Circ.* **2020**, *10*, 2045894020905510. [CrossRef] [PubMed]
7. Sanchez, O.; Helley, D.; Couchon, S.; Roux, A.; Delaval, A.; Trinquart, L.; Collignon, M.A.; Fischer, A.M.; Meyer, G. Perfusion Defects after Pulmonary Embolism: Risk Factors and Clinical Significance. *J. Thromb. Haemost.* **2010**, *8*, 1248–1255. [CrossRef]
8. Ende-Verhaar, Y.M.; Cannegieter, S.C.; Noordegraaf, A.V.; Delcroix, M.; Pruszczyk, P.; Mairuhu, A.T.A.; Huisman, M.V.; Klok, F.A. Incidence of Chronic Thromboembolic Pulmonary Hypertension after Acute Pulmonary Embolism: A Contemporary View of the Published Literature. *Eur. Respir. J.* **2017**, *49*, 1601792. [CrossRef]
9. Humbert, M.; Kovacs, G.; Hoeper, M.M.; Badagliacca, R.; Berger, R.M.F.; Brida, M.; Carlsen, J.; Coats, A.J.S.; Escribano-Subias, P.; Ferrari, P.; et al. 2022 ESC/ERS Guidelines for the Diagnosis and Treatment of Pulmonary Hypertension. *Eur. Respir. J.* **2022**, *61*, 2200879. [CrossRef]
10. Klok, F.A.; Ageno, W.; Ay, C.; Bäck, M.; Barco, S.; Bertoletti, L.; Becattini, C.; Carlsen, J.; Delcroix, M.; van Es, N.; et al. Optimal Follow-up after Acute Pulmonary Embolism: A Position Paper of the European Society of Cardiology Working Group on Pulmonary Circulation and Right Ventricular Function, in Collaboration with the European Society of Cardiology Working Group on Atherosclerosis and Vascular Biology, Endorsed by the European Respiratory Society. *Eur. Heart J.* **2022**, *43*, 183–189. [CrossRef]
11. Alonso-Martínez, J.L.; Anniccherico-Sánchez, F.J.; Urbieta-Echezarreta, M.A. The Post-Pulmonary Embolism (Post-PE Syndrome). *Eur. J. Intern. Med.* **2020**, *76*, 127–129. [CrossRef] [PubMed]
12. Valerio, L.; Mavromanoli, A.C.; Barco, S.; Abele, C.; Becker, D.; Bruch, L.; Ewert, R.; Faehling, M.; Fistera, D.; Gerhardt, F.; et al. Chronic Thromboembolic Pulmonary Hypertension and Impairment after Pulmonary Embolism: The FOCUS Study. *Eur. Heart J.* **2022**, *43*, 3387–3398. [CrossRef] [PubMed]
13. Coquoz, N.; Weilenmann, D.; Stolz, D.; Popov, V.; Azzola, A.; Fellrath, J.-M.; Stricker, H.; Pagnamenta, A.; Ott, S.; Ulrich, S.; et al. Multicentre Observational Screening Survey for the Detection of CTEPH Following Pulmonary Embolism. *Eur. Respir. J.* **2018**, *51*, 1702505. [CrossRef] [PubMed]
14. Kim, N.H.; Lang, I.M. Risk Factors for Chronic Thromboembolic Pulmonary Hypertension. *Eur. Respir. Rev.* **2012**, *21*, 27–31. [CrossRef] [PubMed]
15. Konstantinides, S.V.; Vicaut, E.; Danays, T.; Becattini, C.; Bertoletti, L.; Beyer-Westendorf, J.; Bouvaist, H.; Couturaud, F.; Dellas, C.; Duerschmied, D.; et al. Impact of Thrombolytic Therapy on the Long-Term Outcome of Intermediate-Risk Pulmonary Embolism. *J. Am. Coll. Cardiol.* **2017**, *69*, 1536–1544. [CrossRef]
16. Pengo, V.; Lensing, A.W.A.; Prins, M.H.; Marchiori, A.; Davidson, B.L.; Tiozzo, F.; Albanese, P.; Biasiolo, A.; Pegoraro, C.; Iliceto, S.; et al. Incidence of Chronic Thromboembolic Pulmonary Hypertension after Pulmonary Embolism. *N. Engl. J. Med.* **2004**, *350*, 2257–2264. [CrossRef]
17. Kim, N.H.; Delcroix, M.; Jais, X.; Madani, M.M.; Matsubara, H.; Mayer, E.; Ogo, T.; Tapson, V.F.; Ghofrani, H.-A.; Jenkins, D.P. Chronic Thromboembolic Pulmonary Hypertension. *Eur. Respir. J.* **2019**, *53*, 1801915. [CrossRef]
18. Pesavento, R.; Filippi, L.; Palla, A.; Visonà, A.; Bova, C.; Marzolo, M.; Porro, F.; Villalta, S.; Ciammaichella, M.; Bucherini, E.; et al. Impact of Residual Pulmonary Obstruction on the Long-Term Outcome of Patients with Pulmonary Embolism. *Eur. Respir. J.* **2017**, *49*, 1601980. [CrossRef]
19. Pepke-Zaba, J.; Delcroix, M.; Lang, I.; Mayer, E.; Jansa, P.; Ambroz, D.; Treacy, C.; D'Armini, A.M.; Morsolini, M.; Snijder, R.; et al. Chronic Thromboembolic Pulmonary Hypertension (CTEPH): Results from an International Prospective Registry. *Circulation* **2011**, *124*, 1973–1981. [CrossRef]

20. Hunter, R.; Noble, S.; Lewis, S.; Bennett, P. Long-Term Psychosocial Impact of Venous Thromboembolism: A Qualitative Study in the Community. *BMJ Open* **2019**, *9*, e024805. [CrossRef]
21. Kirchberger, I.; Ruile, S.; Linseisen, J.; Haberl, S.; Meisinger, C.; Berghaus, T.M. The Lived Experience with Pulmonary Embolism: A Qualitative Study Using Focus Groups. *Respir. Med.* **2020**, *167*, 105978. [CrossRef]
22. Chow, V.; Reddel, C.; Pennings, G.; Chung, T.; Ng, A.C.C.; Curnow, J.; Kritharides, L. Persistent Global Hypercoagulability in Long-Term Survivors of Acute Pulmonary Embolism. *Blood Coagul. Fibrinolysis* **2015**, *26*, 537–544. [CrossRef]
23. Diehl, P.; Aleker, M.; Helbing, T.; Sossong, V.; Germann, M.; Sorichter, S.; Bode, C.; Moser, M. Increased Platelet, Leukocyte and Endothelial Microparticles Predict Enhanced Coagulation and Vascular Inflammation in Pulmonary Hypertension. *J. Thromb. Thrombolysis* **2011**, *31*, 173–179. [CrossRef] [PubMed]
24. Lang, I.M.; Pesavento, R.; Bonderman, D.; Yuan, J.X.-J. Risk Factors and Basic Mechanisms of Chronic Thromboembolic Pulmonary Hypertension: A Current Understanding. *Eur. Respir. J.* **2013**, *41*, 462–468. [CrossRef] [PubMed]
25. Morris, T.A.; Marsh, J.J.; Chiles, P.G.; Auger, W.R.; Fedullo, P.F.; Woods, V.L. Fibrin Derived from Patients with Chronic Thromboembolic Pulmonary Hypertension Is Resistant to Lysis. *Am. J. Respir. Crit. Care Med.* **2006**, *173*, 1270–1275. [CrossRef]
26. Oka, M.; McMurtry, I.F.; Oshima, K. How Does Pulmonary Endarterectomy Cure CTEPH: A Clue to Cure PAH? *Am. J. Physiol. —Lung Cell. Mol. Physiol.* **2016**, *311*, L766–L769. [CrossRef] [PubMed]
27. Galiè, N.; Kim, N.H.S. Pulmonary Microvascular Disease in Chronic Thromboembolic Pulmonary Hypertension. *Proc. Am. Thorac. Soc.* **2006**, *3*, 571–576. [CrossRef] [PubMed]
28. Lang, I.M.; Dorfmüller, P.; Noordegraaf, A.V. The Pathobiology of Chronic Thromboembolic Pulmonary Hypertension. *Am. Thorac. Soc.* **2016**, *13*, S215–S221. [CrossRef]
29. Eagleton, M.J.; Henke, P.K.; Luke, C.E.; Hawley, A.E.; Bedi, A.; Knipp, B.S.; Wakefield, T.W.; Greenfield, L.J. Inflammation and Intimal Hyperplasia Associated with Experimental Pulmonary Embolism. *J. Vasc. Surg.* **2002**, *36*, 581–588. [CrossRef]
30. Konstantinides, S.V.; Meyer, G.; Becattini, C.; Bueno, H.; Geersing, G.-J.; Harjola, V.-P.; Huisman, M.V.; Humbert, M.; Jennings, C.S.; Jiménez, D.; et al. 2019 ESC Guidelines for the Diagnosis and Management of Acute Pulmonary Embolism Developed in Collaboration with the European Respiratory Society (ERS): The Task Force for the Diagnosis and Management of Acute Pulmonary Embolism of the European Society of Cardiology (ESC). *Eur. Respir. J.* **2019**, *54*, 1901647. [CrossRef]
31. Boon, G.J.A.M.; Ende-Verhaar, Y.M.; Bavalia, R.; Bouazzaoui, L.H.E.; Delcroix, M.; Dzikowska-Diduch, O.; Huisman, M.V.; Kurnicka, K.; Mairuhu, A.T.A.; Middeldorp, S.; et al. Non-Invasive Early Exclusion of Chronic Thromboembolic Pulmonary Hypertension after Acute Pulmonary Embolism: The InShape II Study. *Thorax* **2021**, *76*, 1002–1009. [CrossRef]
32. Furfaro, D.; Azadi, J.; Housten, T.; Kolb, T.M.; Damico, R.L.; Hassoun, P.M.; Chin, K.; Mathai, S.C. Discordance between Imaging Modalities in the Evaluation of Chronic Thromboembolic Pulmonary Hypertension: A Combined Experience from Two Academic Medical Centers. *Ann. Am. Thorac. Soc.* **2019**, *16*, 277–280. [CrossRef] [PubMed]
33. Den Exter, P.L.; Van Es, J.; Kroft, L.J.M.; Erkens, P.M.G.; Douma, R.A.; Mos, I.C.M.; Jonkers, G.; Hovens, M.M.C.; Durian, M.F.; Cate, H.T.; et al. Thromboembolic Resolution Assessed by CT Pulmonary Angiography after Treatment for Acute Pulmonary Embolism. *Thromb. Haemost.* **2015**, *114*, 26–34. [CrossRef] [PubMed]
34. Roach, P.J.; Schembri, G.P.; Bailey, D.L. V/Q Scanning Using SPECT and SPECT/CT. *J. Nucl. Med.* **2013**, *54*, 1588–1596. [CrossRef]
35. Gopalan, D.; Delcroix, M.; Held, M. Diagnosis of Chronic Thromboembolic Pulmonary Hypertension. *Eur. Respir. Rev.* **2017**, *26*, 160108. [CrossRef]
36. Morris, T.A.; Fernandes, T.M.; Channick, R.N. Evaluation of Dyspnea and Exercise Intolerance After Acute Pulmonary Embolism. *Chest* **2023**, *163*, 933–941. [CrossRef] [PubMed]
37. Held, M.; Grün, M.; Holl, R.; Hübner, G.; Kaiser, R.; Karl, S.; Kolb, M.; Schäfers, H.J.; Wilkens, H.; Jany, B. Cardiopulmonary Exercise Testing to Detect Chronic Thromboembolic Pulmonary Hypertension in Patients with Normal Echocardiography. *Respiration* **2014**, *87*, 379–387. [CrossRef] [PubMed]
38. Delcroix, M.; Torbicki, A.; Gopalan, D.; Sitbon, O.; Klok, F.A.; Lang, I.; Jenkins, D.; Kim, N.H.; Humbert, M.; Jais, X.; et al. ERS Statement on Chronic Thromboembolic Pulmonary Hypertension. *Eur. Respir. J.* **2021**, *57*, 2002828. [CrossRef]
39. Jevnikar, M.; Solinas, S.; Brenot, P.; Lechartier, B.; Kularatne, M.; Montani, D.; Savale, L.; Garcia-Alonso, C.; Sitbon, O.; Beurnier, A.; et al. Sequential Multimodal Therapy in Chronic Thromboembolic Pulmonary Hypertension with Mixed Anatomical Lesions: A Proof of Concept. *Eur. Respir. J.* **2023**, *62*, 2300517. [CrossRef]
40. Stevens, S.M.; Woller, S.C.; Kreuziger, L.B.; Bounameaux, H.; Doerschug, K.; Geersing, G.-J.; Huisman, M.V.; Kearon, C.; King, C.S.; Knighton, A.J.; et al. Antithrombotic Therapy for VTE Disease: Second Update of the CHEST Guideline and Expert Panel Report. *Chest* **2021**, *160*, e545–e608. [CrossRef]
41. Ortel, T.L.; Neumann, I.; Ageno, W.; Beyth, R.; Clark, N.P.; Cuker, A.; Hutten, B.A.; Jaff, M.R.; Manja, V.; Schulman, S.; et al. American Society of Hematology 2020 Guidelines for Management of Venous Thromboembolism: Treatment of Deep Vein Thrombosis and Pulmonary Embolism. *Blood Adv.* **2020**, *4*, 4693–4738. [CrossRef] [PubMed]
42. Bunclark, K.; Newnham, M.; Chiu, Y.-D.; Ruggiero, A.; Villar, S.S.; Cannon, J.E.; Coghlan, G.; Corris, P.A.; Howard, L.; Jenkins, D.; et al. A Multicenter Study of Anticoagulation in Operable Chronic Thromboembolic Pulmonary Hypertension. *J. Thromb. Haemost.* **2020**, *18*, 114–122. [CrossRef] [PubMed]
43. Humbert, M.; Simonneau, G.; Pittrow, D.; Delcroix, M.; Pepke-Zaba, J.; Langleben, D.; Mielniczuk, L.M.; Subias, P.E.; Snijder, R.J.; Barberà, J.A.; et al. Oral Anticoagulants (NOAC and VKA) in Chronic Thromboembolic Pulmonary Hypertension. *J. Heart Lung Transplant.* **2022**, *41*, 716–721. [CrossRef] [PubMed]

44. Lankeit, M.; Krieg, V.; Hobohm, L.; Kölmel, S.; Liebetrau, C.; Konstantinides, S.; Hamm, C.W.; Mayer, E.; Wiedenroth, C.B.; Guth, S. Pulmonary Endarterectomy in Chronic Thromboembolic Pulmonary Hypertension. *J. Heart Lung Transplant.* **2018**, *37*, 250–258. [CrossRef] [PubMed]
45. Madani, M.M.; Auger, W.R.; Pretorius, V.; Sakakibara, N.; Kerr, K.M.; Kim, N.H.; Fedullo, P.F.; Jamieson, S.W. Pulmonary Endarterectomy: Recent Changes in a Single Institution's Experience of More than 2700 Patients. *Ann. Thorac. Surg.* **2012**, *94*, 97–103, discussion 103. [CrossRef]
46. Lewczuk, J.; Piszko, P.; Jagas, J.; Porada, A.; Sobkowicz, B.; Wrabec, K.; Wójciak, S. Prognostic Factors in Medically Treated Patients With Chronic Pulmonary Embolism. *Chest* **2001**, *119*, 818–823. [CrossRef]
47. De Perrot, M.; Donahoe, L.; McRae, K.; Thenganatt, J.; Moric, J.; Chan, J.; McInnis, M.; Jumaa, K.; Tan, K.T.; Mafeld, S.; et al. Outcome after Pulmonary Endarterectomy for Segmental Chronic Thromboembolic Pulmonary Hypertension. *J. Thorac. Cardiovasc. Surg.* **2022**, *164*, 696–707.e4. [CrossRef]
48. de Perrot, M.; McRae, K.; Donahoe, L.; Abdelnour-Berchtold, E.; Thenganatt, J.; Granton, J. Pulmonary Endarterectomy in Severe Chronic Thromboembolic Pulmonary Hypertension: The Toronto Experience. *Ann. Cardiothorac. Surg.* **2022**, *11*, 133–142. [CrossRef]
49. Casaclang-Verzosa, G.; McCully, R.B.; Oh, J.K.; Miller, F.A.; McGregor, C.G.A. Effects of Pulmonary Thromboendarterectomy on Right-Sided Echocardiographic Parameters in Patients with Chronic Thromboembolic Pulmonary Hypertension. *Mayo Clin. Proc.* **2006**, *81*, 777–782. [CrossRef]
50. Matsuda, H.; Ogino, H.; Minatoya, K.; Sasaki, H.; Nakanishi, N.; Kyotani, S.; Kobayashi, J.; Yagihara, T.; Kitamura, S. Long-Term Recovery of Exercise Ability After Pulmonary Endarterectomy for Chronic Thromboembolic Pulmonary Hypertension. *Ann. Thorac. Surg.* **2006**, *82*, 1338–1343. [CrossRef]
51. Taboada, D.; Pepke-Zaba, J.; Jenkins, D.P.; Berman, M.; Treacy, C.M.; Cannon, J.E.; Toshner, M.; Dunning, J.J.; Ng, C.; Tsui, S.S.; et al. Outcome of Pulmonary Endarterectomy in Symptomatic Chronic Thromboembolic Disease. *Eur. Respir. J.* **2014**, *44*, 1635–1645. [CrossRef] [PubMed]
52. Olgun Yıldızeli, Ş. Pulmonary Endarterectomy for Chronic Thromboembolic Disease. *Anatol. J. Cardiol.* **2018**, *19*, 273–278. [CrossRef] [PubMed]
53. Lang, I.M.; Andreassen, A.K.; Andersen, A.; Bouvaist, H.; Coghlan, G.; Escribano-Subias, P.; Jansa, P.; Kopec, G.; Kurzyna, M.; Matsubara, H.; et al. Balloon Pulmonary Angioplasty for Chronic Thromboembolic Pulmonary Hypertension: A Clinical Consensus Statement of the ESC Working Group on Pulmonary Circulation and Right Ventricular Function. *Eur. Heart J.* **2023**, *44*, 2659–2671. [CrossRef]
54. Räber, L.; Ueki, Y.; Lang, I. Balloon Pulmonary Angioplasty for the Treatment of Chronic Thromboembolic Pulmonary Hypertension. Available online: https://eurointervention.pcronline.com/article/balloon-pulmonary-angioplasty-for-the-treatment-of-chronic-thromboembolic-pulmonary-hypertension (accessed on 31 August 2024).
55. Ogawa, A.; Satoh, T.; Fukuda, T.; Sugimura, K.; Fukumoto, Y.; Emoto, N.; Yamada, N.; Yao, A.; Ando, M.; Ogino, H.; et al. Balloon Pulmonary Angioplasty for Chronic Thromboembolic Pulmonary Hypertension: Results of a multicenter registry. *Circ. Cardiovasc. Qual. Outcomes* **2017**, *10*, e004029. [CrossRef]
56. Brenot, P.; Jaïs, X.; Taniguchi, Y.; Garcia Alonso, C.; Gerardin, B.; Mussot, S.; Mercier, O.; Fabre, D.; Parent, F.; Jevnikar, M.; et al. French Experience of Balloon Pulmonary Angioplasty for Chronic Thromboembolic Pulmonary Hypertension. *Eur. Respir. J.* **2019**, *53*, 1802095. [CrossRef] [PubMed]
57. Olsson, K.M.; Wiedenroth, C.B.; Kamp, J.-C.; Breithecker, A.; Fuge, J.; Krombach, G.A.; Haas, M.; Hamm, C.; Kramm, T.; Guth, S.; et al. Balloon Pulmonary Angioplasty for Inoperable Patients with Chronic Thromboembolic Pulmonary Hypertension: The Initial German Experience. *Eur. Respir. J.* **2017**, *49*, 1602409. [CrossRef]
58. Bashir, R.; Noory, A.; Oliveros, E.; Romero, C.M.; Maruthi, R.; Mirza, A.; Lakhter, V.; Zhao, H.; Brisco-Bacik, M.; Vaidya, A.; et al. Refined Balloon Pulmonary Angioplasty in Chronic Thromboembolic Pulmonary Hypertension. *JACC Adv.* **2023**, *2*, 100291. [CrossRef]
59. Jaïs, X.; Brenot, P.; Bouvaist, H.; Jevnikar, M.; Canuet, M.; Chabanne, C.; Chaouat, A.; Cottin, V.; De Groote, P.; Favrolt, N.; et al. Balloon Pulmonary Angioplasty versus Riociguat for the Treatment of Inoperable Chronic Thromboembolic Pulmonary Hypertension (RACE): A Multicentre, Phase 3, Open-Label, Randomised Controlled Trial and Ancillary Follow-up Study. *Lancet Respir. Med.* **2022**, *10*, 961–971. [CrossRef]
60. Kawakami, T.; Matsubara, H.; Shinke, T.; Abe, K.; Kohsaka, S.; Hosokawa, K.; Taniguchi, Y.; Shimokawahara, H.; Yamada, Y.; Kataoka, M.; et al. Balloon Pulmonary Angioplasty versus Riociguat in Inoperable Chronic Thromboembolic Pulmonary Hypertension (MR BPA): An Open-Label, Randomised Controlled Trial. *Lancet Respir. Med.* **2022**, *10*, 949–960. [CrossRef]
61. Ghofrani, H.-A.; D'Armini, A.M.; Grimminger, F.; Hoeper, M.M.; Jansa, P.; Kim, N.H.; Mayer, E.; Simonneau, G.; Wilkins, M.R.; Fritsch, A.; et al. Riociguat for the Treatment of Chronic Thromboembolic Pulmonary Hypertension. *N. Engl. J. Med.* **2013**, *369*, 319–329. [CrossRef]
62. Simonneau, G.; D'Armini, A.M.; Ghofrani, H.-A.; Grimminger, F.; Hoeper, M.M.; Jansa, P.; Kim, N.H.; Wang, C.; Wilkins, M.R.; Fritsch, A.; et al. Riociguat for the Treatment of Chronic Thromboembolic Pulmonary Hypertension: A Long-Term Extension Study (CHEST-2). *Eur. Respir. J.* **2015**, *45*, 1293–1302. [CrossRef] [PubMed]

63. Ghofrani, H.-A.; Simonneau, G.; D'Armini, A.M.; Fedullo, P.; Howard, L.S.; Jaïs, X.; Jenkins, D.P.; Jing, Z.-C.; Madani, M.M.; Martin, N.; et al. Macitentan for the Treatment of Inoperable Chronic Thromboembolic Pulmonary Hypertension (MERIT-1): Results from the Multicentre, Phase 2, Randomised, Double-Blind, Placebo-Controlled Study. *Lancet Respir. Med.* **2024**, *12*, 262–263. [CrossRef]
64. Jaïs, X.; D'Armini, A.M.; Jansa, P.; Torbicki, A.; Delcroix, M.; Ghofrani, H.A.; Hoeper, M.M.; Lang, I.M.; Mayer, E.; Pepke-Zaba, J.; et al. Bosentan for Treatment of Inoperable Chronic Thromboembolic Pulmonary Hypertension: BENEFiT (Bosentan Effects in iNopErable Forms of chronIc Thromboembolic Pulmonary Hypertension), a Randomized, Placebo-Controlled Trial. *J. Am. Coll. Cardiol.* **2008**, *52*, 2127–2134. [CrossRef]
65. Sadushi-Kolici, R.; Jansa, P.; Kopec, G.; Torbicki, A.; Skoro-Sajer, N.; Campean, I.-A.; Halank, M.; Simkova, I.; Karlocai, K.; Steringer-Mascherbauer, R.; et al. Subcutaneous Treprostinil for the Treatment of Severe Non-Operable Chronic Thromboembolic Pulmonary Hypertension (CTREPH): A Double-Blind, Phase 3, Randomised Controlled Trial. *Lancet Respir. Med.* **2019**, *7*, 239–248. [CrossRef] [PubMed]
66. Guth, S.; D'Armini, A.M.; Delcroix, M.; Nakayama, K.; Fadel, E.; Hoole, S.P.; Jenkins, D.P.; Kiely, D.G.; Kim, N.H.; Lang, I.M.; et al. Current Strategies for Managing Chronic Thromboembolic Pulmonary Hypertension: Results of the Worldwide Prospective CTEPH Registry. *ERJ Open Res.* **2021**, *7*, 00850–02020. [CrossRef]
67. Delcroix, M.; Lang, I.; Pepke-Zaba, J.; Jansa, P.; D'Armini, A.M.; Snijder, R.; Bresser, P.; Torbicki, A.; Mellemkjaer, S.; Lewczuk, J.; et al. Long-Term Outcome of Patients with Chronic Thromboembolic Pulmonary Hypertension. *Circulation* **2016**, *133*, 859–871. [CrossRef] [PubMed]
68. Noack, F.; Schmidt, B.; Amoury, M.; Stoevesandt, D.; Gielen, S.; Pflaumbaum, B.; Girschick, C.; Völler, H.; Schlitt, A. Feasibility and Safety of Rehabilitation after Venous Thromboembolism. *Vasc. Health Risk Manag.* **2015**, *11*, 397–401. [CrossRef] [PubMed]
69. Cires-Drouet, R.S.; Mayorga-Carlin, M.; Toursavadkohi, S.; White, R.; Redding, E.; Durham, F.; Dondero, K.; Prior, S.J.; Sorkin, J.D.; Lal, B.K. Safety of Exercise Therapy after Acute Pulmonary Embolism. *Phlebology* **2020**, *35*, 824–832. [CrossRef]
70. Amoury, M.; Noack, F.; Kleeberg, K.; Stoevesandt, D.; Lehnigk, B.; Bethge, S.; Heinze, V.; Schlitt, A. Prognosis of Patients with Pulmonary Embolism after Rehabilitation. *Vasc. Health Risk Manag.* **2018**, *14*, 183–187. [CrossRef]
71. Lakoski, S.G.; Savage, P.D.; Berkman, A.M.; Penalosa, L.; Crocker, A.; Ades, P.A.; Kahn, S.R.; Cushman, M. The Safety and Efficacy of Early-initiation Exercise Training after Acute Venous Thromboembolism: A Randomized Clinical Trial. *J. Thromb. Haemost.* **2015**, *13*, 1238–1244. [CrossRef]
72. Nopp, S.; Klok, F.A.; Moik, F.; Petrovic, M.; Derka, I.; Ay, C.; Zwick, R.H. Outpatient Pulmonary Rehabilitation in Patients with Persisting Symptoms after Pulmonary Embolism. *J. Clin. Med.* **2020**, *9*, 1811. [CrossRef] [PubMed]
73. Boon, G.J.A.M.; Janssen, S.M.J.; Barco, S.; Bogaard, H.J.; Ghanima, W.; Kroft, L.J.M.; Meijboom, L.J.; Ninaber, M.K.; Nossent, E.J.; Spruit, M.A.; et al. Efficacy and Safety of a 12-Week Outpatient Pulmonary Rehabilitation Program in Post-PE Syndrome. *Thromb. Res.* **2021**, *206*, 66–75. [CrossRef] [PubMed]
74. Nagel, C.; Prange, F.; Guth, S.; Herb, J.; Ehlken, N.; Fischer, C.; Reichenberger, F.; Rosenkranz, S.; Seyfarth, H.-J.; Mayer, E.; et al. Exercise Training Improves Exercise Capacity and Quality of Life in Patients with Inoperable or Residual Chronic Thromboembolic Pulmonary Hypertension. *PLoS ONE* **2012**, *7*, e41603. [CrossRef]

Disclaimer/Publisher's Note: The statements, opinions and data contained in all publications are solely those of the individual author(s) and contributor(s) and not of MDPI and/or the editor(s). MDPI and/or the editor(s) disclaim responsibility for any injury to people or property resulting from any ideas, methods, instructions or products referred to in the content.

Review

Age-Adjusted and Clinical Probability Adapted D-Dimer Cutoffs to Rule Out Pulmonary Embolism: A Narrative Review of Clinical Trials

Marc Righini [1,*], Helia Robert-Ebadi [1] and Grégoire Le Gal [2,3]

[1] Division of Angiology and Hemostasis, Geneva University Hospitals and Faculty of Medicine, 1205 Geneva, Switzerland; helia.robert-ebadi@hcuge.ch
[2] Department of Medicine, Ottawa Hospital Research Institute, University of Ottawa, Ottawa, ON K1H 8L6, Canada; glegal@toh.ca
[3] EA3878, University of Brest, 29200 Brest, France
* Correspondence: marc.righini@hug.ch; Tel.: +41-22-372-92-92

Abstract: Diagnosis of pulmonary embolism remains a challenge for clinicians as its differential diagnosis is wide. The use of sequential diagnostic strategies based on the assessment of clinical probability, D-dimer measurement, and computed tomography pulmonary angiography have been validated in large prospective outcome studies. D-dimer measurement at a standard cutoff of 500 µg/L has gained wide acceptance to rule out pulmonary embolism in around 20 to 30% of patients with a clinically suspected pulmonary embolism. To improve the efficiency of D-dimer measurement, different ways of selecting a higher, albeit safe cutoff were explored: the age-adjusted D-dimer cutoff and the clinical adapted D-dimer cutoff. While both have been prospectively validated in large studies, some differences do exist. In particular, the prevalence of pulmonary embolism in these different validation studies was very different. Overall, the age-adjusted cutoff seems to be safer and less efficient, while the clinical probability adapted cutoff seems more efficient and less safe. Here, we report the available data regarding these two different ways to increase the diagnostic yield of D-dimer. Also, well beyond the accuracy of these adjusted/adapted cutoffs, some external factors, such as the prevalence of pulmonary embolism in the tested population and the clinical setting, have an important impact of the negative predictive value and on the overall efficiency of these cutoffs. Therefore, we also discuss which cutoff should be used according to the expected prevalence of the disease and according to the clinical setting.

Keywords: diagnosis; pulmonary embolism; D-dimer; age-adjusted D-dimer cutoff; clinical probability adapted D-dimer cutoff

1. Introduction

Pulmonary embolism (PE) is a frequently suspected diagnosis in the emergency room (ER) in patients presenting with shortness of breath and/or chest pain without any obvious cause identified. Modern PE diagnosis relies on diagnostic strategies, including sequential evaluation of clinical probability, measurement of plasma D-dimer levels, and, most often, CT pulmonary angiography (CTPA) rather than a standalone test. The initial step is the assessment of pre-test clinical probability, either by gestalt or by validated clinical prediction rules (Wells rule of Geneva score) [1–3]. This allows separating patients into different groups of PE prevalence, and thus directly influencing the negative and positive predictive values of the diagnostic tests used in these patients [4].

Plasma D-dimer measurement has been extensively evaluated for the exclusion of PE in outpatients. The diagnostic usefulness of the D-dimers lies in their high sensitivity and hence in their capacity to exclude PE when below a certain cutoff ("negative D-dimer") without further investigations. Indeed, in patients with a non-high clinical probability (low and intermediate groups in a three-level score or unlikely group in a dichotomic score), a highly sensitive negative D-dimer test safely excludes PE without any additional investigation [4]. Sensitive D-dimer tests include those performed by the ELISA technique (median sensitivity 99%; VIDAS® (bioMérieux, Marcy L'Etoile, France), Stratus® (Siemens, Munich, Germany), AxSYM® (Abbott Diagnostics, Abbott Park, IL, USA) and by quantitative latex methods (median sensitivity 96%; STA Liatest® (Stago, Asnières sur Seine, France), Tinaquant® (Roche Diagnostics, Basel, Switzerland)) [5]. In patients with high clinical probability or likely PE, the negative predictive value of even a highly sensitive D-dimer test may be insufficient to exclude PE. D-dimer measurement is thus not used in these patients.

The specificity of the ELISA and quantitative latex D-dimer tests for venous thromboembolism (VTE) is limited, ranging from 35 to 40%. Indeed, D-dimer levels increase in various clinical situations, such as cancer, post-operative periods, infectious/inflammatory states, pregnancy, and with age, leading to a reduced specificity of the test in elderly patients [6,7]. In other words, the probability of having a negative test result is reduced, and the number of patients needed to test (NNT) to exclude one PE without further investigations is higher. Whereas PE can be ruled out in the presence of non-high clinical probability and a negative D-dimer in one out of three outpatients in the emergency room with suspected PE [8], it can be excluded in only one out of twenty patients > 80 years. As current diagnostic strategies include imaging (most often CTPA) in patients with positive D-dimers, a lack of specificity of D-dimers in the elderly can lead to a high proportion of these patients undergoing CTPA.

2. The Age-Adjusted D-Dimer Cutoff

The question of a higher D-dimer cutoff in elderly patients was raised many years ago [7], but studies confirming the potential security of such a strategy by retrospectively applying age-adjusted cutoffs to large prospective cohorts of consecutive patients with suspected VTEs were published between 2010 and 2012 [9–13] and confirmed the safety of using an age-adjusted cutoff on an overall population of several thousands of patients.

A progressive age-adjusted D-dimer cutoff (age $\times$ 10 µg/L in patients > 50 years) was retrospectively derived and validated in a sample of 1712 patients with suspected PE [9]. The retrospective validation study showed that the age-adjusted cutoff could increase the number of patients in whom the D-dimer test was considered negative by around 20%, without increasing the proportion of false-negative results when compared to the standard cutoff (<500 µg/L). The increase in the diagnostic yield of the D-dimer was particularly pronounced in patients over 80 years, as the age-adjusted cutoff allowed for an increase in the proportion of "negative" D-dimers from 9% to 21% [9], without any false-negative results.

3. The ADJUST-PE Study

This progressive age-adjusted D-dimer cutoff was prospectively validated in the ADJUST-PE study, a large multicenter multinational management outcome study [14]. Consecutive patients who presented to the emergency department with clinically suspected PE were assessed by a sequential diagnostic work-up using clinical probability assessment (by one of the two following scores: simplified Geneva score or the two-level Wells score) [2,3,15], highly sensitive D-dimer measurement (ELISA or immuno-turbidimetric assays), and CTPA. Patients with a D-dimer level below their age-adjusted cutoff did not undergo further investigations and were thus left without anticoagulant treatment and followed-up for a period of 3 months [14].

This study included a total of 3346 patients with suspected PE. The subgroup of particular interest for answering the question raised in the ADJUST-PE study was of course patients having D-dimer levels between 500 µg/L and their age-adjusted cutoff (n = 337). None of these patients were lost to follow-up, and 6 patients received therapeutic anticoagulation for another indication than VTE. Of the remaining 331, 7 died and 7 had suspected VTE. Only one of these fourteen events was adjudicated as confirmed VTEs (nonfatal PE). The so-called "failure rate" of the age-adjusted cutoff was thus very low at 1/331 (0.3%; 95% CI 0.1–1.7%).

Increasing the proportion of patients in whom PE can be ruled out based on a clinical probability assessment and D-dimer measurement without further testing is particularly interesting in older patients. Indeed, the higher prevalence of renal failure in this population increases the potential risk of contrast-induced nephropathy related to CTPA or even contraindicates this test, and ventilation/perfusion lung scan (which can be performed in patients with severe renal failure) provides a high proportion of inconclusive results in older patients [6]. Moreover, ruling out PE based on clinical probability and a simple blood test could contribute to reducing the time spent in the emergency department and the costs related to PE diagnostic work-ups. Indeed, a previous study had shown that D-the dimer measurement with a conventional cutoff was highly cost-saving in patients less than 80 years, but not in patients over 80 years. Using an age-adjusted D-dimer cutoff dramatically increases the proportion of patients in whom PE can be ruled out and it has been shown to reduce the costs of PE diagnosis in the emergency department. In the ADJUST-PE study, six different D-dimer assays were used depending on the site of inclusion of patients. Therefore, the number of patients with a negative D-dimer, but a value between 500 and their age-adjusted cutoff, was rather limited for each individual test.

4. The RELAX-PE Study

The RELAX-PE study was a real-life study including 1507 patients, which confirmed the safety of the age-adjusted cutoff [16]. Outpatients with suspected PE in whom PE was excluded by a non-high probability and a negative age-adjusted D-dimer, i.e., D-dimer < 500 µg/L up to 50 years, and D-dimer < (age × 10) µg/L in patients above 50 years, were included and followed for three months. The primary outcome was the rate of adjudicated venous thromboembolic events (VTEs).

The 3-month VTE risk in patients left untreated after a negative work-up was 1/1421 (0.07%, 95% CI 0.01–0.40%) in patients with a D-dimer < 500 µg/L and 0/269 (0.0%; 95% CI 0.0–1.41%) after a D-dimer $\geq$ 500 µg/L but < (age × 10) µg/L. Using the age-adjusted cutoff substantially increased the proportion of patients in whom PE could be excluded without imaging by 20% in the whole cohort and by 67% in patients 75 years or older. Six different D-dimer tests were used: the VIDAS D-dimer exclusion test (bioMérieux, Marcy L'Etoile, France), the Innovance D-dimer (Siemens, Munich, Germany), the Liatest D-dimer (Stago, Asnières sur Seine, France), the AxSYM D-dimer (Abbott Diagnostics, Abbott Park, IL, USA), the HemosIL DD HS (Instrumentation Laboratory, Lexington, MA, USA), and the DPC Immulite 2000 test (Siemens, Munich, Germany).

5. Extending the Kind of D-Dimer Assays That Can Be Used with an Age-Adjusted Cutoff

In the ADJUST-PE study, six different D-dimer assays were used depending on the site of inclusion of patients. Table 1 shows the breakdown of the different tests used and the proportion of patients having negative D-dimer results, separated into D-dimer < 500 µg/L and DD $\geq$ 500 µg/L but < patient's age-adjusted cutoff. For some of the D-dimer tests used, the number of patients with a value between 500 and their age-adjusted cutoff was rather limited. Therefore, the next step would be to further validate the safety of the age-adjusted D-dimer cutoff by using frozen samples stored during the ADJUST-PE study. Therefore, some other tests (Innovance D-dimer test® (Siemens) on an Atellica COAG 360 automat, the STA Liatest® (Stago) on a STA R Max automat, and a point-of-care LumiraDx®) are currently being evaluated on frozen samples arising from the ADJUST-PE study. The analysis is still ongoing, but it should further extend the number of D-dimer tests that can be used to rule out PE with the age-adjusted cutoff.

Table 1. Main results of studies using age-adjusted or clinically adapted D-dimer cutoffs.

D-Dimer Cutoff	Description of the D-Dimer Use in the Diagnostic Strategy	PE Prevalence	Percentage of CTPA Avoided When Compared with Usual Cutoff	3-Mo TE Rate
Conventional cutoff (500 µg/L) [2,3,8]	D-dimer cutoff: 500 µg/L PE ruled out if negative D-dimer in patients with a low/intermediate or unlikely PTP	20%	-	0.1 (0.0–0.7)
Age-adjusted cutoff (ADJUST PE study) [14]	D-dimer cutoff: age × 10 in patients aged 50 or older, normal cutoff in patients less than 50 years. PE ruled out if negative D-dimer in patients with a low/intermediate or unlikely PTP	19%	12%	0.3 (0.1–1.7)
Age-adjusted cutoff (RELAX-PE study) [16]	D-dimer cutoff: age × 10 in patients aged 50 or older, normal cutoff in patients less than 50 years. PE ruled out if negative D-dimer in patients with a low/intermediate PTP	NA	20%	0.07% (95% CI: 0.01–0.4)
Clinical probability adapted cutoff (YEARS study) [17]	Three criteria from the Wells score: signs of DVT, hemoptysis, PE most likely diagnosis. D-dimer cutoff: 1000 µg/L if no criteria, 500 µg/L if ≥1 criteria	13%	14%	0.8 (0.4–1.5)
Clinical probability adapted cutoff (PEGeD study) [18]	D-dimer cutoff: 1000 µg/L if Wells 0–4 points, 500 µg/L if Wells 4.5–6 points	7.4%	17.6%	0.05 (0.01–0.3)

Abbreviations: PE: pulmonary embolism; PTP: pre-test probability; 3-Mo TE rate: three-month thromboembolic rate.

6. The Clinical Probability Adapted D-Dimer Cutoff

In the first algorithms for PE diagnosis, a D-dimer cutoff set at 500 µg/L allowed to rule out PE in 20–30% of patients without performing CTPA, with an overall failure rate of less than 1%. The age-adjusted cutoff discussed above increases to around 40% the proportion of outpatients in whom PE can be ruled out with a very low failure rate. However, this adjusted cutoff also has limitations. Particularly, it increases the yield of D-dimers only in patients aged 50 years or older, and specifically in those older than 75 years. Therefore, other options were developed by researchers.

7. The YEARS Model and the YEARS Study

On the basis of a post hoc derivation and validation study (ref), three items of the original Wells' clinical decision rule—i.e., clinical signs of deep vein thrombosis, hemoptysis, and whether pulmonary embolism is the most likely diagnosis—were the most predictive for pulmonary embolism [19]. They allowed the use of a differential D-dimer threshold based on the presence of one of these items, without losing sensitivity. Hence, this algorithm involves the simultaneous assessment of only the three above-mentioned items and a D-dimer test threshold of 500 µg/L in the presence and 1000 µg/L in the absence of one of the YEARS items.

This simplified diagnostic strategy was used in the YEARS study [17], which showed a 14% absolute reduction in the use of CTPA imaging in comparison with a conventional strategy, without altering the safety outcome, i.e., the rate of venous thromboembolic events (VTE) at three months, which was 0.61 (95% CI: 0.3–0.96%). An external validation study including 3314 patients reported that 42.9% of patients would have PE excluded without the need for imaging, with an overall failure rate of 1.2% (95% CI: 0.8–1.9%), confirming the safety of this strategy. However, among the 272 patients with no YEARS criteria and a D-dimer < 1000 µg/L but above their age-adjusted D-dimer cutoff, PE was diagnosed in 6.3% of them (CI 3.9–9.8%). Therefore, some caution may be needed in this category of patients.

8. Another Clinical Probability Adapted D-Dimer Cutoff: The PEGeD Study

In the PEGeD study [18], a simplified diagnostic strategy was proposed in which a modified Wells score was used along with differential D-dimer cutoff values. Pulmonary embolism was ruled out without further testing in patients with a low clinical probability and a D-dimer less than 1000 µg/L as well as in patients with an intermediate clinical probability and a D-dimer less than 500 µg/L. This algorithm was prospectively evaluated in a multicentric Canadian study and resulted in a 17.6% absolute reduction in the use of CTPA imaging in comparison with a conventional strategy [17], without altering the safety outcome, i.e., the rate of venous thromboembolic events (VTEs) at three months, which was 0.05 (95% CI:0.01–0.3%).

An external validation study of the PEGeD algorithm, including 3302 patients, reported that 1621 (49.0%) of patients would have had PE excluded without the need for imaging. Of these patients, 38 (2.3%; 95% CI 1.7–3.2%) had symptomatic PE at initial testing or during the three-month follow-up. Therefore, this external validation study suggested that the algorithm was safe. Upon further analysis, 36 patients out of the 38 patients in whom PE was ruled out based on a low clinical probability and a D-dimer less than 1000 µg/L had a positive age-adjusted D-dimer. Therefore, the risk of VTEs among the 414 patients with a D-dimer below 1000 µg/L but above the age-adjusted D-dimer cutoff was 36/414 (8.7%; 95% CI 6.4–11.8%), suggesting that some caution might be needed in these patients. Table 1 summarizes the data of studies using age-adjusted and clinical probability adapted D-dimer cutoffs.

9. Which Cutoff Should We Choose?

A systematic review and individual-patient data meta-analysis was performed on more than 20,000 patients initially included in 16 prospective studies [20]. Overall, D-dimer levels fell below 500 μg/L in 26% to 30% of cases, and below the higher cutoffs in 41% to 47% of cases. Failure rates (missed PE diagnosis) ranged from 1% with a 500-μg/L cutoff to 2.8% with higher cutoffs. When the age-adjusted D-dimer threshold was used, the predicted failure rate varied between 0.76% (95% CI: 0.5–1.1%) and 1.1% (95% CI: 0.8–1.5%). For strategies applying the D-dimer threshold dependent on pretest probability, the predicted failure rate varied between 1.8% (95% CI: 1.4–2.4%) and 2.8% (95% CI: 2.3 to 3.5%). The predicted overall efficiency (PE considered as excluded) was highest for strategies applying a D-dimer threshold dependent on pretest probability and varied from 41% to 47%. The predicted efficiencies for the strategies using the age-adjusted D-dimer threshold varied between 32 and 37%. Overall, these data suggest that the age-adjusted cutoff is safer but less efficient than the clinical probability adapted cutoff to rule out PE.

Another systematic review and individual-patient data meta-analysis performed on more than 20,000 patients analyzed the diagnostic performances of these different D-dimer cutoffs across different healthcare settings. The performance of diagnostic strategies varied considerably across different healthcare settings due to the difference in patient characteristics and the prevalence of PE. For example, the proportion of patients reported to have a thromboembolic event during the 3-month follow-up after a negative age-adjusted D-dimer cutoff was 0.47% (95% CI: 0.18–1.23%) in primary healthcare, 0.65% (95% CI: 0.43–0.99%) in referred secondary care, and 1.7% (95% CI: 0.65–4.25%) in hospitalized patients or nursing home care. The figures with a negative clinical adapted D-dimer cutoff were 0.4 (95% CI: 0.16–1.19%) in primary healthcare, 3.0% (95% CI: 2.47–3.78%) in referred secondary care, and 4.1% (95% CI: 2.54–6.61%) in hospitalized patients or nursing home care.

Regarding efficiency, i.e., the proportion of patients in whom PE could be safely ruled by the clinical probability assessment and D-dimer was as follows: in primary care, 43.5% (95% CI: 29.14–59.03%) for the age-adjusted cutoff and 61.7% (95% CI: 8.33–73.62%) for the clinical probability adapted cutoff; in referred secondary care, 30.46% (95% CI:26.75–34.44%) for the age-adjusted cutoff and 48.75% (95% CI: 43.64–53.94%) for the clinical probability adapted cutoff; in hospitalized patients or nursing home care, 14.8% (95% CI:11.66–18.79%) for the age-adjusted cutoff and 19.4% (95% CI: 15.58–23.99%) for the clinical probability adapted cutoff. Overall, these figures confirm that the safety and diagnostic yield vary according to the clinical settings.

10. Conclusions

Both the age-adjusted D-dimer cutoff and the clinical probability adapted cutoff were validated in robust prospective outcome studies. However, some differences exist regarding safety and the diagnostic yield. The age-adjusted cutoff is safer and less efficient; the clinical adapted cutoff is less safe but more efficient. The presented data should help clinicians to balance the trade-off between missing PE cases and decreasing unnecessary CTPA. While the expected prevalence of PE is not always known, it has also an important impact on the safety and efficacy of our diagnostic strategies. Overall, as the age-adjusted cutoff is safer, it seems wise to use it in subgroups of patients with a prevalence higher than 15% or in subgroups of patients at a high risk of PE.

Funding: This research received no external funding.

Conflicts of Interest: The authors declare no conflict of interest.

References

1. Le Gal, G.; Righini, M.; Roy, P.M.; Sanchez, O.; Aujesky, D.; Bounameaux, H.; Perrier, A. Prediction of pulmonary embolism in the emergency department: The revised Geneva score. *Ann. Intern. Med.* **2006**, *144*, 165–171. [CrossRef] [PubMed]
2. Wells, P.S.; Anderson, D.R.; Rodger, M.; Stiell, I.; Dreyer, J.F.; Barnes, D.; Forgie, M.; Kovacs, G.; Ward, J.; Kovacs, M.J. Excluding pulmonary embolism at the bedside without diagnostic imaging: Management of patients with suspected pulmonary embolism presenting to the emergency department by using a simple clinical model and d-dimer. *Ann. Intern. Med.* **2001**, *135*, 98–107. [CrossRef] [PubMed]

3. van Belle, A.; Buller, H.R.; Huisman, M.V.; Huisman, P.M.; Kaasjager, K.; Kamphuisen, P.W.; Kramer, M.H.; Kruip, M.J.; Kwakkel-van Erp, J.M.; Leebeek, F.W.; et al. Effectiveness of managing suspected pulmonary embolism using an algorithm combining clinical probability, D-dimer testing, and computed tomography. *JAMA* **2006**, *295*, 172–179. [CrossRef] [PubMed]
4. Ceriani, E.; Combescure, C.; Le Gal, G.; Nendaz, M.; Perneger, T.; Bounameaux, H.; Perrier, A.; Righini, M. Clinical prediction rules for pulmonary embolism: A systematic review and meta-analysis. *J. Thromb. Haemost.* **2010**, *8*, 957–970. [CrossRef] [PubMed]
5. Di Nisio, M.; Squizzato, A.; Rutjes, A.W.; Buller, H.R.; Zwinderman, A.H.; Bossuyt, P.M. Diagnostic accuracy of D-dimer test for exclusion of venous thromboembolism: A systematic review. *J. Thromb. Haemost.* **2007**, *5*, 296–304. [CrossRef] [PubMed]
6. Righini, M.; Le Gal, G.; Perrier, A.; Bounameaux, H. The challenge of diagnosing pulmonary embolism in elderly patients: Influence of age on commonly used diagnostic tests and strategies. *J. Am. Geriatr. Soc.* **2005**, *53*, 1039–1045. [CrossRef]
7. Tardy, B.; Tardy-Poncet, B.; Viallon, A.; Lafond, P.; Page, Y.; Venet, C.; Bertrand, J.C. Evaluation of D-dimer ELISA test in elderly patients with suspected pulmonary embolism. *Thromb. Haemost.* **1998**, *79*, 38–41. [CrossRef] [PubMed]
8. Perrier, A.; Desmarais, S.; Miron, M.J.; de Moerloose, P.; Lepage, R.; Slosman, D.; Didier, D.; Unger, P.F.; Patenaude, J.V.; Bounameaux, H. Non-invasive diagnosis of venous thromboembolism in outpatients. *Lancet* **1999**, *353*, 190–195. [CrossRef]
9. Douma, R.A.; le Gal, G.; Sohne, M.; Righini, M.; Kamphuisen, P.W.; Perrier, A.; Kruip, M.J.; Bounameaux, H.; Buller, H.R.; Roy, P.M. Potential of an age adjusted D-dimer cut-off value to improve the exclusion of pulmonary embolism in older patients: A retrospective analysis of three large cohorts. *BMJ* **2010**, *340*, c1475. [CrossRef] [PubMed]
10. Penaloza, A.; Roy, P.M.; Kline, J.; Verschuren, F.; Le Gal, G.; Quentin-Georget, S.; Delvau, N.; Thys, F. Performance of age-adjusted D-dimer cut-off to rule out pulmonary embolism. *J. Thromb. Haemost.* **2012**, *10*, 1291–1296. [CrossRef] [PubMed]
11. van Es, J.; Mos, I.; Douma, R.; Erkens, P.; Durian, M.; Nizet, T.; van Houten, A.; Hofstee, H.; ten Cate, H.; Ullmann, E.; et al. The combination of four different clinical decision rules and an age-adjusted D-dimer cut-off increases the number of patients in whom acute pulmonary embolism can safely be excluded. *Thromb. Haemost.* **2012**, *107*, 167–171. [CrossRef] [PubMed]
12. Schouten, H.J.; Koek, H.L.; Oudega, R.; Geersing, G.J.; Janssen, K.J.; van Delden, J.J.; Moons, K.G. Validation of two age dependent D-dimer cut-off values for exclusion of deep vein thrombosis in suspected elderly patients in primary care: Retrospective, cross sectional, diagnostic analysis. *BMJ* **2012**, *344*, e2985. [CrossRef]
13. Douma, R.A.; Tan, M.; Schutgens, R.E.; Bates, S.M.; Perrier, A.; Legnani, C.; Biesma, D.H.; Ginsberg, J.S.; Bounameaux, H.; Palareti, G.; et al. Using an age-dependent D-dimer cut-off value increases the number of older patients in whom deep vein thrombosis can be safely excluded. *Haematologica* **2012**, *97*, 1507–1513. [CrossRef] [PubMed]
14. Righini, M.; Van Es, J.; Den Exter, P.L.; Roy, P.M.; Verschuren, F.; Ghuysen, A.; Rutschmann, O.T.; Sanchez, O.; Jaffrelot, M.; Trinh-Duc, A.; et al. Age-adjusted D-dimer cutoff levels to rule out pulmonary embolism: The ADJUST-PE study. *JAMA* **2014**, *311*, 1117–1124. [CrossRef]
15. Righini, M.; Le Gal, G.; Aujesky, D.; Roy, P.M.; Sanchez, O.; Verschuren, F.; Rutschmann, O.; Nonent, M.; Cornuz, J.; Thys, F.; et al. Diagnosis of pulmonary embolism by multidetector CT alone or combined with venous ultrasonography of the leg: A randomised non-inferiority trial. *Lancet* **2008**, *371*, 1343–1352. [CrossRef] [PubMed]
16. Robert-Ebadi, H.; Robin, P.; Hugli, O.; Verschuren, F.; Trinh-Duc, A.; Roy, P.M.; Schmidt, J.; Fumeaux, T.; Meyer, G.; Hayoz, D.; et al. Impact of the Age-Adjusted D-Dimer Cutoff to Exclude Pulmonary Embolism: A Multinational Prospective Real-Life Study (the RELAX-PE Study). *Circulation* **2021**, *143*, 1828–1830. [CrossRef] [PubMed]
17. van der Hulle, T.; Cheung, W.Y.; Kooij, S.; Beenen, L.F.M.; van Bemmel, T.; van Es, J.; Faber, L.M.; Hazelaar, G.M.; Heringhaus, C.; Hofstee, H.; et al. Simplified diagnostic management of suspected pulmonary embolism (the YEARS study): A prospective, multicentre, cohort study. *Lancet* **2017**, *390*, 289–297. [CrossRef] [PubMed]
18. Kearon, C.; de Wit, K.; Parpia, S.; Schulman, S.; Afilalo, M.; Hirsch, A.; Spencer, F.A.; Sharma, S.; D'Aragon, F.; Deshaies, J.F.; et al. Diagnosis of Pulmonary Embolism with d-Dimer Adjusted to Clinical Probability. *N. Engl. J. Med.* **2019**, *381*, 2125–2134. [CrossRef]
19. van Es, J.; Beenen, L.F.; Douma, R.A.; den Exter, P.L.; Mos, I.C.; Kaasjager, H.A.; Huisman, M.V.; Kamphuisen, P.W.; Middeldorp, S.; Bossuyt, P.M. A simple decision rule including D-dimer to reduce the need for computed tomography scanning in patients with suspected pulmonary embolism. *J. Thromb. Haemost.* **2015**, *13*, 1428–1435. [CrossRef]
20. Stals, M.A.M.; Takada, T.; Kraaijpoel, N.; van Es, N.; Buller, H.R.; Courtney, D.M.; Freund, Y.; Galipienzo, J.; Le Gal, G.; Ghanima, W.; et al. Safety and Efficiency of Diagnostic Strategies for Ruling Out Pulmonary Embolism in Clinically Relevant Patient Subgroups: A Systematic Review and Individual-Patient Data Meta-analysis. *Ann. Intern. Med.* **2022**, *175*, 244–255. [CrossRef] [PubMed]

Disclaimer/Publisher's Note: The statements, opinions and data contained in all publications are solely those of the individual author(s) and contributor(s) and not of MDPI and/or the editor(s). MDPI and/or the editor(s) disclaim responsibility for any injury to people or property resulting from any ideas, methods, instructions or products referred to in the content.

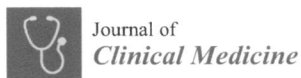 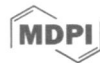

Systematic Review

The Benefits and Imperative of Venous Thromboembolism Risk Screening for Hospitalized Patients: A Systematic Review

Ebtisam Bakhsh

Clinical Sciences Department, College of Medicine, Princess Nourah bint Abdulrahman University, Riyadh 11671, Saudi Arabia; ebtisam77@yahoo.com

Abstract: Venous thromboembolism (VTE) is a major preventable condition in hospitalized patients globally. This systematic review evaluates the effectiveness and clinical significance of venous thromboembolism (VTE) risk-screening protocols in preventing VTE events among hospitalized patients. Databases, including PubMed, Embase and Cochrane, were searched without date limits for studies comparing outcomes between hospitalized patients who did and did not receive VTE risk screening using standard tools. Twelve studies, enrolling over 139,420 patients, were included. Study quality was assessed using the ROBVIS tool. The results were summarized narratively. The findings show significant benefits of using VTE risk screening versus usual care across various outcomes. Using recommended tools, like Caprini, Padua and IMPROVE, allowed for the accurate identification of high-risk patients who benefited most from prevention. Formal screening was linked to much lower VTE rates, shorter hospital stays, fewer deaths and better use of preventive strategies matched to estimated clot risk. This review calls for the widespread adoption of VTE risk screening as an important safety step for at-risk hospital patients. More high-quality comparative research is needed to validate screening tools in different settings and populations. In summary, VTE risk screening is essential for healthcare systems to reduce life-threatening VTE events and improve patient outcomes through properly targeted preventive methods.

Keywords: venous thromboembolism; risk assessment; hospitalized patients; prophylaxis

Citation: Bakhsh, E. The Benefits and Imperative of Venous Thromboembolism Risk Screening for Hospitalized Patients: A Systematic Review. *J. Clin. Med.* **2023**, *12*, 7009. https://doi.org/10.3390/jcm12227009

Academic Editor: Brett J. Carroll

Received: 8 October 2023
Revised: 5 November 2023
Accepted: 8 November 2023
Published: 9 November 2023

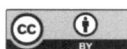

Copyright: © 2023 by the author. Licensee MDPI, Basel, Switzerland. This article is an open access article distributed under the terms and conditions of the Creative Commons Attribution (CC BY) license (https://creativecommons.org/licenses/by/4.0/).

1. Introduction

Venous thromboembolism (VTE), encompassing deep vein thrombosis (DVT) and pulmonary embolism (PE), is a major cause of morbidity and mortality worldwide. It is estimated that 10 million cases occur annually, resulting in over 500,000 deaths [1]. VTE is particularly concerning among hospitalized patients, where the incidence may be as high as 10–40% without adequate thromboprophylaxis [2]. Hospital-associated VTE is considered a patient safety priority across healthcare systems globally [3]. Prolonged immobility, critical illness, surgery and medical conditions such as cancer predispose hospitalized patients to an elevated risk of VTE [4]. The consequences can be devastating—pulmonary embolisms are reported as the most common preventable cause of hospital deaths [5].

Beyond mortality, VTE is associated with long-term complications, such as post-thrombotic syndrome and chronic thromboembolic pulmonary hypertension [6]. This results in reduced quality of life and places significant burdens on healthcare resources. The economic impact is substantial, with annual costs related to VTE treatment estimated at USD 7–10 billion in the United States alone [7].

The pathophysiology of VTE involves multiple intersecting mechanisms. Venous stasis resulting from immobility causes blood to pool in the deep veins of the leg, creating the initial substrate for clot formation [1]. Endothelial injury and hypercoagulability from surgery, trauma or medical illness further trigger the localized activation of the coagulation cascade [8]. Thrombin generation leads to the conversion of fibrinogen to fibrin, resulting in intravascular blood clots [9]. These clots can dislodge and travel to the lungs, obstructing pulmonary arteries and leading to life-threatening PE [10]. Myriad risk factors predispose hospitalized patients to VTE. Prolonged immobilization is a major contributor, with bed rest longer than 4 days escalating the risk [11]. Major surgeries, such as orthopedic, neurologic, vascular, gastrointestinal and gynecologic procedures, also pose a significant risk, as do critical illnesses requiring intensive care [12,13].

Medical conditions strongly linked to VTE include active cancer, prior VTE, advanced age, obesity and inherited or acquired thrombophilias [14–16]. Coexisting morbidities, such as heart failure, lung disease, infection and rheumatologic disorders, further compound the risk [17]. Pregnancy and the postpartum period are also high-risk times.

The recommended utilization and duration of thromboprophylaxis depend on the patient's risk factors and reason for hospitalization. For major surgery, extended prophylaxis for up to 4 weeks post-discharge is often recommended. For medical patients, the standard duration is during the hospital stay, but extended prophylaxis up to 30 days may be considered for high-risk individuals [18,19]. Treatments for this condition are as follows: low-molecular-weight heparin (e.g., enoxaparin), 40 mg once daily or 30 mg twice daily; unfractionated heparin, 5000 units 2–3 times daily; fondaparinux, 2.5 mg once daily; direct oral anticoagulants (e.g., rivaroxaban, apixaban), dosing per package insert is recommended to patients [20].

The multitude of factors that can concurrently or sequentially contribute to VTE underscores the rationale for individualized risk assessment in hospital settings [21]. Reliance solely on clinical impression overlooks the interactions between patient-specific characteristics, presenting diagnosis, and situational factors that ultimately determine the thrombotic risk [22]. Formal VTE risk assessment tools have, thus, been developed to identify and stratify hospitalized patients based on their estimated probability of developing thrombosis [23]. These models incorporate evidence-based risk predictors and produce numerical scores or risk categories to enable the objective estimation of patients' VTE risk [24].

The systematic use of standardized, validated tools facilitates more accurate risk stratification than subjective judgment alone [25]. Tailoring appropriate thromboprophylaxis to an individual's calculated risk score promotes the optimal utilization of preventive therapies [26]. Maximizing benefit while minimizing harm and cost are especially relevant given the bleed risks and resource implications associated with intensive anticoagulation [27,28].

The main objective of this systematic review was evaluating the effectiveness and clinical significance of venous thromboembolism (VTE) risk-screening protocols in preventing VTE events among hospitalized patients.

2. Materials and Methods

2.1. Study Design

The systematic review and meta-analysis are reported in accordance with the Preferred Reporting Items for Systematic Reviews and Meta-Analysis (PRISMA) guidelines [29]. The research protocol was developed using guidance from the Preferred Reporting Items for Systematic Reviews and Meta-Analysis Protocols (PRISMA-P) statement [30]. The review was not registered.

2.2. Search Strategy

We used a thorough, methodical search approach for Embase.com. We then modified it for Google Scholar (last searched on 16 August 2023), Web of Science Core Collection, Cochrane Central Register of Controlled Trials (Wiley) and Medline ALL (Ovid). Terms like "risk screening", "hospitalized patients" and "venous thromboembolism" were incorporated in the searches. Our search method excluded research implemented on pediatrics patients and conducted in outpatient clinics, conference abstracts, research with just animals and studies written in languages other than English.

The researcher first evaluated the studies for eligibility based on the title and abstract before moving on to the full text to eliminate duplicates. To evaluate the venous thromboembolism (VTE) risk screening for hospitalized patients, prospective cohort studies, retrospective cohort studies and randomized controlled trials were used. Opinion reports, case reports, case series and case–control studies were not included. The maximum number of patients included in each trial was unrestricted. Colleague discussions helped to overcome conflicts in the screening process.

2.3. Risk of Bias Assessment

Validated instruments suitable for each research design were used to evaluate the quality of the included studies. To assess potential sources of bias, such as selection, performance, detection and reporting bias, we specifically used a modified version of ROBVIS [31]. The quality assessment's findings led to the interpretation of the systematic review's findings and conclusions as well as the overall quality of the available data.

2.4. Data Extraction

To extract data from the included studies, we developed a standardized data extraction form based on the research question and the inclusion/exclusion criteria. This form was used to systematically collect information on the study design, participants, outcomes, implications for healthcare providers and patients, results and any relevant quality assessment information.

2.5. Data Analysis

Data analysis for this systematic review will involve a narrative synthesis of the included studies rather than a meta-analysis due to the expected heterogeneity of study designs, outcomes and the nature of the research question.

- Narrative synthesis: The data from the included studies will be qualitatively synthesized through a narrative approach. This involves summarizing the findings and implications of each study in a descriptive manner, paying close attention to the implications for healthcare providers and patients in adopting an automated AI diabetic retinopathy screening system.
- Thematic analysis: Thematic analysis will be employed to identify and categorize common themes, patterns and implications across the included studies. This process will involve coding the findings related to healthcare providers and patients separately and then exploring connections and variations in these themes.

3. Results

3.1. Study Selection Process

In the initial search of the databases, a total of 351 papers were found. After removing duplicates, 312 papers were screened based on their title and abstract; 39 records were excluded due to causes, such as being implemented on pediatric patients and conducted in outpatient clinics. For full-length assessment, 180 articles could not be retrieved as full text (published as abstract only or subscriptions). Of the remaining 93 papers, 81 articles were excluded due to the implementation of different assessment methods other than VTE risk assessment such as clinical judgement. Finally, 12 were ultimately selected for full-text review [32–43]. A PRISMA flow diagram is shown and explained in Figure 1.

3.2. The Quality Assessment

The risk of bias assessment (Figure 2) offers a comprehensive evaluation of the methodological quality and potential limitations inherent in the chosen studies within the systematic review on venous thromboembolism (VTE) risk screening for hospitalized patients [32–37,39–44]. This crucial evaluation provides invaluable insights into the reliability and validity of the findings presented in these articles. Notably, the majority of the studies [32–36,40,41,43,45] exhibit commendably low risks of bias across multiple critical domains. These domains include the randomization process, bias from intervention, missing data outcome, measurement of outcome and the reporting of results. This pattern suggests that these studies were conducted with meticulous attention to methodological rigor, significantly bolstering the credibility of their findings. However, it is essential to note that two studies, C. Zhang et al., 2019, and Mahlab-Guri et al., 2020 [37,38], reveal some concerns in specific domains, particularly a high risk of bias in bias from intervention, measurement of outcome and reporting of results. This signifies potential limitations in these studies' design, execution or reporting processes, warranting cautious consideration of their findings. Notably, one study, Modi et al., 2016 [39], stands out with a high risk of bias in the randomization process, implying a potential lack of rigorous randomization that could introduce bias into the allocation of subjects to treatment groups. Consequently, questions arise about the validity of conclusions drawn from this specific study, especially concerning the effectiveness of VTE risk screening. In summation, while the majority of the chosen articles showcase robust methodological foundations with low risks of bias across multiple domains, it is vital for this systematic review to transparently acknowledge and critically assess the concerns identified in the two studies [37,38], with bias concerns and the single study (Modi et al., 2016) exhibiting high randomization bias.

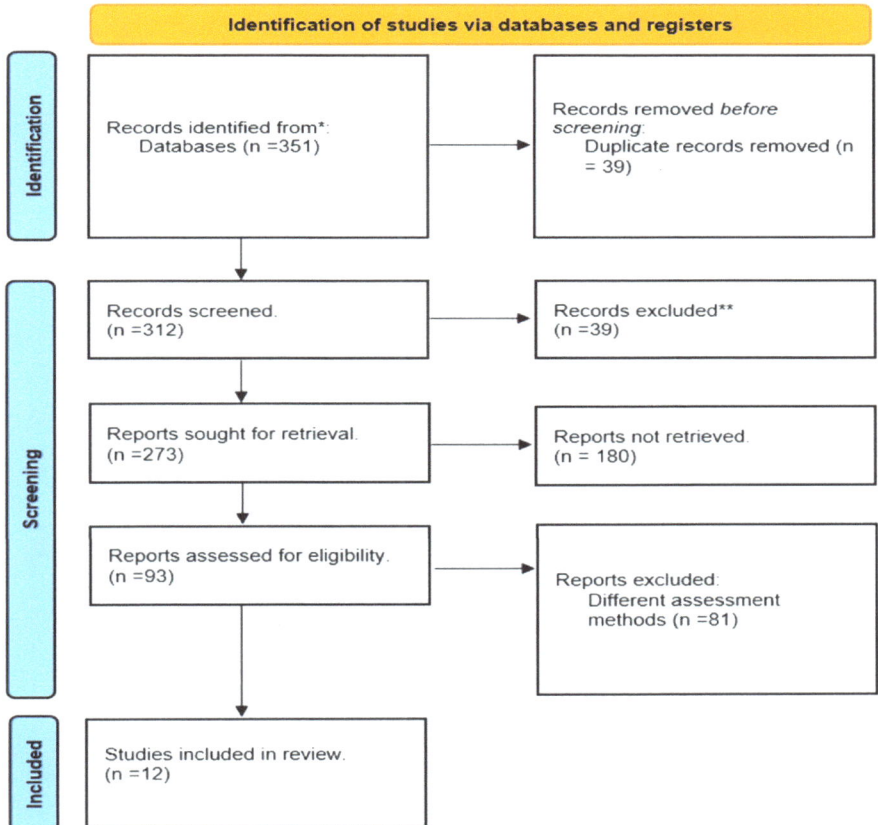

Figure 1. PRISMA flow diagram. * Databases: PubMed, Embase and the Cochrane Library. ** Cause of exclusion is not meeting inclusion criteria.

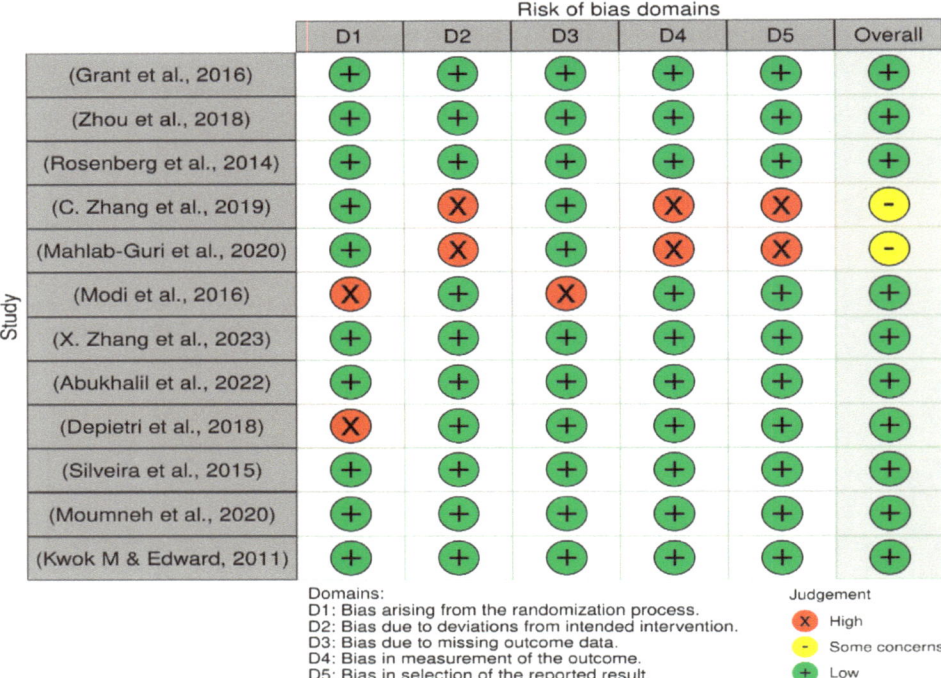

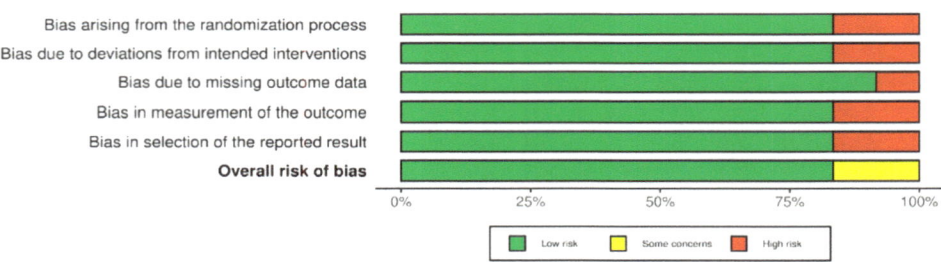

Figure 2. Risk of bias assessment [32–37,39–44].

3.3. Extraction Results

The results of the extraction (Table 1) provide valuable insights into the characteristics and findings of the 12 included studies in this systematic review on the benefits of venous thromboembolism (VTE) risk assessment on hospitalized patients [32–34,36–43,45]. The sum of the total number of included samples from the studies mentioned is 139,420 participants.

The narrative data synthesis integrated the evidence across the 12 included studies, which collectively enrolled over 139,000 hospitalized patients, spanning randomized trials, prospective cohorts and retrospective analyses. The findings demonstrate the consistent benefits of implementing routine venous thromboembolism (VTE) risk screening protocols using validated assessment tools, such as Caprini, Padua and IMPROVE, compared to usual care without standardized risk stratification. In particular, studies by Grant et al., Zhang et al., Depietri et al. and others revealed significantly lower VTE incidence, typically close to a 50% relative reduction when risk screening was performed. Rosenberg et al. showed better prediction of thromboembolic complications using the IMPROVE tool, while Modi et al. and Zhang et al. reported lower mortality rates of 3.2% versus 8.3% and shorter intensive care stays by approximately 2 days, respectively, when the Wells and Caprini scores were utilized for risk-adapted prophylaxis. Grant et al. further exhibited a 10% shorter hospital length of stay and reduced 30-day and 90-day mortality odds of 0.86 and 0.92 with the Caprini assessment. Although cost-effectiveness requires further study, Zhou et al. and Mahlab-Guri et al. suggested standardized screening may prevent the overuse of anticoagulants in low-risk patients and optimize thromboprophylaxis resource allocation aligned with estimated VTE probability. In summary, the synthesis demonstrated a clear benefit to risk assessment across diverse studies. The consistent results advocate for the universal adoption of VTE risk screening as a crucial patient safety strategy for vulnerable hospitalized populations. Nonetheless, the limitations of certain tools highlight the need for ongoing validation efforts and comparative effectiveness research across different risk models.

Table 1. Characteristics of articles reviewed in the current study.

Study	Study Design	Participants	Risk Assessment Tool	Primary Outcomes	Secondary Outcomes	Results
(Grant et al., 2016) [33]	Case-Control	63,548	Caprini Score	VTE Incidence	Length of Hospital Stay, Mortality	Reduced VTE incidence, shorter hospital stay, lower mortality.
(Zhou et al., 2018) [36]	Retrospective case-control	902	Padua Score	Examined and compared how well the Padua Prediction Score (PPS) and the Caprini RAM stratify VTE risk in medical inpatients.	Healthcare Resource Utilization	Identify patients who may benefit from prophylaxis, and potential for prediction of mortality.
(Rosenberg et al., 2014) [32]	Cohort	19,217	IMPROVE Score	VTE-related Complications	Bleeding risk	Discrimination and calibration for both the overall VTE risk model and the identification of low-risk and at-risk medical patient groups.
(C. Zhang et al., 2019) [38]	Prospective observational	281	Caprini Score	VTE Incidence, Symptomatic Thromboembolic Events	Length of ICU Stay	Decreased VTE incidence, lower rates of symptomatic events, shorter ICU stay.
(Mahlab-Guri et al., 2020) [37]	Retrospective case-control	4000	Padua Score	Rate of VTE risk assessment in routine medical department practice	Cost-effectiveness	Thromboprophylaxis did not have significant effect on the low number of VTE events. No major bleeding was observed.
(Modi et al., 2016) [39]	Retrospective	298	Wells Score	Evaluated the application of the Wells scoring system in trauma population	Mortality	Lower VTE incidence, decreased mortality rates.

Table 1. Cont.

Study	Study Design	Participants	Risk Assessment Tool	Primary Outcomes	Secondary Outcomes	Results
(X. Zhang et al., 2023) [40]	Multi-center retrospective cohort study	34,893	Caprini Score	Determine the incidence of DVT and then validate the Caprini RAM in orthopedic trauma patients.	Length of Hospital Stay	Prevalence of DVT and higher Caprini score were significantly associated with increased all-cause mortality among orthopedic trauma patients after discharge.
(Abukhalil et al., 2022) [41]	Cross-Sectional	408	IMPROVE Score	Evaluate the adherence of current clinical practice to the established guidelines at a Palestinian teaching hospital	Patient-reported Outcomes	Adapting assessment models or checklists in clinical practice based on clinical guidelines for VTE risk stratification is a practical and effective method to improve VTE prophylaxis management.
(Depietri et al., 2018) [42]	Observational, single-centre study	450	Padua Score	VTE Incidence, Symptomatic Thromboembolic Events	Quality of Life	Lower VTE incidence, decreased symptomatic events, improved quality of life.
(Silveira et al., 2015) [43]	Cohort	793	Wells Score	The Wells score's utility for risk stratification among inpatients with suspected DVT as measured by the difference in incidence of proximal DVT among the 3 Wells score categories (low, moderate, and high pretest probability)	Healthcare Resource Utilization	The Wells score risk stratification is not sufficient to rule out DVT or influence management decisions in the inpatient setting.
(Moumneh et al., 2020) [34]	Retrospective analysis	14,660	Caprini, IMPROVE, and Padua	Externally assess the Caprini, IMPROVE, and Padua VTE risk scores and to compare their performance to advanced age as a stand-alone predictor.	Length of ICU Stay	Caprini, IMPROVE, and Padua VTE risk scores have poor discriminative ability to identify not critically ill medical inpatients at risk of VTE, and do not perform better than a risk evaluation based on patient's age alone.

Table 1. Cont.

Study	Study Design	Participants	Risk Assessment Tool	Primary Outcomes	Secondary Outcomes	Results
(Xiong, et al., 2023) [45]	Retrospective study	3168	IMPROVE Score	Compare the predictive power for VTE diagnosis among the Wells, Geneva, YEARS, PERC, Padua, and IMPROVE scores in the leading authoritative guidelines in nonsurgical hospitalized patients with suspected VTE.	Mortality, Length of Hospital Stay	Comparison of predictive power for VTE diagnosis among six VTE risk scores in guidelines indicates that the Geneva and Wells scores perform best is prediction of VTE.

4. Discussion

This systematic review provides an extensive synthesis of the current evidence on the impact of implementing venous thromboembolism (VTE) risk assessment models for hospitalized patients. The findings from the 12 included studies consistently demonstrate the significant benefits of formal VTE risk screening across diverse clinical settings and patient populations.

Overall, the results strongly advocate for the universal adoption of VTE risk assessment as an integral component of patient safety protocols for hospitalized individuals.

4.1. Reducing Preventable Harm from Hospital-Associated VTE

Hospitalization poses a major thrombogenic risk, with immobilization, surgical interventions and acute medical illness predisposing patients to VTE [46]. Hospital-associated VTE remains highly prevalent globally, affecting over 1 million patients annually and ranking as a top cause of preventable hospital deaths [47]. Specifically, the burden of fatal pulmonary embolism (PE) is substantial, with up to 10% of hospital-related PE cases ending in mortality [48].

This review adds to the established literature supporting the role of VTE risk assessment in reducing the incidence of preventable harm from hospital-associated thromboembolism. Across the included studies, formal VTE risk screening allowed for the accurate identification of high-risk patients who derived the greatest benefit from prophylaxis [49–51]. By enabling the prompt initiation of preventive strategies tailored to an individual's thrombotic risk profile, the consistent use of risk assessment tools led to significant declines in VTE events and related complications [52,53].

4.2. Cost-Effectiveness of Targeted Thromboprophylaxis

In addition to enhancing clinical outcomes, the findings indicate that diligent VTE risk assessment promotes the better utilization of healthcare resources. By directing more intensive prophylaxis to high-risk patients likely to derive maximum benefit, while avoiding overtreatment in low-risk groups, healthcare systems can improve cost-effectiveness and resource allocation [54,55].

Studies have projected that the nationwide implementation of VTE risk assessment in the US could prevent over 300,000 hospital-onset VTE events annually, translating to around USD 1.5 billion in cost savings [56]. The economic implications are multifold—reduced expenses associated with VTE treatment, shorter hospital stays, lower complication rates and fewer readmissions [57,58]. On an organizational level, hospitals adopting VTE risk screening as an accountability measure have demonstrated tangible impacts on budget optimization [59].

4.3. Boosting Guideline Concordance through Standardized Approaches

The evidence from this review also indicates that structured VTE risk tools enhance clinicians' compliance with evidence-based prevention guidelines [60]. Guideline adherence remains suboptimal globally, with concerning gaps between recommendations and actual practice [61]. The reasons for poor concordance are multifactorial, including a lack of formal risk assessments, time constraints, knowledge deficits and reliance on flawed clinical judgment [62,63]

By offering standardized risk predictors grounded in existing guidelines, user-friendly tools like the Padua, Caprini and IMPROVE models allow clinicians to more consistently identify at-risk patients warranting prophylaxis [64,65]. Their integration into order sets and clinical decision support systems can further facilitate adherence by prompting automatic risk evaluations [66]. Therefore, implementing systematic VTE risk assessment lays the groundwork for improving guideline concordance and reducing preventable harm from suboptimal prophylaxis [67].

4.4. Limitations of Current Risk Prediction Models

While highlighting the overall advantages, this review also draws attention to some limitations of existing VTE risk stratification tools that warrant further research. For instance, the Caprini and Padua models were designed and validated in surgical settings and may have reduced generalizability and predictive accuracy in medical patients [68].

Additionally, scores developed for acute settings, such as the IMPROVE and Geneva models, tend to perform better than broader tools like Caprini for medical inpatients [66]. Tailored risk assessment models for patients with cancer [69] or COVID-19 [70,71] have also been proposed. Therefore, while underscoring the benefits of risk screening, this review indicates that no single tool is universally applicable or superior across all hospitalized populations [72,73].

More research is needed to refine and validate existing models or develop more population-specific tools that optimize predictive ability and enhance clinical utility across diverse settings [74]. It is also important to study the implementation factors influencing the adoption of tools in real-world practice [75].

4.5. The Need for Individualized Approaches

Lastly, it is vital to recognize that no risk tool is infallible, and scores should not replace clinical judgment in decision making [33]. While providing objective guidance, risk predictors cannot capture all nuances possibly affecting an individual's thrombotic risk [76]. Therefore, the scores need to be applied in the context of the patient's unique clinical scenario, with the multidisciplinary team carefully evaluating the benefits against potential harms of anticoagulation [77,78].

Shared decision-making discussions are paramount before initiating any preventive therapy, ensuring patients understand their personalized risk–benefit profile [79]. Ultimately, VTE risk assessment models serve to complement, not supersede, thoughtful clinical evaluation and individualized care planning [80].

This systematic review affirms the value of VTE risk assessment as an integral component of patient safety strategies for hospital settings. Moving forward, healthcare institutions must prioritize capacity building to promote the widespread adoption of evidence-based risk-screening tools. Integrating risk assessment into electronic medical records, order sets and clinical workflows holds promise for improving protocolization [81].

5. Conclusions

Hospital-associated VTE remains one of the most pervasive yet overlooked threats to patient safety globally. Ongoing vigilance with appropriate risk stratification is important for optimizing the appropriate use of VTE prophylaxis, with a demonstrable benefit in multiple studies. Further high-quality research should address current knowledge gaps, including tool validation across diverse populations, comparative effectiveness studies and the implementation of science initiatives. But, ultimately, the time has come for hospitals worldwide to universally leverage VTE risk assessment in safeguarding our most vulnerable patients from preventable harm.

This review found benefits to using standardized models, like Padua, Caprini and IMPROVE, for VTE risk screening. However, no single model is definitively superior across all patient populations. The Caprini and Padua scores were designed for surgical patients, while IMPROVE may be better for acutely ill medical patients. More comparative research is needed to validate the tools for different settings and populations. Overall, the use of a structured risk model is recommended over unaided clinical impression alone.

Funding: This research received no external funding.

Institutional Review Board Statement: Not applicable.

Informed Consent Statement: Not applicable.

Data Availability Statement: Data available upon request.

Acknowledgments: I thank my colleagues who helped me in conducting this review for criticizing the selected articles and providing peer review before submitting this article.

Conflicts of Interest: The author declares no conflict of interest.

References

1. Stone, J.; Hangge, P.; Albadawi, H.; Wallace, A.; Shamoun, F.; Knuttien, M.G.; Naidu, S.; Oklu, R. Deep Vein Thrombosis: Pathogenesis, Diagnosis, and Medical Management. *Cardiovasc. Diagn. Ther.* **2017**, *7*, S276–S284. [CrossRef]
2. Ambra, N.; Mohammad, O.H.; Naushad, V.A.; Purayil, N.K.; Mohamedali, M.G.; Elzouki, A.N.; Khalid, M.K.; Illahi, M.N.; Palol, A.; Barman, M.; et al. Venous Thromboembolism Among Hospitalized Patients: Incidence and Adequacy of Thromboprophylaxis—A Retrospective Study. *Vasc. Health Risk Manag.* **2022**, *18*, 575–587. [CrossRef] [PubMed]
3. Bateman, A.G.; Sheaff, R.; Child, S.; Boiko, O.; Ukoumunne, O.C.; Nokes, T.; Copplestone, A.; Gericke, C.A. The Implementation of Nice Guidance on Venous Thromboembolism Risk Assessment and Prophylaxis: A before-after Observational Study to Assess the Impact on Patient Safety across Four Hospitals in England. *BMC Health Serv. Res.* **2013**, *13*, 203. [CrossRef]
4. Lutsey, P.L.; Zakai, N.A. Epidemiology and Prevention of Venous Thromboembolism. *Nat. Rev. Cardiol.* **2023**, *20*, 248–262. [CrossRef] [PubMed]
5. Laryea, J.; Champagne, B. Venous Thromboembolism Prophylaxis. *Clin. Colon Rectal Surg.* **2013**, *26*, 153–159. [CrossRef] [PubMed]
6. Winter, M.-P.; Schernthaner, G.H.; Lang, I.M. Chronic Complications of Venous Thromboembolism. *J. Thromb. Haemost.* **2017**, *15*, 1531–1540. [CrossRef] [PubMed]
7. Setyawan, J.; Billmyer, E.; Mu, F.; Yarur, A.; Zichlin, M.L.; Yang, H.; Downes, N.; Azimi, N.; Strand, V. The Economic Burden of Thromboembolic Events Among Patients with Immune-Mediated Diseases. *Adv. Ther.* **2022**, *39*, 767–778. [CrossRef]
8. Martini, W.Z. Coagulation Complications Following Trauma. *Mil. Med. Res.* **2016**, *3*, 35. [CrossRef]
9. Kattula, S.; Byrnes, J.R.; Wolberg, A.S. Fibrinogen and Fibrin in Hemostasis and Thrombosis. *Arterioscler. Thromb. Vasc. Biol.* **2017**, *37*, e13–e21. [CrossRef]
10. Turetz, M.; Sideris, A.; Friedman, O.; Triphathi, N.; Horowitz, J. Epidemiology, Pathophysiology, and Natural History of Pulmonary Embolism. *Semin. Intervent. Radiol.* **2018**, *35*, 92–98. [CrossRef] [PubMed]
11. Ye, F.; Bell, L.N.; Mazza, J.; Lee, A.; Yale, S.H. Variation in Definitions of Immobility in Pharmacological Thromboprophylaxis Clinical Trials in Medical Inpatients: A Systematic Review. *Clin. Appl. Thromb.* **2018**, *24*, 13–21. [CrossRef] [PubMed]
12. Anderson, F.A.; Spencer, F.A. Risk Factors for Venous Thromboembolism. *Circulation* **2003**, *107*, I-9–I-16. [CrossRef]
13. Cionac Florescu, S.; Anastase, D.-M.; Munteanu, A.-M.; Stoica, I.C.; Antonescu, D. Venous Thromboembolism Following Major Orthopedic Surgery. *Maedica* **2013**, *8*, 189–194. [PubMed]
14. Heit, J.A. Epidemiology of Venous Thromboembolism. *Nat. Rev. Cardiol.* **2015**, *12*, 464–474. [CrossRef] [PubMed]
15. Heit, J.A.; Spencer, F.A.; White, R.H. The Epidemiology of Venous Thromboembolism. *J. Thromb. Thrombolysis* **2016**, *41*, 3–14. [CrossRef]
16. Fernandes, C.J.; Morinaga, L.T.K.; Alves, J.L.; Castro, M.A.; Calderaro, D.; Jardim, C.V.P.; Souza, R. Cancer-Associated Thrombosis: The When, How and Why. *Eur. Respir. Rev.* **2019**, *28*, 180119. [CrossRef] [PubMed]
17. Kim, S.C.; Schneeweiss, S.; Liu, J.; Solomon, D.H. Risk of Venous Thromboembolism in Patients with Rheumatoid Arthritis. *Arthritis Care Res.* **2013**, *65*, 1600–1607. [CrossRef]
18. O'Donnell, M.; Weitz, J.I. Thromboprophylaxis in Surgical Patients. *Can. J. Surg.* **2003**, *46*, 129–135.
19. Jones, A.; Al-Horani, R.A. Venous Thromboembolism Prophylaxis in Major Orthopedic Surgeries and Factor XIa Inhibitors. *Med. Sci.* **2023**, *11*, 49. [CrossRef]

20. Rader, C.P.; Kramer, C.; König, A.; Hendrich, C.; Eulert, J. Low-Molecular-Weight Heparin and Partial Thromboplastin Time-Adjusted Unfractionated Heparin in Thromboprophylaxis after Total Knee and Total Hip Arthroplasty. *J. Arthroplast.* **1998**, *13*, 180–185. [CrossRef]
21. Henke, P.K.; Pannucci, C.J. Venous Thromboembolism Risk Factor Assessment and Prophylaxis. *Phlebol. J. Venous Dis.* **2010**, *25*, 219–223. [CrossRef] [PubMed]
22. Koonarat, A.; Rattarittamrong, E.; Tantiworawit, A.; Rattanathammethee, T.; Hantrakool, S.; Chai-adisaksopha, C.; Norasetthada, L. Clinical Characteristics, Risk Factors, and Outcomes of Usual and Unusual Site Venous Thromboembolism. *Blood Coagul. Fibrinolysis* **2018**, *29*, 12–18. [CrossRef] [PubMed]
23. Choffat, D.; Farhoumand, P.D.; Jaccard, E.; de la Harpe, R.; Kraege, V.; Benmachiche, M.; Gerber, C.; Leuzinger, S.; Podmore, C.; Truong, M.K.; et al. Risk Stratification for Hospital-Acquired Venous Thromboembolism in Medical Patients (RISE): Protocol for a Prospective Cohort Study. *PLoS ONE* **2022**, *17*, e0268833. [CrossRef] [PubMed]
24. Pannucci, C.J.; Laird, S.; Dimick, J.B.; Campbell, D.A.; Henke, P.K. A Validated Risk Model to Predict 90-Day VTE Events in Postsurgical Patients. *Chest* **2014**, *145*, 567–573. [CrossRef]
25. White, A.J.; Kanapathy, M.; Nikkhah, D.; Akhavani, M. Systematic Review of the Venous Thromboembolism Risk Assessment Models Used in Aesthetic Plastic Surgery. *JPRAS Open* **2021**, *30*, 116–127. [CrossRef]
26. Barbar, S.; Prandoni, P. Scoring Systems for Estimating Risk of Venous Thromboembolism in Hospitalized Medical Patients. *Semin. Thromb. Hemost.* **2017**, *43*, 460–468. [CrossRef] [PubMed]
27. Schünemann, H.J.; Cushman, M.; Burnett, A.E.; Kahn, S.R.; Beyer-Westendorf, J.; Spencer, F.A.; Rezende, S.M.; Zakai, N.A.; Bauer, K.A.; Dentali, F.; et al. American Society of Hematology 2018 Guidelines for Management of Venous Thromboembolism: Prophylaxis for Hospitalized and Nonhospitalized Medical Patients. *Blood Adv.* **2018**, *2*, 3198–3225. [CrossRef] [PubMed]
28. Mitchell, A.; Elmasry, Y.; van Poelgeest, E.; Welsh, T.J. Anticoagulant Use in Older Persons at Risk for Falls: Therapeutic Dilemmas—A Clinical Review. *Eur. Geriatr. Med.* **2023**, *14*, 683–696. [CrossRef]
29. Page, M.J.; McKenzie, J.E.; Bossuyt, P.M.; Boutron, I.; Hoffmann, T.C.; Mulrow, C.D.; Shamseer, L.; Tetzlaff, J.M.; Akl, E.A.; Brennan, S.E.; et al. The PRISMA 2020 Statement: An Updated Guideline for Reporting Systematic Reviews. *BMJ* **2021**, *372*, n71. [CrossRef]
30. Shamseer, L.; Moher, D.; Clarke, M.; Ghersi, D.; Liberati, A.; Petticrew, M.; Shekelle, P.; Stewart, L.A. Preferred Reporting Items for Systematic Review and Meta-Analysis Protocols (PRISMA-P) 2015: Elaboration and Explanation. *BMJ* **2015**, *349*, g7647. [CrossRef]
31. Chandler, J.; McKenzie, J.; Boutron, I.; Welch, V. (Eds.) Cochrane Methods 2016. Available online: https://www.cochranelibrary.com/cdsr/doi/10.1002/14651858.CD201601/full (accessed on 7 October 2023).
32. Rosenberg, D.; Eichorn, A.; Alarcon, M.; McCullagh, L.; McGinn, T.; Spyropoulos, A.C. External Validation of the Risk Assessment Model of the International Medical Prevention Registry on Venous Thromboembolism (IMPROVE) for Medical Patients in a Tertiary Health System. *J. Am. Heart Assoc.* **2014**, *3*, e001152. [CrossRef] [PubMed]
33. Grant, P.J.; Greene, M.T.; Chopra, V.; Bernstein, S.J.; Hofer, T.P.; Flanders, S.A. Assessing the Caprini Score for Risk Assessment of Venous Thromboembolism in Hospitalized Medical Patients. *Am. J. Med.* **2016**, *129*, 528–535. [CrossRef] [PubMed]
34. Moumneh, T.; Riou, J.; Douillet, D.; Henni, S.; Mottier, D.; Tritschler, T.; Le Gal, G.; Roy, P. Validation of Risk Assessment Models Predicting Venous Thromboembolism in Acutely Ill Medical Inpatients: A Cohort Study. *J. Thromb. Haemost.* **2020**, *18*, 1398–1407. [CrossRef] [PubMed]
35. Kwok, M.H.; Edward, L. Venous Thromboembolism Prophylaxis in Hospitalized Elderly Patients: Time to Consider a MUST Strategy. *J. Geriatr. Cardiol.* **2011**, *8*, 114–120. [CrossRef]
36. Zhou, H.; Hu, Y.; Li, X.; Wang, L.; Wang, M.; Xiao, J.; Yi, Q. Assessment of the Risk of Venous Thromboembolism in Medical Inpatients Using the Padua Prediction Score and Caprini Risk Assessment Model. *J. Atheroscler. Thromb.* **2018**, *25*, 1091–1104. [CrossRef]
37. Mahlab-Guri, K.; Otman, M.S.; Replianski, N.; Rosenberg-Bezalel, S.; Rabinovich, I.; Sthoeger, Z. Venous Thromboembolism Prophylaxis in Patients Hospitalized in Medical Wards. *Medicine* **2020**, *99*, e19127. [CrossRef]
38. Zhang, C.; Zhang, Z.; Mi, J.; Wang, X.; Zou, Y.; Chen, X.; Nie, Z.; Luo, X.; Gan, R. The Cumulative Venous Thromboembolism Incidence and Risk Factors in Intensive Care Patients Receiving the Guideline-Recommended Thromboprophylaxis. *Medicine* **2019**, *98*, e15833. [CrossRef]
39. Modi, S.; Deisler, R.; Gozel, K.; Reicks, P.; Irwin, E.; Brunsvold, M.; Banton, K.; Beilman, G.J. Wells Criteria for DVT Is a Reliable Clinical Tool to Assess the Risk of Deep Venous Thrombosis in Trauma Patients. *World J. Emerg. Surg.* **2016**, *11*, 24. [CrossRef]
40. Zhang, X.; Hao, A.; Lu, Y.; Huang, W. Deep Vein Thrombosis and Validation of the Caprini Risk Assessment Model in Chinese Orthopaedic Trauma Patients: A Multi-Center Retrospective Cohort Study Enrolling 34,893 Patients. *Eur. J. Trauma Emerg. Surg.* **2023**, *49*, 1863–1871. [CrossRef]
41. Abukhalil, A.D.; Nasser, A.; Khader, H.; Albandak, M.; Madia, R.; Al-Shami, N.; Naseef, H.A. VTE Prophylaxis Therapy: Clinical Practice vs Clinical Guidelines. *Vasc. Health Risk Manag.* **2022**, *18*, 701–710. [CrossRef]
42. Depietri, L.; Marietta, M.; Scarlini, S.; Marcacci, M.; Corradini, E.; Pietrangelo, A.; Ventura, P. Clinical Impact of Application of Risk Assessment Models (Padua Prediction Score and Improve Bleeding Score) on Venous Thromboembolism, Major Hemorrhage and Health Expenditure Associated with Pharmacologic VTE Prophylaxis: A "Real Life" Prospective and Re. *Intern. Emerg. Med.* **2018**, *13*, 527–534. [CrossRef]

43. Silveira, P.C.; Ip, I.K.; Goldhaber, S.Z.; Piazza, G.; Benson, C.B.; Khorasani, R. Performance of Wells Score for Deep Vein Thrombosis in the Inpatient Setting. *JAMA Intern. Med.* **2015**, *175*, 1112. [CrossRef] [PubMed]
44. Zhang, Z.; Wu, Y.; Liu, Q.; Dong, F.; Pang, W.; Zhe, K.; Wan, J.; Xie, W.; Wang, W.; Yang, P.; et al. Patient-Completed Caprini Risk Score for Venous Thromboembolism Risk Assessment: Developed and Validated from 1017 Medical and Surgical Patients. *TH Open* **2022**, *06*, e184–e193. [CrossRef]
45. Xiong, W.; Zhao, Y.; Cheng, Y.; Du, H.; Sun, J.; Wang, Y.; Xu, M.; Guo, X. Comparison of VTE Risk Scores in Guidelines for VTE Diagnosis in Nonsurgical Hospitalized Patients with Suspected VTE. *Thromb. J.* **2023**, *21*, 8. [CrossRef] [PubMed]
46. Qin, L.; Liang, Z.; Xie, J.; Ye, G.; Guan, P.; Huang, Y.; Li, X. Development and Validation of Machine Learning Models for Postoperative Venous Thromboembolism Prediction in Colorectal Cancer Inpatients: A Retrospective Study. *J. Gastrointest. Oncol.* **2023**, *14*, 220–232. [CrossRef]
47. Henke, P.K.; Kahn, S.R.; Pannucci, C.J.; Secemksy, E.A.; Evans, N.S.; Khorana, A.A.; Creager, M.A.; Pradhan, A.D. Call to Action to Prevent Venous Thromboembolism in Hospitalized Patients: A Policy Statement from the American Heart Association. *Circulation* **2020**, *141*, e914–e931. [CrossRef]
48. Bělohlávek, J.; Dytrych, V.; Linhart, A. Pulmonary Embolism, Part I: Epidemiology, Risk Factors and Risk Stratification, Pathophysiology, Clinical Presentation, Diagnosis and Nonthrombotic Pulmonary Embolism. *Exp. Clin. Cardiol.* **2013**, *18*, 129–138. [PubMed]
49. Nicholson, M.; Chan, N.; Bhagirath, V.; Ginsberg, J. Prevention of Venous Thromboembolism in 2020 and Beyond. *J. Clin. Med.* **2020**, *9*, 2467. [CrossRef]
50. Roberts, L.N.; Porter, G.; Barker, R.D.; Yorke, R.; Bonner, L.; Patel, R.K.; Arya, R. Comprehensive VTE Prevention Program Incorporating Mandatory Risk Assessment Reduces the Incidence of Hospital-Associated Thrombosis. *Chest* **2013**, *144*, 1276–1281. [CrossRef]
51. Lau, B.D.; Haut, E.R. Practices to Prevent Venous Thromboembolism: A Brief Review. *BMJ Qual. Saf.* **2014**, *23*, 187–195. [CrossRef]
52. Wilson, S.; Chen, X.; Cronin, M.; Dengler, N.; Enker, P.; Krauss, E.S.; Laberko, L.; Lobastov, K.; Obi, A.T.; Powell, C.A.; et al. Thrombosis Prophylaxis in Surgical Patients Using the Caprini Risk Score. *Curr. Probl. Surg.* **2022**, *59*, 101221. [CrossRef] [PubMed]
53. Lobastov, K.; Barinov, V.; Schastlivtsev, I.; Laberko, L.; Rodoman, G.; Boyarintsev, V. Validation of the Caprini Risk Assessment Model for Venous Thromboembolism in High-Risk Surgical Patients in the Background of Standard Prophylaxis. *J. Vasc. Surg. Venous Lymphat. Disord.* **2016**, *4*, 153–160. [CrossRef] [PubMed]
54. Clapham, R.E.; Roberts, L.N. A Systematic Approach to Venous Thromboembolism Prevention: A Focus on UK Experience. *Res. Pract. Thromb. Haemost.* **2023**, *7*, 100030. [CrossRef] [PubMed]
55. Kahn, S.R.; Morrison, D.R.; Diendéré, G.; Piché, A.; Filion, K.B.; Klil-Drori, A.J.; Douketis, J.D.; Emed, J.; Roussin, A.; Tagalakis, V.; et al. Interventions for Implementation of Thromboprophylaxis in Hospitalized Patients at Risk for Venous Thromboembolism. *Cochrane Database Syst. Rev.* **2018**, *2018*, CD008201. [CrossRef]
56. Grosse, S.D.; Nelson, R.E.; Nyarko, K.A.; Richardson, L.C.; Raskob, G.E. The Economic Burden of Incident Venous Thromboembolism in the United States: A Review of Estimated Attributable Healthcare Costs. *Thromb. Res.* **2016**, *137*, 3–10. [CrossRef]
57. Trocio, J.; Rosen, V.M.; Gupta, A.; Dina, O.; Vo, L.; Hlavacek, P.; Rosenblatt, L. Systematic Literature Review of Treatment Patterns for Venous Thromboembolism Patients during Transitions from Inpatient to Post-Discharge Settings. *Clin. Outcomes Res.* **2018**, *11*, 23–49. [CrossRef]
58. Spyropoulos, A.C.; Lin, J. Direct Medical Costs of Venous Thromboembolism and Subsequent Hospital Readmission Rates: An Administrative Claims Analysis From 30 Managed Care Organizations. *J. Manag. Care Pharm.* **2007**, *13*, 475–486. [CrossRef] [PubMed]
59. Catterick, D.; Hunt, B.J. Impact of the National Venous Thromboembolism Risk Assessment Tool in Secondary Care in England. *Blood Coagul. Fibrinolysis* **2014**, *25*, 571–576. [CrossRef]
60. Abboud, J.; Abdel Rahman, A.; Kahale, L.; Dempster, M.; Adair, P. Prevention of Health Care Associated Venous Thromboembolism through Implementing VTE Prevention Clinical Practice Guidelines in Hospitalized Medical Patients: A Systematic Review and Meta-Analysis. *Implement. Sci.* **2020**, *15*, 49. [CrossRef]
61. Pereira, V.C.; Silva, S.N.; Carvalho, V.K.S.; Zanghelini, F.; Barreto, J.O.M. Strategies for the Implementation of Clinical Practice Guidelines in Public Health: An Overview of Systematic Reviews. *Health Res. Policy Syst.* **2022**, *20*, 13. [CrossRef] [PubMed]
62. Wilson, M.; Keeley, J.; Kingman, M.; McDevitt, S.; Brewer, J.; Rogers, F.; Hill, W.; Rideman, Z.; Broderick, M. Clinical Application of Risk Assessment in PAH: Expert Center APRN Recommendations. *Pulm. Circ.* **2022**, *12*, e12106. [CrossRef]
63. Mabey, E.; Ismail, S.; Tailor, F. Improving Venous Thromboembolism Risk Assessment Rates in a Tertiary Urology Department. *BMJ Open Qual.* **2017**, *6*, e000171. [CrossRef] [PubMed]
64. Chamoun, N.; Matta, S.; Aderian, S.S.; Salibi, R.; Salameh, P.; Tayeh, G.; Haddad, E.; Ghanem, H. A Prospective Observational Cohort of Clinical Outcomes in Medical Inpatients Prescribed Pharmacological Thromboprophylaxis Using Different Clinical Risk Assessment Models (COMPT RAMs). *Sci. Rep.* **2019**, *9*, 18366. [CrossRef] [PubMed]
65. Kucher, N.; Koo, S.; Quiroz, R.; Cooper, J.M.; Paterno, M.D.; Soukonnikov, B.; Goldhaber, S.Z. Electronic Alerts to Prevent Venous Thromboembolism among Hospitalized Patients. *N. Engl. J. Med.* **2005**, *352*, 969–977. [CrossRef]

66. Pandor, A.; Tonkins, M.; Goodacre, S.; Sworn, K.; Clowes, M.; Griffin, X.L.; Holland, M.; Hunt, B.J.; de Wit, K.; Horner, D. Risk Assessment Models for Venous Thromboembolism in Hospitalised Adult Patients: A Systematic Review. *BMJ Open* **2021**, *11*, e045672. [CrossRef] [PubMed]
67. Taha, H.; Raji, S.J.; Ellahham, S.; Bashir, N.; Al Hanaee, M.; Boharoon, H.; AlFalahi, M. Improving Venous Thromboembolism Risk Assessment Compliance Using the Electronic Tool in Admitted Medical Patients. *BMJ Qual. Improv. Rep.* **2015**, *4*, u209593.w3965. [CrossRef]
68. Lavon, O.; Tamir, T. Evaluation of the Padua Prediction Score Ability to Predict Venous Thromboembolism in Israeli Non-Surgical Hospitalized Patients Using Electronic Medical Records. *Sci. Rep.* **2022**, *12*, 6121. [CrossRef]
69. Moik, F.; Englisch, C.; Pabinger, I.; Ay, C. Risk Assessment Models of Cancer-Associated Thrombosis—Potentials and Perspectives. *Thromb. Updat.* **2021**, *5*, 100075. [CrossRef]
70. Shaban, M.; Habib, N.; Helmy, I.; Mohammed, H.H. Dehydration Risk Factors and Outcomes in Older People in Rural Areas. *Front. Nurs.* **2022**, *9*, 395–403. [CrossRef]
71. Li, A.; Kuderer, N.M.; Hsu, C.-Y.; Shyr, Y.; Warner, J.L.; Shah, D.P.; Kumar, V.; Shah, S.; Kulkarni, A.A.; Fu, J.; et al. The CoVID-TE Risk Assessment Model for Venous Thromboembolism in Hospitalized Patients with Cancer and COVID-19. *J. Thromb. Haemost.* **2021**, *19*, 2522–2532. [CrossRef]
72. Shaban, M.; Shaban, M.M.; Ramadan, O.; Mohammed, H.H. Omicron: Egyptian Nurses' Knowledge and Attitudes. *J. Integr. Nurs.* **2022**, *4*, 15. [CrossRef]
73. Maynard, G. *Preventing Hospital-Acquired Venous Thromboembolism: A Guide for Effective Quality Improvement*, 2nd ed.; Agency for Healthcare Research and Quality: Rockville, MD, USA, 2016.
74. Van Calster, B.; Wynants, L.; Timmerman, D.; Steyerberg, E.W.; Collins, G.S. Predictive Analytics in Health Care: How Can We Know It Works? *J. Am. Med. Inform. Assoc.* **2019**, *26*, 1651–1654. [CrossRef] [PubMed]
75. Chiasakul, T.; Lam, B.D.; McNichol, M.; Robertson, W.; Rosovsky, R.P.; Lake, L.; Vlachos, I.S.; Adamski, A.; Reyes, N.; Abe, K.; et al. Artificial Intelligence in the Prediction of Venous Thromboembolism: A Systematic Review and Pooled Analysis. *Eur. J. Haematol.* **2023**. [CrossRef]
76. Whittington, R.; Hockenhull, J.; McGuire, J.; Leitner, M.; Barr, W.; Cherry, M.; Flentje, R.; Quinn, B.; Dundar, Y.; Dickson, R. A Systematic Review of Risk Assessment Strategies for Populations at High Risk of Engaging in Violent Behaviour: Update 2002–8. *Health Technol. Assess.* **2013**, *17*, 1–128. [CrossRef]
77. Shaban, M.; Mohammed, H.H.; Hassan, S. Role of Community Health Nurse in the Prevention of Elderly Dehydration: A Mini-Review. *J. Integr. Nurs.* **2022**, *4*, 166–171. [CrossRef]
78. Kalaitzopoulos, D.R.; Panagopoulos, A.; Samant, S.; Ghalib, N.; Kadillari, J.; Daniilidis, A.; Samartzis, N.; Makadia, J.; Palaiodimos, L.; Kokkinidis, D.G.; et al. Management of Venous Thromboembolism in Pregnancy. *Thromb. Res.* **2022**, *211*, 106–113. [CrossRef] [PubMed]
79. Elwyn, G.; Frosch, D.; Thomson, R.; Joseph-Williams, N.; Lloyd, A.; Kinnersley, P.; Cording, E.; Tomson, D.; Dodd, C.; Rollnick, S.; et al. Shared Decision Making: A Model for Clinical Practice. *J. Gen. Intern. Med.* **2012**, *27*, 1361–1367. [CrossRef]
80. Zander, A.L.; Van Gent, J.-M.; Olson, E.J.; Shackford, S.R.; Badiee, J.; Dunne, C.E.; Sise, C.B.; Sise, M.J. Venous Thromboembolic Risk Assessment Models Should Not Solely Guide Prophylaxis and Surveillance in Trauma Patients. *J. Trauma Acute Care Surg.* **2015**, *79*, 194–198. [CrossRef]
81. Buist, D.S.M.; Knight Ross, N.; Reid, R.J.; Grossman, D.C. Electronic Health Risk Assessment Adoption in an Integrated Healthcare System. *Am. J. Manag. Care* **2014**, *20*, 62–69. [PubMed]

Disclaimer/Publisher's Note: The statements, opinions and data contained in all publications are solely those of the individual author(s) and contributor(s) and not of MDPI and/or the editor(s). MDPI and/or the editor(s) disclaim responsibility for any injury to people or property resulting from any ideas, methods, instructions or products referred to in the content.

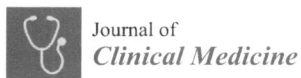 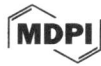

Article

The Obesity Mortality Paradox in Patients with Pulmonary Embolism: Insights from a Tertiary Care Center

Fahad Alkhalfan [1], Syed Bukhari [1], Akiva Rosenzveig [1], Rohitha Moudgal [1], Syed Zamrak Khan [1], Mohamed Ghoweba [1], Pulkit Chaudhury [1], Scott J. Cameron [1,2,3] and Leben Tefera [1,*]

[1] Department of Cardiovascular Medicine, Section of Vascular Medicine, Heart Vascular and Thoracic Institute, Cleveland Clinic Foundation, Cleveland, OH 44195, USA; alkhalf2@ccf.org (F.A.); bukhars6@ccf.org (S.B.); rosenza@ccf.org (A.R.); moudgar@ccf.org (R.M.); khans15@ccf.org (S.Z.K.); ghowebm@ccf.org (M.G.); chaudhp3@ccf.org (P.C.); cameros3@ccf.org (S.J.C.)
[2] Department of Cardiovascular and Metabolic Sciences, Lerner Research Institute, Case Western Reserve University, Cleveland, OH 44120, USA
[3] Department of Hematology, Taussig Cancer Institute, Cleveland Clinic Foundation, Cleveland, OH 44195, USA
* Correspondence: teferal@ccf.org

Abstract: Background: While obesity is associated with an increased risk of venous thromboembolism (VTE), there is some data to suggest that higher BMI is also associated with decreased all-cause mortality in patients with a pulmonary embolism (PE). **Methods:** Using PE Response Team (PERT) activation data from a large tertiary hospital between 27 October 2020 and 28 August 2023, we constructed a multivariate Cox proportional hazards model to assess the association between obesity as a dichotomous variable (defined as BMI $\geq$ 30 vs. BMI 18.5–29.9), BMI as a continuous variable, and 30-day PE-related mortality. **Results:** A total of 248 patients were included in this analysis (150 with obesity and 98 who were in the normal/overweight category). Obesity was associated with a lower risk of 30-day PE-related mortality (adjusted HR 0.29, p = 0.036, 95% CI 0.09–0.92). A higher BMI was paradoxically associated with a lower risk of PE-related mortality (HR = 0.91 per 1 kg/m^2 increase, p = 0.049, 95% CI 0.83–0.999). **Conclusions:** In our contemporary cohort of patients with a PERT activation, obesity was associated with a lower risk of PE-related mortality.

Keywords: pulmonary embolism; obesity; mortality; pulmonary embolism response team

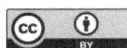

1. Introduction

Pulmonary embolism (PE) is the third most common cause of cardiovascular death in the United States [1] with an estimated mortality approaching 300,000 annually [2]. The advent of the multidisciplinary pulmonary embolism response team (PERT) and novel minimally invasive catheter-based treatments has led to a reduction in mortality [3–5]. Yet, despite the improvements gained, there is a pressing need to identify patients who are at a higher risk of morbidity and mortality.

The prevalence of obesity has been steadily rising, with recent data indicating that 42% of US adults are obese [6]. Obesity is shown to be a significant risk factor of venous thromboembolism (VTE) [7]. A prospective analysis of the Nurses' Health study demonstrated a profound linear association between body mass index (BMI) and the risk of PE, even with modest increases in BMI [8]. The obesity paradox is the concept that despite being a risk factor for various disease states, obesity portends improved outcomes. Although initially described in hemodialysis patients in 1999 [9], it has subsequently been shown in coronary artery disease [10], heart failure [11], and chronic obstructive pulmonary disease (COPD) [12]. A retrospective analysis of PE using the RIETE registry showed a potential signal for reduced all-cause mortality in patients who were overweight [13]. More recently, Keller et al. demonstrated decreased all-cause mortality in class I and II obesity but class III obesity had similar outcomes with non-obese patients [14]. While quite informative, studies to date have been unable to ascertain rates of PE-specific mortality in patients with obesity. In addition, previous studies were performed prior to the era of catheter-based therapies.

Thus, this study sought to identify differences in demographic and treatment characteristics between obese and non-obese patients and to further elucidate the association of obesity with mortality, particularly PE-specific mortality.

2. Methods

This was an analysis of all patients with a PERT activation between 27 October 2020 and 28 August 2023 in a large tertiary care center. Clinical data, including demographics, co-morbidities, hospital course, and relevant outcomes, including mortality, were ascertained from patients' electronic medical records. Patients who were classified as having a low risk of mortality according to the European Society of Cardiology (ESC) were excluded from this analysis as the PE in this situation is not significant enough to cause hemodynamic compromise and unlikely to be contributing to PE mortality.

The primary aim of this analysis was to determine if obesity as a dichotomous variable (BMI of 30 or greater vs. 18.5 to 29.9) was associated with a decreased risk of 30-day PE-related mortality. Patients with a BMI of less than 18.5 were excluded from the study as we did not want to assume that they would have similar event rates as compared to the BMI of 18.5–30 cohort. A death was considered related to the PE if it was believed to occur as a direct complication of the PE (such as worsening hypoxia, cardiogenic shock, or cardiac arrest) or as a result of subsequent treatment (such as anticoagulation leading to a fatal major bleeding event such as intracranial hemorrhage). If the cause of death was unknown or uncertain, it was categorized as not being related to PE. Secondary outcomes included 30-day all-cause mortality, in-hospital major bleeding, and the length of admission. The association between BMI, as a continuous variable, and the previously mentioned outcomes was also assessed.

2.1. Statistical Analysis

Baseline variables were compared between patients who were obese and those who were either in the non-obese or overweight BMI range. Differences in characteristics between the two groups were compared using a t-test or Wilcoxon rank sum for continuous variables depending on the distribution of the values and a Chi-square test for categorical values.

To identify variables that would be included in the final model, we utilized a backward selection approach to identify variables that would be included in our final multivariable Cox proportional hazards model. A p-value of 0.40 was designated as the cut off to exclude variables. This cut off was selected to maximize the number of variables included in the model. We included baseline demographic and clinical variables as potential parameters. This included sex (male vs. female), age, race, ESC PE mortality risk, smoking status (active smoker vs. non-smoker), history of cancer, history of heart disease, history of chronic lung disease, prior VTE, recent COVID infection (a positive test within the last 30 days or history of COVID within the last 30 days), and hypotension (systolic BP < 90 mm Hg). We also re-ran the same model with BMI as a continuous variable.

As for the secondary outcomes of interest, we utilized a multivariable Cox proportional hazards model to assess the association between obesity and all-cause 30-day mortality. We adjusted for the same variables used for our primary outcome of interest. We utilized the Fisher's exact test to assess the association between obesity and major bleeding (all major bleeding, extracranial major bleeding, and intracranial major bleeding separately). We utilized the International Society on Thrombosis and Hemostasis (ISTH) criteria for major bleeding (Fatal bleeding, symptomatic bleeding in a critical organ or a fall in hemoglobin by more than 2 g/dL, or transfusion of at least 2 units of packed red blood cells) [15]. We assessed the difference in the length of hospitalization between the two groups using the Wilcoxon rank sum test. A p-value of <0.05 was determined to be statistically significant.

We did not adjust for multiple comparisons. The analysis was conducted using STATA MP/16.1 (College Station, TX, USA).

2.2. Sensitivity Analysis

To account for the differences between obese and non-obese patients that were not included in our final multivariable Cox proportional hazards model, we included additional variables that were significantly different between the two groups ($p < 0.05$). We also included advanced PE treatments if they had not already been included in the final model. We re-ran two versions of the model: obesity as a dichotomous variable as described previously and BMI as a continuous variable.

3. Results

A total of 248 patients were included in this analysis (150 patients with a BMI $\geq$ 30 and 98 patients with a BMI between 18.5 and 29.9). A comparison of baseline demographics can be seen in Table 1. To summarize, patients who were obese tended to be younger (mean age 59.9 years vs. 65.5, $p = 0.005$), were less likely to have a history of cancer (22.0% vs. 39.8%, $p = 0.003$), and a higher proportion of patients had a recent COVID infection (13.3% vs. 4.1%, $p = 0.016$). There was no significant difference in sex, history of prior VTE, history of heart failure or chronic lung disease, or hypotension at presentation. Additionally, the distribution of intermediate–low-, intermediate–high-, and high-risk patients was similar between the two groups. Finally, the rates of advanced treatments, including catheter-based thrombectomy and systemic thrombolysis, were similar between patients who were obese and those who were non-obese or overweight.

Table 1. Baseline Demographics.

Variable		BMI $\geq$ 30 (N = 150)	BMI 18.5–29.9 (N = 98)	*p*-Value
Male		70 (46.7%)	55 (56.1%)	0.15
Age, mean (SD)		59.9 (15.3)	65.5 (15.2)	0.005
Prior VTE		7 (4.7%)	4 (4.1%)	0.83
Recent COVID infection		20 (13.3%)	4 (4.1%)	0.016
History of cancer		33 (22.0%)	39 (39.8%)	0.003
History of heart failure		26 (17.3%)	15 (15.3%)	0.67
History of chronic lung disease		29 (19.3%)	24 (24.5%)	0.33
Smoking		19 (12.7%)	15 (15.8%)	0.49
Hypoxia (defined as requiring oxygen)		116 (77.3%)	76 (78.4%)	0.85
Hypotension		13 (8.7%)	13 (13.4%)	0.24
European Society of Cardiology PE Mortality Risk	Intermediate–Low	30 (20.0%)	27 (27.6%)	0.38
	Intermediate–High	85 (56.7%)	51 (52.0%)	
	High	35 (23.3%)	20 (20.4%)	
Catheter thrombectomy		80 (53.7%)	46 (46.9%)	0.30
Systemic thrombolysis		13 (8.7%)	8 (8.2%)	0.89

There were 24 deaths from all causes at 30 days (7 (4.8%) in the obesity group and 17 (17.4%) in the non-obese/overweight group). Of those, 15 deaths were determined to be because of a complication of PE or its subsequent treatment (5 in the obesity group (3.4%) and 10 (10.5%) in the normal/overweight group). As seen in Figure 1, the separation occurred relatively early and persisted during the entire follow-up period. In an unadjusted analysis, obesity (as compared to patients in the non-obese/overweight category) was associated with a lower risk of 30-day PE-related mortality (Hazard ratio (HR) 0.31, $p = 0.031$, 95% CI

0.10–0.90) and all-cause mortality (HR 0.25, p = 0.002, 95% CI 0.10–0.61). This association remained significant when BMI was treated as a continuous variable ((PE-related mortality: 0.90, p = 0.023, 95% CI 0.82–0.99); (all-cause mortality: 0.91, p = 0.007, 95% CI 0.85–0.97)).

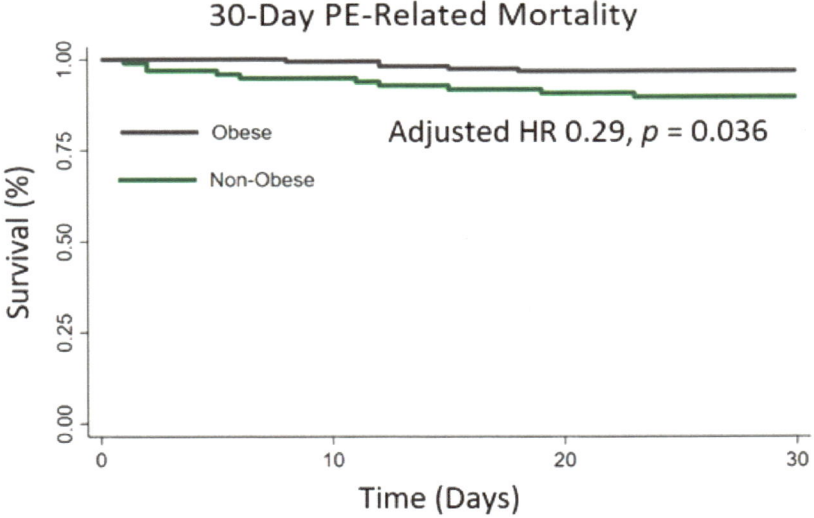

Figure 1. Kaplan–Meier curve for 30-day PE-related mortality.

As seen in Table 2, the final multivariable Cox proportional hazards model adjusted for sex, age, history of heart failure, history of chronic lung disease, recent COVID infection, use of systemic thrombolysis, and ESC PE mortality risk. After adjustment, the association between obesity and 30-day PE-related death remained significant (HR 0.29, p = 0.036, 95% CI 0.09–0.92). This association remained significant when BMI was treated as a continuous variable (HR 0.91, p = 0.049, 95% CI 0.83–0.999) (Table 3). As seen in Supplemental Tables S1 and S2, this pattern remained consistent when assessing for 30-day all-cause mortality (obesity: adjusted HR: 0.25, p = 0.004, 95% CI 0.10–0.64; BMI: adjusted HR 0.92, p = 0.018, 95% CI 0.86–0.99). There was no statistically significant difference in the duration of hospitalization (obesity: median 9 days, IQR 6–18; non-obese/overweight: median 9 days, IQR 6–17; p = 0.66).

Table 2. Final multivariable Cox proportional hazards model for the association between obesity and 30-Day PE-related mortality.

	Hazard Ratio	p-Value	95% Confidence Interval
Obesity (BMI ≥ 30 vs. BMI 18.5–29.9)	0.29	0.04	0.09–0.92
Male	0.54	0.27	0.18–1.60
Age (per 1 year)	1.02	0.27	0.98–1.06
History of Heart Failure	1.98	0.23	0.65–6.04
History of Chronic Lung Disease	2.09	0.18	0.72–6.05
Recent COVID Infection	2.56	0.25	0.52–12.6
Systemic Thrombolysis	3.14	0.12	0.76–13.0
ESC Mortality Risk (Baseline: Intermediate–Low Risk)			
Intermediate–High Risk	0.29	0.06	0.08–1.06
High Risk	0.61	0.46	0.17–2.22

Table 3. Final multivariable Cox proportional hazards model for the association between body mass index and 30-day PE-related mortality.

	Hazard Ratio	p-Value	95% Confidence Interval
BMI (per 1 kg/m^2)	0.91	0.049	0.83–0.999
Male	0.53	0.30	0.16–1.74
Age (per 1 year)	1.01	0.47	0.98–1.05
History of Heart Failure	2.40	0.14	0.75–7.72
History of Chronic Lung Disease	2.04	0.23	0.64–6.50
Recent COVID Infection	2.58	0.25	0.52–12.9
Systemic Thrombolysis	3.09	0.12	0.75–12.7
ESC Mortality Risk (Baseline: Intermediate–Low Risk)			
Intermediate–High Risk	0.43	0.22	0.11–1.66
High Risk	0.64	0.53	0.16–2.59

The sensitivity analysis included history of cancer and catheter-related thrombectomy as additional parameters. The association between obesity as a dichotomous variable and PE-related mortality remained statistically significant (HR 0.29, p = 0.039, 95% CI 0.09–0.94). However, the association between BMI as a continuous outcome and PE-related death was no longer significant (HR 0.91, p = 0.063, 95% CI 0.83–1.01).

As for our other secondary outcomes of interest, the overall rate of major bleeding was lower in the obesity group, but this did not reach statistical significance (six (4.1%) vs. eight (8.8%), p = 0.16). However, when stratified by extracranial vs. intracranial major bleeding, there was a significantly lower rate of extracranial major bleeding in the obese group (1 (0.7%) vs. 8 (8.8%), p = 0.002) with no statistically significant difference in the rate of intracranial bleeding (4 (2.7%) vs. 0 (0.0%), p = 0.30).

4. Discussion

Our study found that obesity was associated with a lower risk of PE-related mortality and all-cause mortality in PERT patients who had an intermediate or high risk of mortality. Additionally, overall major bleeding rates and the length of hospitalization was similar between obese and non-obese individuals. However, obesity was associated with lower rates of extracranial major bleeding.

Obesity has a well-known association with increased risk of PE, owing in part to increased platelet reactivity [16]. However, paradoxically, patients with obesity have better survival rates with PE compared to non-obese patients—a phenomenon known as obesity paradox. Keller et al. studied the German national database of >345,000 patients with acute PE and demonstrated that obesity was associated with lower all-cause in-hospital mortality rate regardless of age, sex, comorbidities, and reperfusion treatment [14]. Stein et al. used Nationwide Inpatient Sample to demonstrate that all-cause mortality in patients with PE is lower in patients with obesity than in non-obese/under-weight patients, with the greatest effects seen in women and older patients [17].

While the exact mechanism is unknown and it is unclear whether obesity paradox is related to protective effect of increased body fat, few pathophysiologic hypotheses regarding the "obesity paradox" in PE have been proposed. Patients with obesity tend to have greater right ventricular (RV) mass and higher RV volume compared with non-obese, which could potentiate their ability to cope with acute increases in RV overload [18]. Patients with obesity also have greater left ventricular (LV) mass and thicker interventricular septum that can make them more resistant to septal bowing, and potentially mitigate the risk of developing obstructive shock [19]. Some argue that obesity paradox does not necessarily reflect the protective effect of obesity but instead reflects the case of metabolically healthy obese individuals, a frequent and common finding in modern societies. These individuals have a better metabolic reserve, better smoking profile, and/or less disease-associated weight loss [20]. Non-PE-based studies have highlighted that cardiopulmonary fitness is an often-overlooked potential modifier of obesity paradox, and levels of fitness can significantly alter the inverse association between obesity and mortality [21]. The alternative explanation may be that BMI is not be the ideal definition of obesity [22]. In a study from the UK Biobank, waist–hip ratio was found to have the strongest association with all-cause mortality when compared with BMI and fat mass index [23].

Our study demonstrates some important findings that have not been reported previously. Firstly, unlike other studies that have reported all-cause mortality as the primary outcome while evaluating the impact of obesity in PE patients, we investigated PE-related deaths as the primary outcome. This helped us to mitigate the influence of confounders on our study analysis such as malignancy, congestive heart failure, etc. that are common non-PE-related causes of death in PE patients. Secondly, our patient population comprised intermediate to high-risk subjects from PERT registry, signifying sicker population with greater disease burden compared with previously reported cohorts. Thirdly, a higher utilization of catheter thrombectomy in our study population makes our study more compatible with the contemporary real-world practices and gives more credence to our results. As seen in Table 1, there was no statistically significant difference in the rates of advanced treatments, including catheter thrombectomy or systemic thrombolysis, between the two groups. Also, we conducted a sensitivity analysis to adjust for variables that were not chosen as part of our backward selection method but were still believed to be clinically significant, such as age and catheter thrombectomy. Finally, ~10% of our patients had a recent COVID infection, making them more vulnerable to thrombotic events. Earlier studies have indicated that obesity paradox is not applicable in patients with COVID, as patients with COVID and obesity exhibit more severe disease, are admitted to the intensive care unit more frequently, and have a higher mortality [7,8]. In our study, the obese group had significantly larger number of patients with recent COVID infection compared to the non-obese group, and yet had lower mortality, potentially signaling that obesity paradox may be applicable in patients with COVID and PE. However, we did adjust for COVID infection in our models.

Our study has some limitations. Firstly, being a single-center study, it lacks external generalizability. Additionally, considering the observational nature of this study, association does not imply causation. We attempted to mitigate this bias by performing multivariable analyses adjusting for difference in baseline characteristics; however, the presence of other confounders that were not accounted for could not be excluded (such as diabetes). Also, as we were only looking at PE-related mortality, the event rate was relatively low, and we were likely overfitting the model. However, we were still able to show that obesity was associated with a statistically significant reduction in PE mortality in both the univariate and multivariable models. We also did not adjust for multiple comparisons. Finally, baseline functional status of these patients could not be accurately assessed, which itself is a predictor of mortality. There remains a need for larger, multicentered studies to better evaluate the impact of obesity on morbidity and mortality in PE patients.

5. Conclusions

In our cohort of contemporary patients who had a PERT activation and an intermediate or high mortality risk, obesity was associated with a significant reduction in PE-related and all-cause mortality. Additionally, there was no statistically significant difference in major bleeding rates and the length of admission between obese individuals and those in the non-obese/overweight category.

Supplementary Materials: The following supporting information can be downloaded at: https://www.mdpi.com/article/10.3390/jcm13082375/s1, Table S1: Multivariable Cox-Proportional Hazards Model for the Association Between Obesity and 30-Day All-Cause Mortality, Table S2: Multivariable Cox-Proportional Hazards Model for the Association Between BMI and 30-Day All-Cause Mortality, Table S3: Sensitivity Analysis: Multivariable Cox-Proportional Hazards Model for the Association

Between Obesity and 30-Day PE-Related Mortality, Table S4: Sensitivity Analysis: Multivariable Cox-Proportional Hazards Model for the Association between BMI and 30-Day PE-Related Mortality.

Author Contributions: L.T. and F.A. designed the project. S.J.C., S.B., A.R., R.M., S.Z.K., P.C., F.A., M.G. and L.T. wrote, revised, and finalized the manuscript. All authors have read and agreed to the published version of the manuscript.

Funding: We gratefully acknowledge financial support by L30H165499 to L.T.

Institutional Review Board Statement: The study was conducted in accordance with the Declaration of Helsinki and approved by the Institutional Review Board of Cleveland Clinic (23-888 28 September 2023).

Informed Consent Statement: Not applicable.

Data Availability Statement: The data presented in this study are available on request from the corresponding author. The data are not publicly available due to institutional policy.

Conflicts of Interest: SC is a safety committee consultant for Sanofi, and has received an educational grant from Inari Inc. All other authors have reported that they have no relationships relevant to the contents of this paper to disclose.

References

1. Virani, S.S.; Alonso, A.; Aparicio, H.J.; Benjamin, E.J.; Bittencourt, M.S.; Callaway, C.W.; Carson, A.P.; Chamberlain, A.M.; Cheng, S.; Delling, F.N.; et al. Heart Disease and Stroke Statistics-2021 Update: A Report From the American Heart Association. *Circulation* **2021**, *143*, e254–e743. [CrossRef] [PubMed]
2. Wendelboe, A.M.; Raskob, G.E. Global Burden of Thrombosis: Epidemiologic Aspects. *Circ. Res.* **2016**, *118*, 1340–1347. [CrossRef] [PubMed]
3. Wright, C.; Goldenberg, I.; Schleede, S.; McNitt, S.; Gosev, I.; Elbadawi, A.; Pietropaoli, A.; Barrus, B.; Chen, Y.L.; Mazzillo, J.; et al. Effect of a Multidisciplinary Pulmonary Embolism Response Team on Patient Mortality. *Am. J. Cardiol.* **2021**, *161*, 102–107. [CrossRef]
4. Chaudhury, P.; Gadre, S.K.; Schneider, E.; Renapurkar, R.D.; Gomes, M.; Haddadin, I.; Heresi, G.A.; Tong, M.Z.; Bartholomew, J.R. Impact of Multidisciplinary Pulmonary Embolism Response Team Availability on Management and Outcomes. *Am. J. Cardiol.* **2019**, *124*, 1465–1469. [CrossRef] [PubMed]
5. Fleitas Sosa, D.; Lehr, A.L.; Zhao, H.; Roth, S.; Lakhther, V.; Bashir, R.; Cohen, G.; Panaro, J.; Maldonado, T.S.; Horowitz, J.; et al. Impact of pulmonary embolism response teams on acute pulmonary embolism: A systematic review and meta-analysis. *Eur. Respir. Rev.* **2022**, *31*, 220023. [CrossRef]
6. Hales, C.M.; Carroll, M.D.; Fryar, C.D.; Ogden, C.L. Prevalence of Obesity and Severe Obesity Among Adults: United States, 2017–2018. *NCHS Data Brief* **2020**, 1–8.
7. Gregson, J.; Kaptoge, S.; Bolton, T.; Pennells, L.; Willeit, P.; Burgess, S.; Bell, S.; Sweeting, M.; Rimm, E.B.; Kabrhel, C.; et al. Cardiovascular Risk Factors Associated with Venous Thromboembolism. *JAMA Cardiol.* **2019**, *4*, 163–173. [CrossRef] [PubMed]
8. Kabrhel, C.; Varraso, R.; Goldhaber, S.Z.; Rimm, E.B.; Camargo, C.A. Prospective study of BMI and the risk of pulmonary embolism in women. *Obesity* **2009**, *17*, 2040–2046. [CrossRef] [PubMed]
9. Fleischmann, E.; Teal, N.; Dudley, J.; May, W.; Bower, J.D.; Salahudeen, A.K. Influence of excess weight on mortality and hospital stay in 1346 hemodialysis patients. *Kidney Int.* **1999**, *55*, 1560–1567. [CrossRef] [PubMed]
10. Lavie, C.J.; De Schutter, A.; Patel, D.A.; Romero-Corral, A.; Artham, S.M.; Milani, R.V. Body composition and survival in stable coronary heart disease: Impact of lean mass index and body fat in the "obesity paradox". *J. Am. Coll. Cardiol.* **2012**, *60*, 1374–1380. [CrossRef] [PubMed]
11. Horwich, T.B.; Fonarow, G.C.; Clark, A.L. Obesity and the Obesity Paradox in Heart Failure. *Prog. Cardiovasc. Dis.* **2018**, *61*, 151–156. [CrossRef] [PubMed]
12. Chittal, P.; Babu, A.S.; Lavie, C.J. Obesity paradox: Does fat alter outcomes in chronic obstructive pulmonary disease? *COPD* **2015**, *12*, 14–18. [CrossRef] [PubMed]
13. Barba, R.; Zapatero, A.; Losa, J.E.; Valdés, V.; Todolí, J.A.; Di Micco, P.; Monreal, M. Body mass index and mortality in patients with acute venous thromboembolism: Findings from the RIETE registry. *J. Thromb. Haemost. JTH* **2008**, *6*, 595–600. [CrossRef] [PubMed]
14. Keller, K.; Hobohm, L.; Münzel, T.; Ostad, M.A.; Espinola-Klein, C.; Lavie, C.J.; Konstantinides, S.; Lankeit, M. Survival Benefit of Obese Patients with Pulmonary Embolism. *Mayo Clin. Proc.* **2019**, *94*, 1960–1973. [CrossRef] [PubMed]
15. Schulman, S.; Kearon, C. Definition of major bleeding in clinical investigations of antihemostatic medicinal products in non-surgical patients. *J. Thromb. Haemost. JTH* **2005**, *3*, 692–694. [CrossRef] [PubMed]
16. Barrachina, M.N.; Hermida-Nogueira, L.; Moran, L.A.; Casas, V.; Hicks, S.M.; Sueiro, A.M.; Di, Y.; Andrews, R.K.; Watson, S.P.; Gardiner, E.E.; et al. Phosphoproteomic Analysis of Platelets in Severe Obesity Uncovers Platelet Reactivity and Signaling Pathways Alterations. *Arterioscler. Thromb. Vasc. Biol.* **2021**, *41*, 478–490. [CrossRef] [PubMed]

17. Stein, P.D.; Matta, F.; Goldman, J. Obesity and pulmonary embolism: The mounting evidence of risk and the mortality paradox. *Thromb. Res.* **2011**, *128*, 518–523. [CrossRef] [PubMed]
18. Chahal, H.; McClelland, R.L.; Tandri, H.; Jain, A.; Turkbey, E.B.; Hundley, W.G.; Barr, R.G.; Kizer, J.; Lima, J.A.C.; Bluemke, D.A.; et al. Obesity and right ventricular structure and function: The MESA-Right Ventricle Study. *Chest* **2012**, *141*, 388–395. [CrossRef] [PubMed]
19. Chowdhury, J.M.; Zhao, H.; Moores, L.K.; Rali, P. Obesity Paradox in VTE Outcomes: An Evolving Concept. *Chest* **2020**, *158*, 1290–1291. [CrossRef] [PubMed]
20. Wang, S.; Ren, J. Obesity Paradox in Aging: From Prevalence to Pathophysiology. *Prog. Cardiovasc. Dis.* **2018**, *61*, 182–189. [CrossRef] [PubMed]
21. McAuley, P.A.; Beavers, K.M. Contribution of cardiorespiratory fitness to the obesity paradox. *Prog. Cardiovasc. Dis.* **2014**, *56*, 434–440. [CrossRef] [PubMed]
22. Goldhaber, S.Z. Obesity and Pulmonary Embolism: Can We Dismantle the "Obesity Paradox". *Thromb. Haemost.* **2023**, *124*, 058–060. [CrossRef] [PubMed]
23. Khan, I.; Chong, M.; Le, A.; Mohammadi-Shemirani, P.; Morton, R.; Brinza, C.; Kiflen, M.; Narula, S.; Akhabir, L.; Mao, S.; et al. Surrogate Adiposity Markers and Mortality. *JAMA Netw. Open* **2023**, *6*, e2334836. [CrossRef] [PubMed]

Disclaimer/Publisher's Note: The statements, opinions and data contained in all publications are solely those of the individual author(s) and contributor(s) and not of MDPI and/or the editor(s). MDPI and/or the editor(s) disclaim responsibility for any injury to people or property resulting from any ideas, methods, instructions or products referred to in the content.

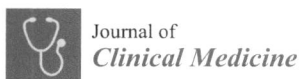 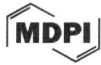

Systematic Review

The Outcomes of Surgical Pulmonary Embolectomy for Pulmonary Embolism: A Meta-Analysis

Mohamed Rahouma [1,2,*,†], Shaikha Al-Thani [1], Haitham Salem [3], Alzahraa Mahmoud [4], Sherif Khairallah [1,2], David Shenouda [5], Batool Sultan [6], Laila Khalil [7], Mohammad Alomari [8], Mostafa Ali [8], Ian A. Makey [8], John C. Haney [8], Stephanie Mick [1] and Magdy M. El-Sayed Ahmed [8,9,*,†]

1. Cardiothoracic Surgery Department, Weill Cornell Medicine, New York, NY 10065, USA; sma9023@med.cornell.edu (S.A.-T.); smk4005@med.cornell.edu (S.K.); slmick@med.cornell.edu (S.M.)
2. Surgical Oncology Department, National Cancer Institute, Cairo University, Cairo 11796, Egypt
3. Ain Shams University Hospital, Ain Shams University, Cairo 11517, Egypt; haithamsalem.md@gmail.com
4. Faculty of Medicine, Beni Suef University, Beni Suef 2721562, Egypt; alzahraamah@gmail.com
5. New York Institute of Technology, New York, NY 10023, USA; shenoudadavid17@gmail.com
6. Rak Medical and Health Sciences University, Ras al Khaimah 11172, United Arab Emirates; batoolsultan77@gmail.com
7. Weill Cornell Medicine, Doha 24144, Qatar; ltk4001@qatar-med.cornell.edu
8. Cardiothoracic Surgery Department, Mayo Clinic, Jacksonville, FL 32224, USA; alomari.mohammad@mayo.edu (M.A.); ali.mostafa@mayo.edu (M.A.); makey.ian@mayo.edu (I.A.M.); haney.john@mayo.edu (J.C.H.)
9. Surgery Department, Faculty of Medicine, Zagazig University, Zagazig 44519, Egypt
* Correspondence: mhmdrahouma@gmail.com or mmr2011@med.cornell.edu (M.R.); elgoharymagdy@yahoo.com or ahmed.magdy@mayo.edu (M.M.E.-S.A.)
† These authors contributed equally to this work.

Citation: Rahouma, M.; Al-Thani, S.; Salem, H.; Mahmoud, A.; Khairallah, S.; Shenouda, D.; Sultan, B.; Khalil, L.; Alomari, M.; Ali, M.; et al. The Outcomes of Surgical Pulmonary Embolectomy for Pulmonary Embolism: A Meta-Analysis. *J. Clin. Med.* **2024**, *13*, 4076. https://doi.org/10.3390/jcm13144076

Academic Editor: Brett J. Carroll

Received: 7 June 2024
Revised: 4 July 2024
Accepted: 6 July 2024
Published: 12 July 2024

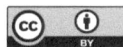

Copyright: © 2024 by the authors. Licensee MDPI, Basel, Switzerland. This article is an open access article distributed under the terms and conditions of the Creative Commons Attribution (CC BY) license (https://creativecommons.org/licenses/by/4.0/).

Abstract: Objectives: The purpose of this study is to assess the efficacy, short- and long-term cardiovascular and non-cardiovascular mortalities and postoperative morbidities of surgical pulmonary embolectomy (SPE) for patients with massive or submassive pulmonary embolism. Methods: A comprehensive literature review was performed to identify articles reporting SPE for pulmonary embolism. The outcomes included in-hospital and long-term mortality in addition to postoperative morbidities. The random effect inverse variance method was used. Cumulative meta-analysis, leave-one-out sensitivity analysis, subgroup analysis and meta-regression were performed. **Results:** Among the 1949 searched studies in our systematic literature search, 78 studies met our inclusion criteria, including 6859 cases. The mean age ranged from 42 to 65 years. The percentage of males ranged from 25.6% to 86.7%. The median rate of preoperative cardiac arrest was 27.6%. The percentage of contraindications to preoperative systemic thrombolysis was 30.4%. The preoperative systemic thrombolysis use was 11.5%. The in-hospital mortality was estimated to be 21.96% (95% CI: 19.21–24.98); in-hospital mortality from direct cardiovascular causes was estimated to be 16.05% (95% CI: 12.95–19.73). With a weighted median follow-up of 3.05 years, the late cardiovascular and non-cardiovascular mortality incidence rates were 0.39 and 0.90 per person-year, respectively. The incidence of pulmonary bleeding, gastrointestinal bleeding, surgical site bleeding, non-surgical site bleeding and wound complications was 0.62%, 4.70%, 4.84%, 5.80% and 7.2%, respectively. Cumulative meta-analysis showed a decline in hospital mortality for SPE from 42.86% in 1965 to 20.56% in 2024. Meta-regression revealed that the publication year and male sex were associated with lower in-hospital mortality, while preoperative cardiac arrest, the need for inotropes or vasopressors and preoperative mechanical ventilation were associated with higher in-hospital mortality. **Conclusions:** This study demonstrates acceptable perioperative mortality rates and late cardiovascular and non-cardiovascular mortality in patients who undergo SPE for massive or submassive pulmonary embolism.

Keywords: surgical pulmonary embolectomy; pulmonary embolism; hospital mortality; pulmonary bleeding; thrombolysis

1. Introduction

Venous thromboembolisms, such as pulmonary embolisms (PEs), are the third most common cardiovascular (CV) syndrome, with increasing incidence in the aging population [1,2]. PE has been reported in the literature to have a high mortality rate [3]. The clinical presentation of PE is often non-specific and can range from incidental findings on a computed tomographic chest scan with no clinical symptoms to patients presenting with hemodynamic instability, defined as individuals who are hypotensive needing pressor support and develop end organ hypoperfusion, and sudden death. Nevertheless, presentation in extremes accounts for only 5% of PE cases.

The primary mode of treatment for acute PE is anticoagulation (1). According to the European Society of Cardiology guidelines, surgical pulmonary embolectomy (SPE) for the treatment of PE should be reserved for individuals who deteriorate hemodynamically while being on rescue thrombolytic therapies, for those with contraindications for thrombolytic therapies or for failed catheter-directed thrombolysis [1,2]. SPE usually included the performance of cardiopulmonary bypass (CPB), and the literature has demonstrated varying outcomes following surgical intervention [3]. Therefore, we performed a systematic review and meta-analysis to assess the efficacy and short- and long-term CV and non-CV mortalities for patients that present with PE.

2. Materials and Methods

This meta-analysis was performed in concordance with the Preferred Reporting Items for Systematic Reviews and Meta-Analyses (PRISMA) statement [4] and AMSTAR (A MeaSurement Tool to Assess systemic Reviews) Guideline.

2.1. Search Strategy

On 14 March 2024, the PubMed and Scopus databases were systematically searched for publications on SPE. The search terms in subject headings and main keywords included the following: "Pulmonary Embolectomy", "surgical embolectomy", "surgical pulmonary embolectomy", "surgical intervention", and "pulmonary embolism". This review was registered with the PROSPERO register of systematic reviews (ID: 542752). There was no individual patient involvement in this study; as such, research ethics board approval was not required.

2.2. Study Selection and Inclusion Criteria

Two investigators (HS, SA) independently performed data extraction. Database searches were conducted, and article de-duplication and screening were performed by these two reviewers. A third independent reviewer (MR) confirmed the adequacy of the studies based on the predefined inclusion and exclusion criteria. Articles were included if they were in full-text English on human subjects that included five or more patients with reported CV or non-CS mortality or morbidity outcomes following SPE. We included studies with the largest sample size and the most comprehensive follow-up period for each outcome of cumulative or longitudinal results in more than one publication. Studies were excluded if they were in a non-English language, did not include SPE, did not specify the number or proportion of mortality or morbidity or had a small case series with less than 5 patients.

The full article text of the screened studies was retrieved for the second round of eligibility screening. Prior meta-analyses and systematic reviews were searched to confirm the inclusion of all eligible studies (i.e., backward snowballing). A PRISMA flow diagram illustrating the study selection process is available in the Supplementary Materials (Supplementary Figure S1). The Newcastle–Ottawa scale (NOS) for assessing the quality of Cohort Studies was used for the critical appraisal of eligible studies. Studies with scores of six or more were included [5].

2.3. Clinical Outcomes/Definitions

The primary outcome of interest was SPE hospital mortality. Secondary outcomes included CV and non-CV mortality, postoperative pulmonary bleeding, gastrointestinal (GI) bleeding, surgical site bleeding, non-surgical site bleeding and wound complication.

Subgroup analysis for the primary outcome was conducted based on continents.

2.4. Data Extraction and Statistical Analysis

Extracted variables included the following: study name, publication year, study design, mean age, percentage of males, mean follow-up in years, percentage of individuals with a contraindication to systemic thrombolytic therapy, percent of preoperative cardiac arrest, preoperative mechanical ventilation, percent of individuals that underwent CPB or extracorporeal membrane oxygenation (ECMO) support, percent of right ventricular (RV) dysfunction, the need for inotropes or vasopressors, systemic thrombolysis, use of myocardial protective techniques and aortic cross-clamping.

Measurement data were reported as the mean and standard deviation or as the median and interquartile range based on the reported studies. The proportion per 100 observations with a 95% confidence interval (95% CI) was calculated for each binary outcome. For late mortality following SPE, the incidence rate with a constant event rate was used to account for different follow-up times of the various studies with the total number of events observed within the treatment group out of the total person-year of the follow-up.

Meta-regression was used to assess the effect of publication year, sex, systemic thrombolysis, contraindication to systemic thrombolytics, preoperative cardiac arrest, inotrope or vasopressor use, preoperative mechanical ventilation, use of CPB, myocardial protective techniques, use of intraoperative hypothermia and aortic cross-clamping percent on hospital mortality after SPE. Heterogeneity among the included studies was assessed using the Cochran Q statistic and the I^2 test. For the primary outcome, if heterogeneity was significant ($I^2 > 75\%$), a leave-one-out sensitivity analysis was performed. The publication bias was assessed using a funnel plot and Egger's regression test. We used a random effect model (inverse variance method) for the entire analysis. The hypothesis testing for equivalence was set at a two-tailed value of 0.05. Analyses were performed using R (version 4.3.3 R Project for Statistical Computing), using the following statistical packages: "meta" and "metafor" within RStudio (2023.12.1+402 "Ocean Storm" Release for windows; Postit: Boston, MA, USA).

3. Results

Among the 1949 searched studies in our systematic literature search, 78 studies met our inclusion criteria including 6859 cases that underwent an SPE intervention [6–83]. A PRISMA flowchart is shown in Supplementary Figure S1.

The criteria of all included studies are presented in Table 1. The mean age of included patients ranged from 42 to 65 years. The percentage of males ranged from 25.6% to 86.7%. Preoperative cardiac arrest was reported in 57 studies and ranged from 0% to 87.2% of operations with a median preoperative cardiac arrest of 27.6%. The percentage of contraindications to preoperative systemic thrombolysis was reported by 29 studies with a median percent of 30.4% (interquartile range 20.00–45.50) in these studies. The preoperative systemic thrombolysis percent was reported by 35 studies with a median percent of 11.5% (interquartile range 3.65–25.30) in these studies. The use of CPB appeared to be nearly universal (median 100% (IQR: 100–100)). The criteria of the included studies are shown in Table 1.

Table 1. The criteria of the included studies.

	Country	Number of Patients	Age, Years	Mean Follow-Up (Year)	Male Percent
Hartman 2015 [6]	USA	96	57.70	2.50	62.50
Ahmed 2008 [7]	USA	15	59.60		46.70
Alqahtani 2019 [8]	USA	3486	56.00		53.00
Amirghofran 2007 [9]	Iran	11	45.60	3.00	63.60
Argyriou 2024 [10]	England	256	54.00		55.90
Azari 2015 [11]	Iran	30	56.10	3.50	43.33
Barrett 2010 [12]	UK/Sydney	9	62.00		55.60
Bauer 1991 [13]	Switzerland	44	49.00	4.60	54.50
Bennett 2015 [14]	USA	40	50.33		40.00
Berger 1973 [15]	USA	17			52.90
Biglioli 1991 [16]	Italy	11			
Bottzauw 1981 [17]	USA	23	53.00		56.50
Boulafendis 1991 [18]	USA	16	51.50	5.04	62.50
Cale 2002 [19]	Singapore	12			41.70
Clarke 1986 [20]	England	55			45.50
Dauphine 2005 [21]	USA	11	48.50	0.75	45.50
De Weese1976 [22]	Germany	11	42.30		45.50
DiChiacchio 1986 [23]	USA	90	53.56		50.00
Digonnet 2007 [24]	France	21	62.00	4.75	61.90
Doerge 1998 [25]	Germany	41	51.10	10.58	51.20
Dohle 2018 [26]	Germany	175	59.30	4.60	50.00
Edelman 2016 [27]	Australia	37	57.00	0.12	41.00
Estrer 1981 [28]	USA	5	43.60		60.00
Fedorov 2022 [29]	Russia	10	54.60		40.00
Glassford 1981 [30]	USA	20	57.10		40.00
Gray 1988 [31]	England	71	43.10	7.88	31.00
Greelish 2011 [32]	USA	15	57.00	2.00	86.70
Hajizadeh 2017 [33]	Iran	36	50.80	0.50	38.90
Hennig 1974 [34]	Germany	6		1.67	
Jako1995 [35]	Germany	25	57.00		40.00
Jaumin 1986 [36]	Belgium	23			
Keeling 2016 [37]	USA	214	56.00		56.40
Keeling 2016 [38]	USA	44	51.60	2.52	43.20
Khoury 1992 [39]	Australia	61	53.00		32.80
Kieny 1991 [40]	France	134	55.00		55.20
Konstantinov 2007 [41]	Australia	7	46.40	4.17	28.60
Laas 1993 [42]	Germany	34		4.90	
Leacche 2005 [43]	USA	47	59.00	2.25	63.80
Lehnert 2012 [44]	Denmark	33	55.00	5.20	51.50
Lund 1986 [45]	Denmark	25	52.00	3.90	56.00

Table 1. Cont.

	Country	Number of Patients	Age, Years	Mean Follow-Up (Year)	Male Percent
Malekan 2012 [46]	USA	26	59.10	0.08	69.20
Marshall 2012 [47]	Australia	10	49.00	3.25	40.00
Mattox 1982 [48]	USA	39	42.00		25.60
Meyer 1991 [49]	France	96	52.00	4.67	52.10
Meyns 1992 [50]	Belgium	30	47.80	7.25	33.30
Minakawa 2018 [51]	Japan	355	62.10		47.60
Mkalaluh 2019 [52]	Germany	49	58.00	0.08	51.00
Neely 2015 [53]	USA	115	59.00	1.08	62.60
Newcom 2022 [54]	USA	16	53.00		44.00
Osborne 2014 [55]	USA	15	48.50	0.09	46.70
Panholzer 2022 [56]	Germany	103	58.40		
Park 2019 [57]	Korea	27	47.30	0.08	45.00
Pasrij 2017 [58]	USA	30	55.50	0.50	50.00
Pasrij 2018 [59]	USA	55	53.00	1.00	60.00
QiMin 2020 [60]	China	41	65.00	2.00	51.20
Rathore 2020 [61]	Australia	82	60.00	3.18	57.30
Rivas 1975 [62]	Germany	5			
Sa 2007 [63]	Korea	12	46.00	8.50	58.30
Salehi 2013 [64]	Iran	16	53.00	2.00	37.50
Sareyyupoglu 2010 [65]	USA	18	60.00	1.33	72.20
Satter 1980 [66]	Germany	36			44.40
Saylam 1978 [67]	USA	8	58.50		62.50
Shiomi 2016 [68]	Japan	31	58.30	3.98	35.50
Spagnolo 2006 [69]	Italy	21			38.10
Stalpaert 1986 [70]	Germany	30	44.50		30.00
Stulz 1994 [71]	Switzerland	50	53.40		36.00
Takahashi 2012 [72]	Japan	24	59.90	0.57	29.20
Taniguchi 2012 [73]	Japan	32	57.00	0.08	34.40
Thielmann 2012 [74]	Germany	46	50.50	0.08	32.60
Turnier 1973 [75]	USA	8	56.80		50.00
Ullman 1999 [76]	Germany	40	55.00	3.75	42.50
Vohr 2010 [77]	UK	21	55.00	3.17	71.40
Vossschulte 1965 [78]	Germany	7	48.70		57.10
Wu 2013 [79]	Taiwan	25	49.40	1.58	36.00
Yalamanchili 2004 [80]	USA	13	53.70		46.20
Yavuz 2014 [81]	Turkey	13	61.80	2.08	61.50
Zarrabi 2013 [82]	Iran	30			
Zielinski 2023 [83]	Poland	20	53.65	3.83	55.00

A quality assessment of all studies was conducted according to the Newcastle–Ottawa scale (NOS) criteria, as shown in Supplementary Table S2.

3.1. Efficacy Outcomes

Point estimates for hospital and late mortality outcomes are reported in Figure 1A and Supplementary Figure S7. Hospital mortality was reported by all 75 studies involving 6779 cases. The hospital mortality was estimated to be 21.96% (95% CI: 19.21–24.98) (Figure 1A). The CV hospital mortality was reported in 53 studies and was estimated to be 16.05% (95% CI: 12.95–19.73). The non-CV hospital mortality was reported in 35 studies and was estimated to be 8.32% (95% CI: 6.22–11.06).

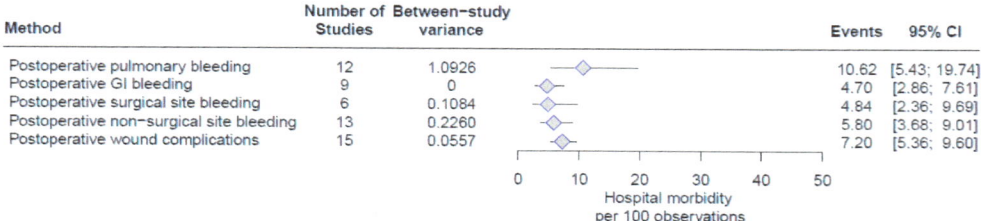

Figure 1. Forest plot of (A) hospital mortality (The * refers to the different subgroups of hospital mortality) and (B) hospital morbidity.

3.2. Late All-Cause Mortality

With a weighted median follow-up of 3.05 years, the late CV and non-CV mortality incidence rates were 0.39 per person-year (95% CI: 0.14–0.65) and 0.90 per person-year (95% CI: 0.40–2.06), respectively. (Supplementary Figure S7).

3.3. Safety Outcomes

Point estimates for pulmonary bleeding, gastrointestinal bleeding, surgical site bleeding, non-surgical site bleeding and wound complications are reported in Figure 1B.

Pulmonary bleeding was reported by 12 studies, and the incidence was estimated to be 10.62% (95% CI: 5.43–19.74%). Gastrointestinal bleeding was reported by nine studies, and the incidence was estimated to be 4.70% (95% CI: 2.86–7.61). Surgical site bleeding was reported in six studies with an estimated incidence of 4.84% (95% CI: 3.36–9.69%), while non-surgical site bleeding was reported in 13 studies with an estimated incidence of 5.80% (95% CI: 3.68–9.01%). Wound complications were reported in 15 studies with an estimated incidence of 7.2% (95% CI: 5.36–9.60%), Figure 1B.

There were 15 cases of GI bleeding reported, and most of them were due to abdominal surgical operations. Clarke et al.'s 1986 study reported that 10 patients had abdominal surgery for malignant tumor resection, and 4 of them had GI bleeding. Cases of GI bleeding and cerebral strokes were contraindicated for thrombolytics and anticoagulants.

3.4. Sensitivity and Subgroup Analyses and Meta-Regression

There is high heterogeneity in hospital mortality with an I2 of 73%. To explore such reasons for heterogeneity, we performed a leave-one-out analysis that showed the robustness of the obtained estimate for hospital mortality (Supplementary Figure S4). Additionally, cumulative meta-analysis showed a decline in hospital mortality for SPE from 42.86% in 1965 to 20.56% in 2024.

Meta-regression analyses were performed to evaluate the impact of different variables on hospital mortality and found that the publication year (Figure 2A) (beta = -0.0288 ± 0.0051, $p < 0.0001$) and percentage of males (Figure 2B) (beta = -0.0232 ± 0.0071, $p = 0.0011$) were associated with lower hospital mortality, while preoperative cardiac arrest (Figure 2C) (beta = -0.0288 ± 0.0051, $p < 0.0001$), the need for inotropes or vasopressors (beta = 0.0137 ± 0.0042, $p = 0.0012$) and preoperative mechanical ventilation (Figure 2D) (beta = 0.0143 ± 0.0061, $p = 0.0196$) were associated with higher hospital mortality (Table 2 and Supplementary Figure S3).

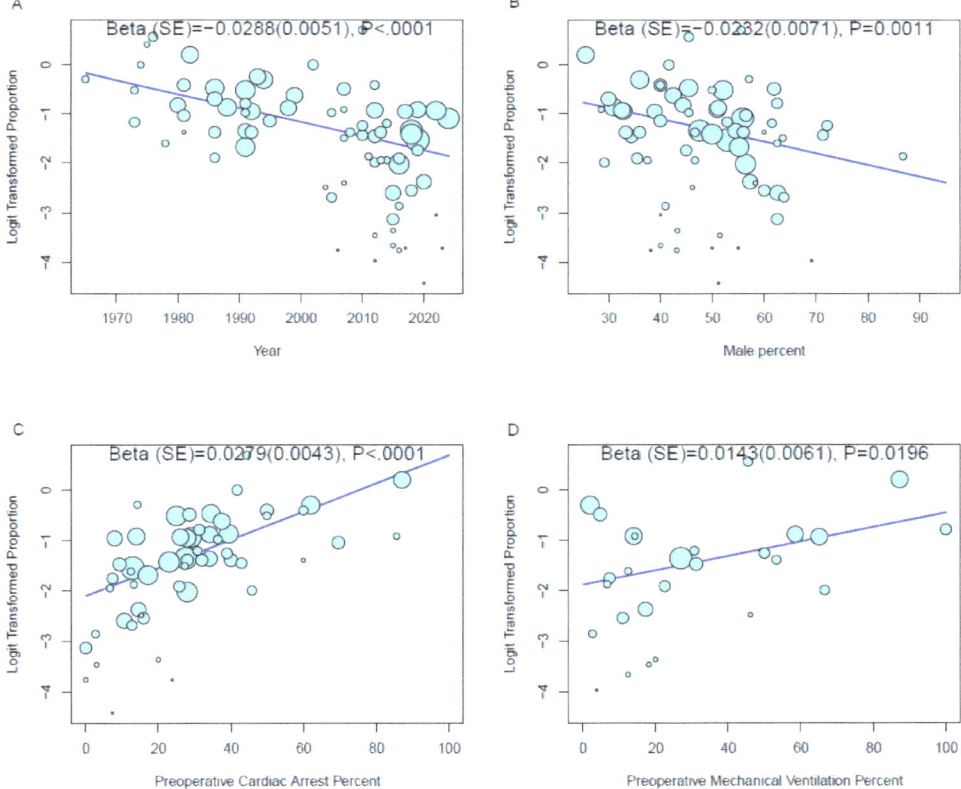

Figure 2. Bubble plots of meta-regression of (**A**) publication year, (**B**) percentage of males, (**C**) preoperative cardiac arrest and (**D**) preoperative mechanical ventilation on hospital mortality outcome.

There was no observed publication bias either visually by inspecting the symmetry of the funnel plot or statistically by using Egger's test (estimate = 0.2246 ± 0.2986, $p = 0.4507$), Supplementary Figure S4.

Table 2. Meta regression of hospital mortality.

Variables	Beta ± SE, p-Value
Year	-0.0288 ± 0.0051, $p < 0.0001$
Male Percent	-0.0232 ± 0.0071, $p = 0.0011$
Systemic Thrombolysis Percent	-0.0136 ± 0.0078, $p = 0.0785$
Systemic Thrombolytics Contraindication Percent	0.0075 ± 0.0062, $p = 0.2261$
Preoperative Cardiac Arrest Percent	0.0279 ± 0.0043, $p < 0.0001$
Need for Inotropes or Vasopressors Percent	0.0137 ± 0.0042, $p = 0.0012$
Preoperative Mechanical Ventilation Percent	0.0143 ± 0.0061, $p = 0.0196$
Use Of Cardiopulmonary Bypass Percent	-0.0060 ± 0.0040, $p = 0.1325$
Use Of Myocardial Protective Techniques Percent	-0.0032 ± 0.0050, $p = 0.5243$
Use Of Intraoperative Hypothermia Percent	0.0013 ± 0.0042, $p = 0.7656$
Use Of Aortic Cross-Clamping Percent	-0.0012 ± 0.0036, $p = 0.7454$

Beta (regression coefficient): the negative value reflects inverse association with the hospital mortality outcome.

4. Discussion

This meta-analysis and systematic review examined the efficacy of SPE, as well as short- and long-term outcomes including CV and non-CV mortality in 78 studies, which included 6859 cases that underwent an SPE. The analysis demonstrated a hospital mortality rate of approximately 22%, with a CV mortality rate of 16%. Additionally, there were long-term CV and non-CV mortality rates of 39 per 100 person-year and 90 deaths per 100 person-year, respectively. The median preoperative cardiac arrest rate was approximately 28%, with the use of CPB universally in patients that underwent SPE.

The in-hospital mortality rates, as well as CV and non-CV mortality rates, reported in this study are similar to the reported mortality rates by Karla et al. who reported an in-hospital mortality rate of 26.3% [4]. A study was conducted by Kilic et al. using a weighted nationwide inpatient sample, which included 1050 participating institutions in 44 states and identified 2709 patients that underwent an SPE for a PE. In this study, they reported an in-hospital mortality rate of 27.2% and identified that the comorbidity index and black race were independently associated with inpatient mortality following SPE [84].

A retrospective study performed by Hartman et al. reported a 30-day mortality rate of 4.2% for all comers but illustrated that patients that were unstable had a higher 30-day mortality rate of 12.5% compared to stable patients who had a 30-day mortality rate of 1.4% [6]. Studies have also shown that mortality rates are higher following cardiac arrest, which could explain the reported in-hospital mortality rate of 27% in this study, given that 28% of patients that underwent SPE had preoperative cardiac arrest. Stein and colleagues reported an operative mortality rate of 59% in patients who had preoperative cardiac arrest compared to a rate of 20% in patients who did not have preoperative cardiac arrest [85].

Furthermore, we found in this study that there is a decline in the in-hospital mortality rate following SPE. It decreased from 42.86% in 1965 to 20.56% in 2024. Studies have previously shown this reduction in mortality over time [86]. This trend is likely due to improvements in the diagnosis of PE, the stabilization of the patient and early intervention. There is also likely a significant selection bias at work, as the dramatic improvement in catheter-based interventions has offered many patients embolectomy in the absence of surgery. This lack of randomization is a major confounder of such a retrospective meta-analysis. This review supports the concept that in appropriately selected patients, surgical embolectomy may be performed safely and with a good outcome; it does not argue against the utility of popular catheter-based techniques/approaches that have rapidly evolved from catheter-directed thrombolysis to ultrasound-augmented thrombolysis and to multiple generations of percutaneous thrombectomy devices.

Among the included studies, there was an apparent trend toward higher inotrope/vasopressor use with RV dysfunction, in studies that reported both variables, but this was statistically insignificant (*p*- for trend = 0.347). The hospital mortality was mainly due to cardiovascular comorbidities which included the need for inotropes or vasopressors, preoperative mechanical ventilation, shock and cardiac arrest. The weighted median follow-up was 3.05 years. Late mortality causes included both CV and non-CV causes. Cardiovascular comorbidities such as hypertension and heart failure and non-CV causes such as malignant neoplasms are the most common causes for late mortality.

Finally, this study has limitations that include the lack of demographic data such as race in the majority of included studies, since previous studies have shown an association between race and in-hospital mortality following SPE. Specifically, the black and African American race was associated with higher mortality rates compared to white Americans [84]. Additionally, hemodynamic information was not present in a reasonable number of the included studies. It would have been interesting to observe if there were differences in hospital mortality following SPE in stable and unstable patients or to understand the baseline presentation of the patient and why that contributed to a hospital mortality rate of approximately 27%; however, we were able to identify some predictors of mortality such as an earlier era of surgery, prior cardiac arrest, need for preoperative mechanical ventilation and the need for vasopressors or inotropes. There is a discernible lack of data on the institution of ECMO among included patients. There is a need to evaluate other late outcomes, such as the rate of development of chronic pulmonary hypertension in patients who undergo SPE for acute PE.

5. Conclusions

In conclusion, this meta-analysis and systematic review demonstrates acceptable perioperative mortality rates and late CV and non-CV mortality in patients who undergo SPE for massive or submassive PE. There is a noticeably reduced mortality rate with more recent studies using SPE.

Supplementary Materials: The following supporting information can be downloaded at https://www.mdpi.com/article/10.3390/jcm13144076/s1. Figure S1: A PRISMA flowchart of the included studies, Figure S2: Forest plot of hospital mortality, Figure S3: Cumulative meta-analysis showing a decrease in hospital mortality for surgical pulmonary embolectomy from 42.86% in 1965 to 20.56% in 2024, Figure S4: Hospital mortality (A) leave-one-out and (B) funnel plot, Figure S5: Forest plot for hospital CV mortality, Figure S6: Forest plot of non-CV hospital mortality, Figure S7: (A) Late cardiovascular (CV) mortality and (B) late non-CV mortality, Figure S8: Forest plot of postoperative pulmonary bleeding, Figure S9: Forest plot of postoperative gastrointestinal (GI) bleeding, Figure S10: Forest plot bleeding at surgical site, Figure S11: Forest plot bleeding at non-surgical site, Figure S12: Wound complications, Table S1: Intraoperative criteria of included studies, Table S2: Newcastle–Ottawa scale for quality assessment of included studies.

Author Contributions: M.R. and M.M.E.-S.A. designed the project, M.R., S.A.-T., H.S., A.M., S.K., D.S., B.S., L.K., M.A. (Mohammad Alomari), M.A. (Mostafa Ali), I.A.M., J.C.H., S.M. and M.M.E.-S.A. wrote, revised and finalized the manuscript. All authors have read and agreed to the published version of the manuscript.

Funding: This research received no external funding.

Institutional Review Board Statement: There was no individual patient involvement in this study; as such, research ethics board approval was not required.

Informed Consent Statement: Not applicable.

Data Availability Statement: The data presented in this study are available on request from the corresponding authors. The data are not publicly available due to institutional policy.

Conflicts of Interest: All authors have reported that they have no relationships relevant to the contents of this paper to disclose.

References

1. Goldhaber, S.Z. Surgical Pulmonary Embolectomy: The Resurrection of an Almost Discarded Operation. *Tex. Heart Inst. J.* **2013**, *40*, 5–8.
2. Konstantinides, S.V.; Meyer, G.; Becattini, C.; Bueno, H.; Geersing, G.-J.; Harjola, V.-P.; Huisman, M.V.; Humbert, M.; Jennings, C.S.; Jiménez, D.; et al. 2019 ESC Guidelines for the Diagnosis and Management of Acute Pulmonary Embolism Developed in Collaboration with the European Respiratory Society (ERS). *Eur. Heart J.* **2020**, *41*, 543–603. [CrossRef]
3. Duffett, L.; Castellucci, L.A.; Forgie, M.A. Pulmonary Embolism: Update on Management and Controversies. *BMJ* **2020**, *370*, m2177. [CrossRef]
4. Kalra, R.; Bajaj, N.S.; Arora, P.; Arora, G.; Crosland, W.A.; McGiffin, D.C.; Ahmed, M.I. Surgical Embolectomy for Acute Pulmonary Embolism: Systematic Review and Comprehensive Meta-Analyses. *Ann. Thorac. Surg.* **2017**, *103*, 982–990. [CrossRef]
5. Wells, G.A.; Shea, B.; O'Connell, D.; Peterson, J.; Welch, V.; Losos, M.; Tugwell, P. The Newcastle-Ottawa Scale (NOS) for Assessing the Quality of Nonrandomised Studies in Meta-Analyses. Available online: https://web.archive.org/web/20210716121605id_/http://www3.med.unipmn.it/dispense_ebm/2009-2010/Corso%20Perfezionamento%20EBM_Faggiano/NOS_oxford.pdf (accessed on 5 July 2024).
6. Hartman, A.R.; Manetta, F.; Lessen, R.; Pekmezaris, R.; Kozikowski, A.; Jahn, L.; Akerman, M.; Lesser, M.L.; Glassman, L.R.; Graver, M.; et al. Acute Surgical Pulmonary Embolectomy: A 9-Year Retrospective Analysis. *Tex. Heart Inst. J.* **2015**, *42*, 25–29. [CrossRef]
7. Ahmed, P.; Khan, A.A.; Smith, A.; Pagala, M.; Abrol, S.; Cunningham, J.N.; Vaynblat, M. Expedient Pulmonary Embolectomy for Acute Pulmonary Embolism: Improved Outcomes. *Interact. Cardiovasc. Thorac. Surg.* **2008**, *7*, 591–594. [CrossRef]
8. Alqahtani, F.; Munir, M.B.; Aljohani, S.; Tarabishy, A.; Almustafa, A.; Alkhouli, M. Surgical Thrombectomy for Pulmonary Embolism: Updated Performance Rates and Outcomes. *Tex. Heart Inst. J.* **2019**, *46*, 172–174. [CrossRef]
9. Amirghofran, A.A.; Emami Nia, A.; Javan, R. Surgical Embolectomy in Acute Massive Pulmonary Embolism. *Asian Cardiovasc. Thorac. Ann.* **2007**, *15*, 149–153. [CrossRef]
10. Argyriou, A.; Vohra, H.; Chan, J.; Ahmed, E.M.; Rajakaruna, C.; Angelini, G.D.; Fudulu, D.P. Incidence and Outcomes of Surgical Pulmonary Embolectomy in the UK. *Br. J. Surg.* **2024**, *111*, znae003. [CrossRef]
11. Azari, A.; Bigdelu, L.; Moravvej, Z. Surgical Embolectomy in the Management of Massive and Sub-Massive Pulmonary Embolism: The Results of 30 Consecutive Ill Patients. *ARYA Atheroscler.* **2015**, *11*, 208–213.
12. Barrett, N.A.; Byrne, A.; Delaney, A.; Hibbert, M.; Ramakrishnan, N. Management of Massive Pulmonary Embolism: A Retrospective Single-Centre Cohort Study. *Crit. Care Resusc.* **2010**, *12*, 242–247. [CrossRef]
13. Bauer, E.; Laske, A.; Segesser, L.; Carrel, T.; Turina, M. Early and Late Results after Surgery for Massive Pulmonary Embolism. *Thorac. Cardiovasc. Surg.* **1991**, *39*, 353–356. [CrossRef]
14. Bennett, J.M.; Pretorius, M.; Ahmad, R.M.; Eagle, S.S. Hemodynamic Instability in Patients Undergoing Pulmonary Embolectomy: Institutional Experience. *J. Clin. Anesth.* **2015**, *27*, 207–213. [CrossRef]
15. Berger, R.L. Pulmonary Embolectomy with Preoperative Circulatory Support. *Ann. Thorac. Surg.* **1973**, *16*, 217–227. [CrossRef]
16. Biglioli, P.; Alamanni, F.; Spirito, R.; Arena, V. From deep venous thrombosis to pulmonary embolism. *Cardiologia* **1991**, *36*, 195–201.
17. Bøttzauw, J.; Vejlsted, H.; Albrechtsen, O. Pulmonary Embolectomy Using Extracorporeal Circulation. *Thorac. Cardiovasc. Surg.* **1981**, *29*, 320–322. [CrossRef]
18. Boulafendis, D.; Bastounis, E.; Panayiotopoulos, Y.P.; Papalambros, E.L. Pulmonary Embolectomy (Answered and Unanswered Questions). *Int. Angiol. J. Int. Union Angiol.* **1991**, *10*, 187–194.
19. Caleb, M.G. Massive Pulmonary Embolism with Haemodynamic Collapse. *Singap. Med. J.* **2002**, *43*, 25–27.
20. Clarke, D.B.; Abrams, L.D. Pulmonary Embolectomy: A 25 Year Experience. *J. Thorac. Cardiovasc. Surg.* **1986**, *92*, 442–445. [CrossRef]
21. Dauphine, C.; Omari, B. Pulmonary Embolectomy for Acute Massive Pulmonary Embolism. *Ann. Thorac. Surg.* **2005**, *79*, 1240–1244. [CrossRef]
22. De Weese, J.A. The Role of Pulmonary Embolectomy in Venous Thromboembolism. *J. Cardiovasc. Surg.* **1976**, *17*, 348–353.
23. DiChiacchio, L.; Pasrija, C.; Boulos, F.M.; Ramani, G.; Jeudy, J.; Deatrick, K.B.; Griffith, B.P.; Kon, Z.N. Occult Chronic Thromboembolic Disease in Patients Presenting for Surgical Pulmonary Embolectomy. *Ann. Thorac. Surg.* **2019**, *108*, 1183–1188. [CrossRef]
24. Digonnet, A.; Moya-Plana, A.; Aubert, S.; Flecher, E.; Bonnet, N.; Leprince, P.; Pavie, A.; Gandjbakhch, I. Acute Pulmonary Embolism: A Current Surgical Approach. *Interdiscip. CardioVascular Thorac. Surg.* **2007**, *6*, 27–29. [CrossRef]
25. Doerge, H.; Schoendube, F.; Voß, M.; Seipelt, R.; Messmer, B. Surgical Therapy of Fulminant Pulmonary Embolism: Early and Late Results. *Thorac. Cardiovasc. Surg.* **1999**, *47*, 9–13. [CrossRef]
26. Dohle, K.; Dohle, D.-S.; El Beyrouti, H.; Buschmann, K.; Emrich, A.L.; Brendel, L.; Vahl, C.-F. Short- and Long-Term Outcomes for the Surgical Treatment of Acute Pulmonary Embolism. *Innov. Surg. Sci.* **2018**, *3*, 271–276. [CrossRef]
27. Edelman, J.J.; Okiwelu, N.; Anvardeen, K.; Joshi, P.; Murphy, B.; Sanders, L.H.; Newman, M.A.; Passage, J. Surgical Pulmonary Embolectomy: Experience in a Series of 37 Consecutive Cases. *Heart Lung Circ.* **2016**, *25*, 1240–1244. [CrossRef]
28. Estrera, A.S.; Platt, M.R.; Mills, L.J. Pulmonary Embolectomy for Massive Pulmonary Embolism. *Tex. Med.* **1981**, *77*, 46–51.

29. Fedorov, S.A.; Pichugin, V.V.; Chiginev, V.A.; Brichkin, Y.D.; Kulkarni, S.V.; Tselousova, L.M.; Kalinina, M.L.; Taranov, E.V.; Domnin, S.E. Domnin Possibilities and Perspectives of Retrograde Pulmonary Artery Perfusion as a Component of Surgical Treatment of Pulmonary Embolism. *Opera Med. Physiol.* **2022**, *9*, 95–102. [CrossRef]
30. Glassford, D.M.; Alford, W.C.; Burrus, G.R.; Stoney, W.S.; Thomas, C.S. Pulmonary Embolectomy. *Ann. Thorac. Surg.* **1981**, *32*, 28–32. [CrossRef]
31. Gray, H.H.; Morgan, J.M.; Paneth, M.; Miller, G.A. Pulmonary Embolectomy for Acute Massive Pulmonary Embolism: An Analysis of 71 Cases. *Heart* **1988**, *60*, 196–200. [CrossRef]
32. Greelish, J.P.; Leacche, M.; Solenkova, N.S.; Ahmad, R.M.; Byrne, J.G. Improved Midterm Outcomes for Type A (Central) Pulmonary Emboli Treated Surgically. *J. Thorac. Cardiovasc. Surg.* **2011**, *142*, 1423–1429. [CrossRef]
33. Hajizadeh, R.; Ghaffari, S.; Habibzadeh, A.; Safaei, N.; Mohammadi, K.; Ranjbar, A.; Ghodratizadeh, S. Outcome of Surgical Embolectomy in Patients with Massive Pulmonary Embolism with and without Cardiopulmonary Resuscitation. *Pol. J. Thorac. Cardiovasc. Surg.* **2017**, *4*, 241–244. [CrossRef]
34. Hennig, K.; Franke, D.; Fenn, K. Pulmonary embolectomy (report on 3 personal cases). *VASA Z. Gefasskrankh.* **1974**, *3*, 342–348.
35. Jakob, H.; Vahl, C.; Lange, R.; Micek, M.; Tanzeem, A.; Hagl, S. Modified Surgical Concept for Fulminant Pulmonary Embolism. *Eur. J. Cardio-Thorac. Surg.* **1995**, *9*, 557–561. [CrossRef]
36. Jaumin, P.; Moriau, M.; el Gariani, A.; Rubay, J.; Baele, P.; Dautrebande, J.; Goenen, M.; Servaye-Kestens, Y.; Ponlot, R. Pulmonary embolectomy. Clinical experience. *Acta Chir. Belg.* **1986**, *85*, 123–125.
37. Keeling, W.B.; Sundt, T.; Leacche, M.; Okita, Y.; Binongo, J.; Lasajanak, Y.; Aklog, L.; Lattouf, O.M. Outcomes After Surgical Pulmonary Embolectomy for Acute Pulmonary Embolus: A Multi-Institutional Study. *Ann. Thorac. Surg.* **2016**, *102*, 1498–1502. [CrossRef]
38. Keeling, W.B.; Leshnower, B.G.; Lasajanak, Y.; Binongo, J.; Guyton, R.A.; Halkos, M.E.; Thourani, V.H.; Lattouf, O.M. Midterm Benefits of Surgical Pulmonary Embolectomy for Acute Pulmonary Embolus on Right Ventricular Function. *J. Thorac. Cardiovasc. Surg.* **2016**, *152*, 872–878. [CrossRef]
39. Khoury, E.; Rabinov, M.; Davis, B.B.; Stirling, G.R. Pulmonary Embolectomy in the Management of Massive Pulmonary Embolism. *Australas. J. Card. Thorac. Surg.* **1992**, *1*, 25–26. [CrossRef]
40. Kieny, R.; Charpentier, A.; Kieny, M.T. What Is the Place of Pulmonary Embolectomy Today? *J. Cardiovasc. Surg.* **1991**, *32*, 549–554.
41. Konstantinov, I.E.; Saxena, P.; Koniuszko, M.D.; Alvarez, J.; Newman, M.A.J. Acute Massive Pulmonary Embolism with Cardiopulmonary Resuscitation: Management and Results. *Tex. Heart Inst. J.* **2007**, *34*, 41–45; discussion 45–46.
42. Laas, J.; Schmid, C.; Albes, J.M.; Borst, H.G. Surgical aspects of fulminant pulmonary embolism. *Z. Kardiol.* **1993**, *82* (Suppl. S2), 25–28.
43. Leacche, M.; Unic, D.; Goldhaber, S.Z.; Rawn, J.D.; Aranki, S.F.; Couper, G.S.; Mihaljevic, T.; Rizzo, R.J.; Cohn, L.H.; Aklog, L.; et al. Modern Surgical Treatment of Massive Pulmonary Embolism: Results in 47 Consecutive Patients after Rapid Diagnosis and Aggressive Surgical Approach. *J. Thorac. Cardiovasc. Surg.* **2005**, *129*, 1018–1023. [CrossRef]
44. Lehnert, P.; Møller, C.H.; Carlsen, J.; Grande, P.; Steinbrüchel, D.A. Surgical Treatment of Acute Pulmonary Embolism—A 12-Year Retrospective Analysis. *Scand. Cardiovasc. J.* **2012**, *46*, 172–176. [CrossRef]
45. Lund, O.; Nielsen, T.; Schifter, S.; Roenne, K. Treatment of Pulmonary Embolism with Full-Dose Heparin, Streptokinase or Embolectomy—Results and Indications. *Thorac. Cardiovasc. Surg.* **1986**, *34*, 240–246. [CrossRef]
46. Malekan, R.; Saunders, P.C.; Yu, C.J.; Brown, K.A.; Gass, A.L.; Spielvogel, D.; Lansman, S.L. Peripheral Extracorporeal Membrane Oxygenation: Comprehensive Therapy for High-Risk Massive Pulmonary Embolism. *Ann. Thorac. Surg.* **2012**, *94*, 104–108. [CrossRef]
47. Marshall, L.; Mundy, J.; Garrahy, P.; Christopher, S.; Wood, A.; Griffin, R.; Shah, P. Surgical Pulmonary Embolectomy: Mid-term Outcomes. *ANZ J. Surg.* **2012**, *82*, 822–826. [CrossRef]
48. Mattox, K.L.; Feldtman, R.W.; Beall, A.C.; DeBAKEY, M.E. Pulmonary Embolectomy for Acute Massive Pulmonary Embolism. *Ann. Surg.* **1982**, *195*, 726–731. [CrossRef]
49. Meyer, G.; Tamisier, D.; Sors, H.; Vouhé, P.; Makowski, S.; Neveux, J.-Y.; Leca, F.; Even, P. Pulmonary Embolectomy: A 20-Year Experience at One Center. *Ann. Thorac. Surg.* **1991**, *51*, 232–236. [CrossRef]
50. Meyns, B.; Sergeant, P.; Flameng, W.; Daenen, W. Surgery for Massive Pulmonary Embolism. *Acta Cardiol.* **1992**, *47*, 487–493.
51. Minakawa, M.; Fukuda, I.; Miyata, H.; Motomura, N.; Takamoto, S.; Taniguchi, S.; Daitoku, K.; Kondo, N.; Japan Cardiovascular Surgery Database Organization. Outcomes of Pulmonary Embolectomy for Acute Pulmonary Embolism. *Circ. J.* **2018**, *82*, 2184–2190. [CrossRef]
52. Mkalaluh, S.; Szczechowicz, M.; Karck, M.; Szabo, G. Twenty-Year Results of Surgical Pulmonary Thromboembolectomy in Acute Pulmonary Embolism. *Scand. Cardiovasc. J.* **2019**, *53*, 98–103. [CrossRef]
53. Neely, R.C.; Byrne, J.G.; Gosev, I.; Cohn, L.H.; Javed, Q.; Rawn, J.D.; Goldhaber, S.Z.; Piazza, G.; Aranki, S.F.; Shekar, P.S.; et al. Surgical Embolectomy for Acute Massive and Submassive Pulmonary Embolism in a Series of 115 Patients. *Ann. Thorac. Surg.* **2015**, *100*, 1245–1252. [CrossRef]
54. Newcomb, G.; Wilson, B.L.; White, R.J.; Goldman, B.; Lachant, N.A.; Lachant, D.J. An Untapped Resource: Characteristics of Thrombus Recovered from Intermediate or High Risk Pulmonary Embolus Patients. *Cardiovasc. Pathol.* **2022**, *57*, 107392. [CrossRef]

55. Osborne, Z.J.; Rossi, P.; Aucar, J.; Dharamsy, S.; Cook, S.; Wheatley, B. Surgical Pulmonary Embolectomy in a Community Hospital. *Am. J. Surg.* **2014**, *207*, 337–341. [CrossRef]
56. Panholzer, B.; Gravert, H.; Borzikowsky, C.; Huenges, K.; Schoettler, J.; Schoeneich, F.; Attmann, T.; Haneya, A.; Frank, D.; Cremer, J.; et al. Outcome after Surgical Embolectomy for Acute Pulmonary Embolism. *J. Cardiovasc. Med.* **2022**, *23*, 519–523. [CrossRef]
57. Park, J.; Lim, S.-H.; Hong, Y.S.; Park, S.; Lee, C.J.; Lee, S.O. Acute Pulmonary Thromboembolism: 14 Years of Surgical Experience. *Korean J. Thorac. Cardiovasc. Surg.* **2019**, *52*, 78–84. [CrossRef]
58. Pasrija, C.; Shah, A.; Sultanik, E.; Rouse, M.; Ghoreishi, M.; Bittle, G.J.; Boulos, F.; Griffith, B.P.; Kon, Z.N. Minimally Invasive Surgical Pulmonary Embolectomy: A Potential Alternative to Conventional Sternotomy. *Innov. Technol. Tech. Cardiothorac. Vasc. Surg.* **2017**, *12*, 406–410. [CrossRef]
59. Pasrija, C.; Kronfli, A.; Rouse, M.; Raithel, M.; Bittle, G.J.; Pousatis, S.; Ghoreishi, M.; Gammie, J.S.; Griffith, B.P.; Sanchez, P.G.; et al. Outcomes after Surgical Pulmonary Embolectomy for Acute Submassive and Massive Pulmonary Embolism: A Single-Center Experience. *J. Thorac. Cardiovasc. Surg.* **2018**, *155*, 1095–1106.e2. [CrossRef]
60. Wang, Q.; Chen, L.; Chen, D.; Qiu, H.; Huang, Z.; Dai, X.; Huang, X.; Lin, F.; Chen, H. Clinical Outcomes of Acute Pulmonary Embolectomy as the First-Line Treatment for Massive and Submassive Pulmonary Embolism: A Single-Centre Study in China. *J. Cardiothorac. Surg.* **2020**, *15*, 321. [CrossRef]
61. Rathore, K.S.; Weightman, W.; Passage, J.; Joshi, P.; Sanders, L.; Newman, M. Risk Stratification Using Serum Lactate in Patients Undergoing Surgical Pulmonary Embolectomy. *J. Cardiothorac. Surg.* **2020**, *35*, 1531–1538. [CrossRef]
62. Rivas, J.; Bircks, W.; Nier, H.; Schneider, E.; Tarbiat, S. Lungenembolie. *DMW—Dtsch. Med. Wochenschr.* **1975**, *100*, 1239–1245. [CrossRef] [PubMed]
63. Sa, Y.; Choi, S.; Lee, J.; Kwon, J.; Moon, S.; Jo, K.; Wang, Y.; Kim, S.; Park, J.; Jung, H. Off-Pump Open Pulmonary Embolectomy for Patients with Major Pulmonary Embolism. *Heart Surg. Forum* **2007**, *10*, E304–E308. [CrossRef] [PubMed]
64. Salehi, R.; Ansarin, K. Surgical Embolectomy in Treating Acute Massive Pulmonary Embolism. *J. Pak. Med. Assoc.* **2013**, *63*, 969–972.
65. Sareyyupoglu, B.; Greason, K.L.; Suri, R.M.; Keegan, M.T.; Dearani, J.A.; Sundt, T.M. A More Aggressive Approach to Emergency Embolectomy for Acute Pulmonary Embolism. *Mayo Clin. Proc.* **2010**, *85*, 785–790. [CrossRef]
66. Satter, P. Pulmonary Embolectomy. Indication and Results. *Ann. Radiol.* **1980**, *23*, 321–324.
67. Saylam, A.; Melo, J.Q.; Ahmad, A.; Chapman, R.D.; Wood, J.A.; Starr, A. Pulmonary Embolectomy. *West. J. Med.* **1978**, *128*, 377–381.
68. Shiomi, D.; Kiyama, H.; Shimizu, M.; Yamada, M.; Shimada, N.; Takahashi, A.; Kaki, N. Surgical Embolectomy for High-Risk Acute Pulmonary Embolism Is Standard Therapy. *Interdiscip. CardioVascular Thorac. Surg.* **2017**, *25*, 297–301. [CrossRef]
69. Spagnolo, S.; Grasso, M.A.; Tesler, U.F. Retrograde Pulmonary Perfusion Improves Results in Pulmonary Embolectomy for Massive Pulmonary Embolism. *Tex. Heart Inst. J.* **2006**, *33*, 473–476.
70. Stalpaert, G.; Suy, R.; Daenen, W.; Flameng, W.; Sergeant, P.; Nevelsteen, A.; Lauwers, P.; De Geest, H.; Van Elst, F. Surgical Treatment of Acute, Massive Lung Embolism. Results and Follow-Up. *Acta Chir. Belg.* **1986**, *86*, 118–122.
71. Stulz, P.; Schlapfer, R.; Feer, R.; Habicht, J.; Gradel, E. Decision Making in the Surgical Treatment of Massive Pulmonary Embolism. *Eur. J. Cardio-Thorac. Surg.* **1994**, *8*, 188–193. [CrossRef]
72. Takahashi, H.; Okada, K.; Matsumori, M.; Kano, H.; Kitagawa, A.; Okita, Y. Aggressive Surgical Treatment of Acute Pulmonary Embolism with Circulatory Collapse. *Ann. Thorac. Surg.* **2012**, *94*, 785–791. [CrossRef]
73. Taniguchi, S.; Fukuda, W.; Fukuda, I.; Watanabe, K.-I.; Saito, Y.; Nakamura, M.; Sakuma, M. Outcome of Pulmonary Embolectomy for Acute Pulmonary Thromboembolism: Analysis of 32 Patients from a Multicentre Registry in Japan. *Interact. Cardiovasc. Thorac. Surg.* **2012**, *14*, 64–67. [CrossRef]
74. Thielmann, M.; Pasa, S.; Wendt, D.; Price, V.; Marggraf, G.; Neuhauser, M.; Piotrowski, A.; Jakob, H. Prognostic Significance of Cardiac Troponin I on Admission for Surgical Treatment of Acute Pulmonary Embolism: A Single-Centre Experience over More than 10 Years. *Eur. J. Cardiothorac. Surg.* **2012**, *42*, 951–957. [CrossRef]
75. Turnier, E.; Hill, J.D.; Kerth, W.J.; Gerbode, F. Massive Pulmonary Embolism. *Am. J. Surg.* **1973**, *125*, 611–622. [CrossRef]
76. Ullmann, M.; Hemmer, W.; Hannekum, A. The Urgent Pulmonary Embolectomy: Mechanical Resuscitation in the Operating Theatre Determines the Outcome. *Thorac. Cardiovasc. Surg.* **1999**, *47*, 5–8. [CrossRef]
77. Vohra, H.A.; Whistance, R.N.; Mattam, K.; Kaarne, M.; Haw, M.P.; Barlow, C.W.; Tsang, G.M.K.; Livesey, S.A.; Ohri, S.K. Early and Late Clinical Outcomes of Pulmonary Embolectomy for Acute Massive Pulmonary Embolism. *Ann. Thorac. Surg.* **2010**, *90*, 1747–1752. [CrossRef]
78. Vossschulte, K.; Stiller, H.; Eisenreich, F. Emergency Embolectomy by the Transsternal Approach in Acute Pulmonary Embolism. *Surgery* **1965**, *58*, 317–323.
79. Wu, M.-Y.; Liu, Y.-C.; Tseng, Y.-H.; Chang, Y.-S.; Lin, P.-J.; Wu, T.-I. Pulmonary Embolectomy in High-Risk Acute Pulmonary Embolism: The Effectiveness of a Comprehensive Therapeutic Algorithm Including Extracorporeal Life Support. *Resuscitation* **2013**, *84*, 1365–1370. [CrossRef]
80. Yalamanchili, K.; Fleisher, A.G.; Lehrman, S.G.; Axelrod, H.I.; Lafaro, R.J.; Sarabu, M.R.; Zias, E.A.; Moggio, R.A. Open Pulmonary Embolectomy for Treatment of Major Pulmonary Embolism. *Ann. Thorac. Surg.* **2004**, *77*, 819–823. [CrossRef]
81. Yavuz, S.; Toktas, F.; Goncu, T.; Eris, C.; Gucu, A.; Ay, D.; Erdolu, B.; Tenekecioglu, E.; Karaagac, K.; Vural, H.; et al. Surgical Embolectomy for Acute Massive Pulmonary Embolism. *Int. J. Clin. Exp. Med.* **2014**, *7*, 5362–5375.

82. Zarrabi, K.; Zolghadrasli, A.; Ostovan, M.A.; Azimifar, A.; Malekmakan, L. Residual Pulmonary Hypertension after Retrograde Pulmonary Embolectomy: Long-Term Follow-up of 30 Patients with Massive and Submassive Pulmonary Embolism. *Interact. Cardiovasc. Thorac. Surg.* **2013**, *17*, 242–246. [CrossRef] [PubMed]
83. Zieliński, D.; Zygier, M.; Dyk, W.; Wojdyga, R.; Wróbel, K.; Pirsztuk, E.; Szostakiewicz, K.; Szatkowski, P.; Darocha, S.; Kurzyna, M.; et al. Acute Pulmonary Embolism with Coexisting Right Heart Thrombi in Transit-Surgical Treatment of 20 Consecutive Patients. *Eur. J. Cardio-Thorac. Surg. Off. J. Eur. Assoc. Cardio-Thorac. Surg.* **2023**, *63*, ezad022. [CrossRef] [PubMed]
84. Kilic, A.; Shah, A.S.; Conte, J.V.; Yuh, D.D. Nationwide Outcomes of Surgical Embolectomy for Acute Pulmonary Embolism. *J. Thorac. Cardiovasc. Surg.* **2013**, *145*, 373–377. [CrossRef] [PubMed]
85. Stein, P.D.; Alnas, M.; Beemath, A.; Patel, N.R. Outcome of Pulmonary Embolectomy. *Am. J. Cardiol.* **2007**, *99*, 421–423. [CrossRef]
86. Poterucha, T.J.; Bergmark, B.; Aranki, S.; Kaneko, T.; Piazza, G. Surgical Pulmonary Embolectomy. *Circulation* **2015**, *132*, 1146–1151. [CrossRef]

Disclaimer/Publisher's Note: The statements, opinions and data contained in all publications are solely those of the individual author(s) and contributor(s) and not of MDPI and/or the editor(s). MDPI and/or the editor(s) disclaim responsibility for any injury to people or property resulting from any ideas, methods, instructions or products referred to in the content.

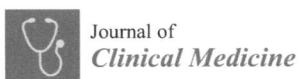

Communication

Predictors of Residual Pulmonary Vascular Obstruction after Acute Pulmonary Embolism Based on Patient Variables and Treatment Modality

Truong-An Andrew Ho [1,*], Jay Pescatore [1], Ka U. Lio [2], Parth Rali [1], Gerard Criner [1] and Shameek Gayen [1]

1. Department of Thoracic Medicine and Surgery, Temple University Hospital, Philadelphia, PA 19140, USA; jay.pescatore@tuhs.temple.edu (J.P.); shameek.gayen@tuhs.temple.edu (S.G.)
2. Department of Medicine, Lewis Katz School of Medicine at Temple University, Philadelphia, PA 19140, USA
* Correspondence: truong-an.ho@tuhs.temple.edu

Abstract: Background: Residual Pulmonary Vascular Obstruction (RPVO) is an area of increasing focus in patients with acute pulmonary embolism (PE) due to its association with long-term morbidity and mortality. The predictive factors and the effect catheter-directed therapies (CDT) have on RPVO are still under investigation. **Methods:** This is a single-center retrospective review between April 2017 and July 2021. Patients with intermediate risk of PE were included. Patient variables associated with RPVO were analyzed and the degree of clot burden was quantified using the Qanadli score. **Results:** A total of 551 patients with acute PE were identified, 288 were intermediate risk and 53 had RPVO based on CT or V/Q scan three months post-PE. Baseline clot burden was higher in patients who received CDT compared to those who received anticoagulation alone (Qanadli score 45.88% vs. 31.94% $p < 0.05$). In univariate analysis, treatment with CDT showed a HR of 0.32 (95% CI 0.21–0.50, $p < 0.001$) when compared with anticoagulation alone. Patient variables including intermediate-high risk, sPESI ≥ 1, elevated biomarkers, RV dysfunction on imaging, malignancy, history of or concurrent DVT were also significantly associated with development of RPVO in univariate analysis. In multivariable analysis, only baseline Qanadli score (HR 13.88, 95% CI 1.42–135.39, $p = 0.02$) and concurrent DVT (HR 2.53, 95% CI 1.01–6.40, $p = 0.04$) were significantly associated with the development of RPVO. **Conclusions:** Catheter-directed therapy may be associated with a reduced risk of RPVO at 3 months; however, quantitative clot burden scores, such as the Qanadli score, may be stronger predictors of the risk of developing RPVO at 3 months. Further prospective studies are required

Keywords: pulmonary embolism; reperfusion; residual pulmonary vascular obstruction; chronic thromboembolic disease; catheter-directed therapy

1. Introduction

Residual Pulmonary Vascular Obstruction (RPVO), defined as persistent vascular obstruction after a pulmonary embolism (PE), has been identified as a key pathophysiologic step in the development of chronic thromboembolic pulmonary hypertension (CTEPH) and chronic thromboembolic disease (CTED) [1]. It has also been associated with an increase in morbidity and mortality after acute pulmonary embolism [2,3], and recurrence of PE [4–6]. Currently, the factors that elevate a patients' risk of RPVO remain under investigation. One study by Raj et al. used the data from the PADIS-PE trial and found that six months after a patients first unprovoked PE, age more than 65, pulmonary vascular obstruction index $\geq 25\%$, elevated factor 8 level, and chronic respiratory disease were predictors of RPVO [7]. Similarly, Sanchez et al. found that age, longer time between symptom onset and diagnosis, initial pulmonary vascular obstruction, and previous VTE (Venous Thromboembolism) were associated [8].

Given the elevated risk of bleeding with systemic thrombolytics, catheter-directed therapies (CDT) have become an increasingly studied treatment modality for intermediate-risk PE, providing an alternative to simple anticoagulation alone [9]. While CDT has been shown to have the potential to improve hemodynamics [10–12], more benefits in terms of patient centered outcomes remains to be seen. The ability for CDT to decrease rates of post PE syndromes such as RPVO is currently lacking in evidence. Defining these long-term benefits becomes increasingly important as the usage of CDT has risen sharply over the recent years and is expected to continue to rise [13].

We hypothesize that the treatment of intermediate-risk PE via CDT is associated with a reduced risk of RPVO after acute PE. Our primary objective was to determine significant and independent associations with the risk of developing RPVO after acute PE.

2. Material and Methods

This is a single-center retrospective review of the electronic medical record between April 2017 and July 2021 for consecutive patients that were collected from the Pulmonary Embolism Response Team database. This study was performed in accordance with the ethical standards of the Helsinki Declaration of 1975 and Western Institutional Review Board (TEMP-9448).

Inclusion criteria included patients with acute pulmonary embolism who were intermediate, low or high, risk based on the European Society of Cardiology guidelines [14]. CT angiogram or ventilation perfusion imaging obtained at least 3 months after treatment were required to identify persistent clot burden. Patient variables identified were risk category per European Society of Cardiology, sPESI, Brain Natriuretic Peptide (BNP), troponin, right ventricular dysfunction on CT angiogram or transthoracic echocardiogram, active malignancy, concurrent deep vein thrombosis (DVT), prior VTE, and initial Qanadli score. The Qanadli score is a validated quantitative clot burden score. It is an additive point scale scoring system in which the maximum score is 40, such that the Qanadli embolism index = (embolism number $\times$ embolism degree)/40 $\times$ 100% [15]. An internal medicine physician was responsible for the calculation of the Qanadli score. Descriptive statistics with univariate and multivariable logistic regression were applied to determine associations with the risk of RPVO. Statistical significance was defined as a p valve less than 0.05 and a confidence interval that did not cross 1. ROC curves were created assessing the performance of the Qanadli score as a predictor of RPVO in patients that received CDT or anticoagulation alone.

3. Results

We identified 551 patients with acute PE that were evaluated during our study period. Of those, 270 were intermediate-low, or high risk and were included in the analysis (Table 1). A total of 51% (n = 138) of patients were female, and mean age was 58.9 with a SD of 15.2. A total of 30% (n = 81) of patients had a history of VTE, and 20.7% (n = 56) had a history of malignancy. A total of 40.7% (n = 110) of patients were intermediate-low risk and 59.3% (n = 160) were intermediate-high risk. On admission, 63.8% (166/260) had an elevated BNP, and 51.7% (139/269) had an elevated troponin. In initial imaging studies, 67.7% (178/263) of patients who underwent CT scan showed RV dysfunction, while 73.8% (194/263) of patients who underwent echocardiogram showed RV dysfunction. A total of 57.4% (143/249) of patients who had lower extremity dopplers performed were positive for DVT.

In regard to treatment, 53% (n = 143) were treated with anticoagulation (AC) alone, 44.8% (n = 121) were treated with AC in conjunction with additional therapy, and 2.2% (n = 6) received no AC. Of those patients that received advanced therapies, 74.2% (n = 89) received CDT, 9.9% (n = 12) received systemic thrombolysis, 16.5% (n = 20) received mechanical thrombectomy, and 2.4% (n = 3) received surgical thrombectomy. There were 53 patients who had RPVO based on either CT or V/Q scan three months after acute PE (Table 1).

Table 1. Baseline demographics of intermediate risk PE patients, stratified by RPVO and treatment modality.

	Intermediate Risk PE n = 270	RPVO (+) n = 53	RPVO (−) n = 217	AC Alone n = 143	CDT n = 89
Demographic data					
Age—years	58.9 ± 15.2	59.2 ± 15.4	58.8 ± 15.2	59.8 ± 15.2	57.4 ± 13
Sex—no. (%)					
Female	138 (51.1)	33 (62.3)	105 (48.4)	64 (44.8)	60 (67.4)
Male	132 (48.9)	20 (37.7)	112 (51.6)	79 (55.2)	29 (32.6)
Race—no. (%)					
Caucasian	147 (54.4)	10 (18.9)	45 (20.7)	23 (16.1)	22 (24.7)
African American	55 (20.4)	33 (62.3)	114 (52.5)	76 (53.1)	48 (53.9)
Asian/Pacific Islander	64 (23.7)	6 (11.3)	58 (26.7)	42 (29.4)	17 (19.1)
Other/unknown	4 (1.5)	4 (7.5)	4 (1.8)	2 (1.4)	2 (2.2)
BMI	34.1 ± 10.5	30.9 ± 7.5	34.8 ± 10.9	32.2 ± 10.78	38.14 ± 9.6
Medical History					
History of DVT—no. (%)	58 (21.5)	8 (15.1)	50 (23)	32 (22.4)	20 (22.5)
History of PE—no. (%)	53 (19.6)	6 (11.3)	47 (21.7)	25 (17.5)	25 (28.1)
History of malignancy—no. (%)	56 (20.7)	10 (18.9)	46 (21.1)	34 (23.8)	11 (12.4)
History of COPD—no. (%)	27 (10)	4 (7.5)	23 (10.6)	19 (13.3)	6 (6.7)
History of recent surgery—no. (%)	29 (10.7)	4 (7.5)	25 (11.5)	19 (13.3)	0 (0)
Clinical Status					
sPESI—mean ± SD	1.58 ± 1.1	1.37 ± 1.07	1.62 ± 1.07	1.71 ± 1.06	1.1 ± 0.85
Intermediate-low risk—no. (%)	110 (40.7)	16 (30.2)	94 (43.3)	90 (63)	9 (10.1)
Intermediate-high risk—no. (%)	160 (59.3)	37 (69.8)	123 (56.7)	53 (37)	80 (89.9)
Oxygen treatment—no. (%)	136 (50.3)	29 (54.7)	107 (49.3)	70 (49)	44 (49.4)
Elevated BNP—no. (%)	166 (61.48)	37 (69.8)	129 (59.4)	78 (54.4)	65 (73)
Elevated troponin—no. (%)	139 (51.5)	31 (58.4)	108 (49.7)	55 (38.5)	60 (67)
RV dysfunction on CT—no. (%)	178 (65.9)	47 (88.7)	131 (60.4)	76 (53.1)	76 (85)
RV dysfunction on ECHO—no. (%)	194 (71.9)	41 (77.4)	153 (70.5)	95 (66.4)	74 (83.1)
Concurrent DVT—no. (%)	143 (57.4)	35 (66)	108 (49.8)	53 (37)	66 (74)
Therapy					
Anticoagulation alone—no. (%)	143 (53)	22 (41.5)	121 (55.5)	143 (100)	0 (0)
Catheter-Directed Thrombolysis—no. (%)	89 (33)	23 (43.3)	66 (30.3)	0 (0)	89 (100)
Mechanical thrombectomy—no. (%)	20 (7.4)	6 (11.3)	14 (6.4)	0 (0)	0 (0)
Systemic thrombolysis—no. (%)	12 (4.4)	2 (3.7)	10 (4.6)	0 (0)	0 (0)
Surgical thrombectomy—no. (%)	3 (1.1)	0 (0)	3 (1.4)	0 (0)	0 (0)
No therapy—no. (%)	6 (2.2)	0 (0)	6 (2.8)	0 (0)	0 (0)
Measurements of clot					
Baseline Qanadli score %	38.87 ± 20.5	51.18 ± 11.9	34.97 ± 21.2	31.94 ± 16.9	45.88 ± 19.5
+RPVO—no. (%)	53 (19.6)	53 (100)	0 (0)	22 (15.4)	23 (25.8)
−RPVO—no. (%)	217 (80.4)	0 (0)	217 (100)	121 (84.6)	66 (74.2)

PE, pulmonary embolism; RPVO, residual pulmonary vascular obstruction; AC, anticoagulation; CDT, catheter directed therapies; BMI, body mass index; DVT, deep vein thrombosis; COPD, chronic obstructive pulmonary disease; sPESI, simplified pulmonary embolism severity index; BNP, brain natriuretic peptide; RV, right ventricular; CT, computed tomography; ECHO, echocardiogram.

For the degree of clot burden, the Qanadli score at baseline for all intermediate-risk PE patients had a mean of 38.87% with a SD of 20.5%. The baseline Qanadli score for patients with RPVO had a mean of 51.18% with a SD of 11.9%, while patients without RPVO had a mean of 34.97% with a SD 21.2%. In patients who underwent CDT, the mean baseline Qanadli score was 45.88% with a of SD 19.6% as compared to the group that received AC alone, which had a Qanadli score of 31.94% with a of SD 16.9%. T-test between mean CDT Qanadli score and anticoagulation group alone was <0.05.

Univariate logistic regression was performed to assess factors associated with RPVO at 3 months post-PE; variables with significant association were then utilized in multivariable logistic regression to determine independent and significant associations with risk of RPVO. Treatment with CDT and AC showed a reduced risk of RPVO development (HR 0.32, 95% CI 0.21–0.50, $p < 0.001$) when compared with AC alone. Patient variables including intermediate-high risk, sPESI greater than or equal to 1, elevated biomarkers (BNP or troponin), RV dysfunction on imaging (CTA or echocardiogram), and concurrent DVT were also significantly associated with development of RPVO in univariate analysis. In multivariable analysis, only the baseline Qanadli score (HR 13.88, 95% CI 1.42–135.39, p = 0.02) and concurrent DVT (HR 2.53, 95% CI 1.01–6.40, p = 0.04) were independently and significantly associated with an increased risk of the development of RPVO (Table 2).

Table 2. Univariate and multivariate analysis of factors predictive of RPVO.

Patient Variables/Interventions	Univariate Analysis	Multivariate Analysis
AC + CDT	**HR 0.32, 95% CI 0.21–0.50, p < 0.001**	HR 0.35, 95% CI 0.11–1.12, p = 0.08
AC + tpa, mechanical thrombectomy	HR 0.40, 95% CI 0.13–1.28, p = 0.12	HR 1.99, 95% CI 0.58–6.77, p = 0.27
Intermediate-high risk	**HR 0.32, 95% CI 0.23–0.46, p < 0.001**	HR 0.98, 95% CI 0.28–3.42, p = 0.97
sPESI	**HR 0.55, 95% CI 0.45–0.66, p < 0.001**	HR 0.74, 95% CI 0.47–1.16, p = 0.19
Elevated biomarkers (BNP or troponin)	**HR 0.26, 95% CI 0.19–0.36, p < 0.001**	HR 0.96, 95% CI 0.29–3.19, p = 0.95
RV dysfunction on imaging (TTE or CTA)	**HR 0.28, 95% CI 0.20–0.39, p < 0.001**	HR 0.55, 95% CI 0.15–2.11, p = 0.39
Concurrent DVT	**HR 0.29, 95% CI 0.20–0.43, p < 0.05**	**HR 2.53, 95% CI 1.01–6.40, p = 0.04**
Baseline Qanadli score	**HR 6.58, 95% CI 1.35–32.17, p < 0.05**	**HR 16.12, 95% CI 2.47–20.84, p < 0.001**

Bolded font is statistically significant hazard ratio (HR). AC, anticoagulation; CDT, catheter directed therapies; tpa, tissue plasminogen activator; sPESI, simplified pulmonary embolism severity index; BNP, brain natriuretic peptide; TTE, transthoracic echocardiogram; CTA, computed tomography angiography; DVT, deep vein thrombosis.

The area under the ROC curve (AUC) was used to compare the ability of the Qanadli score to predict RPVO in patients who received CDT and those who received AC. The AUC for the CDT group was 0.84, p < 0.001 and the AUC for the patients who received AC alone was 0.72, p < 0.001 (Figures 1 and 2).

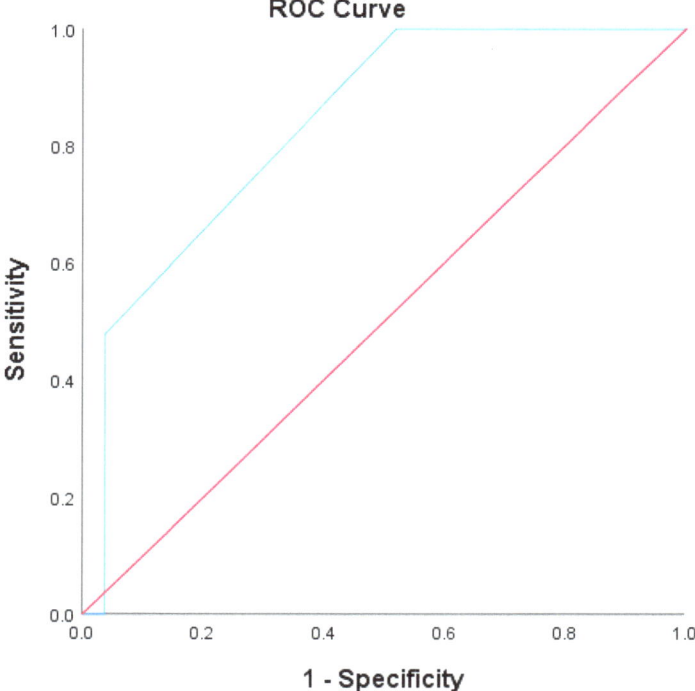

Figure 1. ROC curve assessing the Qanadli score as a predictor of RPVO (Residual Pulmonary Vascular Obstruction) in patients who received CDT (catheter directed therapy). AUC 0.84, p < 0.001.

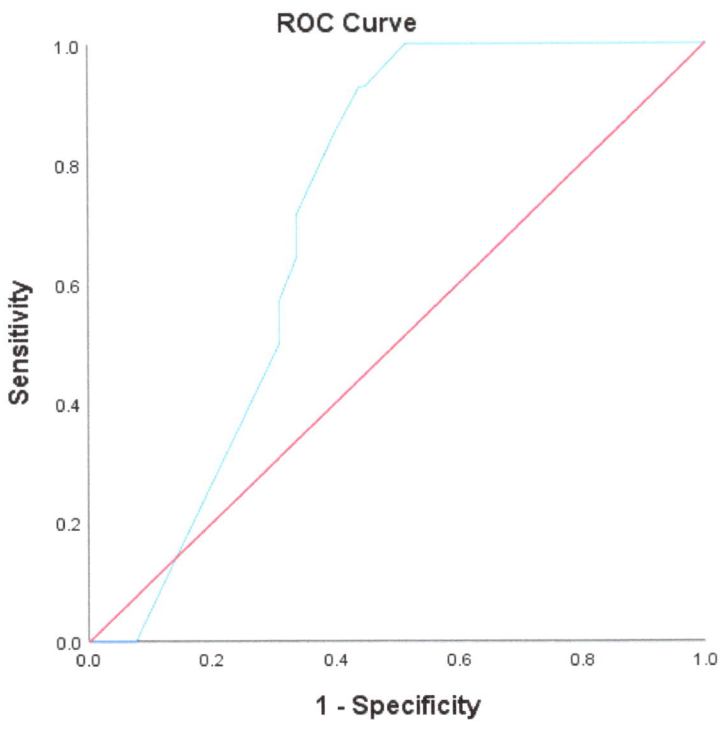

Figure 2. ROC curve assessing the Qanadli score as a predictor of RPVO(Residual Pulmonary Vascular Obstruction) in patients who received AC (anticoagulation) alone. AUC 0.72, $p < 0.001$.

4. Discussion

Post-pulmonary embolism syndromes, including CTEPH, CTED, and RPVO, are an area of increased investigation due to their long-term morbidity and mortality, necessitating studies into predictive factors [2,3]. Many patient characteristics have been associated with clot resolution including initial RV/LV diameter, PE location and size, degree of obstruction, early initiation of treatment, and provoked vs. unprovoked status [16,17]. Our findings noted significantly increased RPVO risk in patients with intermediate-high-risk PE, sPESI greater than or equal to 1, elevated biomarkers, RV dysfunction on imaging, and concurrent DVT. In multivariable analysis, however, only the degree of baseline clot burden, as measured by the Qanadli score and concurrent DVT, remained significantly associated with the development of RPVO. ROC were performed to assess the effectiveness of the Qanadli score and it was shown to perform well as a predictor of RPVO in both the CDT and AC groups, though slightly better in the CDT group.

The degree of initial clot burden has been consistently shown to be a risk factor for lack of clot resolution [7,8,16,17]. This suggests that quantifying the degree of clot burden, whether by Qanadli score, or other objective measurement allows for risk stratification of patients who may go on to develop post-PE syndromes. The Qanadli score is labor intensive, but with increased use of artificial intelligence in the workup of pulmonary embolism, rapid estimation of clot burden may be possible in the future. A small study by Sun et al. in 2020 found that computer-aided interpretation of vascular obstruction, as measured by the Qanadli score, reduced the time for interpretation and reliability of radiologists' findings [18]. PE identification pathways have already seen the integration of artificial intelligence in other ways, outside of clot burden measurements, and has shown synergistic effects when implemented alongside standard radiology practices [19,20]. Larger studies will be needed to see if initial clot burden scores can be integrated into risk stratification.

The increased risk of RPVO in intermediate-risk PE patients with concurrent DVT was also significant in our study. DVT associated with PE has been shown to be associated with increased PE-specific and all-cause mortality [21–23] and has been considered in the risk stratification of PE [24]. In RPVO, however, prior studies have not shown a statistically significant relationship between DVT and residual clot burden [5,6,8]. It is unclear the explanation for this; however, these prior studies assessed all-comers for PE and may have included a subset of patients in which clot resolution occurred without issue, while our intermediate-risk patients may have a higher proportion of patients that have problems resolving clot. We propose that having a DVT at time of diagnosis represents an elevated degree of clot burden, similar to a higher Qanadli score. Further studies will need to reassess the effects of DVT in specific PE populations in respect to RPVO, given the conflicting findings.

The role of CDT in intermediate-risk PE remains under investigation, and current guidelines suggest their use only in patients who have a contraindication or who have failed systemic thrombolysis [14,25]. Small prospective studies have focused on CDT's ability to improve RV dysfunction, as measured by the RV/LV ratio, without increased bleeding [10–12]; however, data showing long term benefit is lacking. A case series in 2022 by Gayen et al. examined three patients who underwent mechanical thrombectomy, and measured pre and post procedure perfusion scores, finding sustained improvements in perfusion immediately post procedure and at 3 months [26]. This suggests that other advanced therapies can improve long-term perfusion, but further studies focused on catheter-directed therapy are needed especially as their usage increases [13].

In our study, while CDT was associated with a reduced risk of RPVO on initial univariate analysis, it was not statistically significant in the multivariable analysis; however, there was a trend towards reduced risk (HR 0.35, 95% CI 0.11–1.12, p = 0.08). One potential explanation for this is that patients selected to undergo CDT had higher initial clot burden as compared to those who did not (Qanadli score 45.88% vs. 31.94%), and it is that initial clot burden that has the highest association with RPVO. Another possibility is that our sample size was too small; however, the potential benefit of CDT in reducing RPVO demonstrated in our analysis is promising. The ROC assessment demonstrated the increased effectiveness of the Qanadli score to predict RPVO in patients who received CDT as compared to AC; however, further studies are warranted (AUC 0.84, p < 0.001 vs. 0.72, p < 0.001) (Figures 1 and 2). To minimize confounders, further studies will require stratifying patients to different treatment arms based on their baseline clot score to truly examine the effects of catheter-directed treatments on long-term, patient-centered outcomes.

Limitations to this study include its retrospective nature, and while we are not able to show causation, our findings are consistent with prior studies evaluating predictive factors of clot nonresolution. Follow-up imaging was not performed at standard time periods; however, all imaging was collected after at least three months of therapy. It may also be significant that the majority of the patients in our study who received advanced therapies received catheter directed thrombolysis (74.2%) and relatively few received mechanical thrombectomy. The composition of clots seen in pulmonary embolism have been shown to evolve over time and have both different macro and micro appearances, with acute clots having higher fibrin content while more chronic clots consist of higher portions of collagen and elastin [1,27]. The chronicity of the clot has also been associated with resistance to fibrinolytics in other populations such as arterial thrombi and deep vein thrombosis [27,28]. This suggests that there may be a subset of patients with more chronic organized clot that may have improved response to mechanical removal given their decreased responsiveness to fibrinolytics; however, that remains to be proven, and improvement in CT imaging ability to distinguish chronicity would be required to stratify patients. The Qanadli score was also calculated by one of the authors, an internal medicine physician. While we believe this limited interoperator variability, future studies, in which a radiologist or artificial intelligence system are utilized, are warranted. Also challenging is how we define post-PE syndromes, such as RPVO, CTED, and CTEPH, with language that continues to evolve. For that reason, our study focuses solely on clot nonresolution, without defining downstream disease processes; however, future studies will be needed.

In conclusion, the degree of baseline clot burden, as measured by the Qanadli score, was the strongest predictor of RPVO after 3 months of therapy. Quantifying clot burden on admission and providing an objective measurement may allow the stratification of patients more likely to develop CTEPH or CTED. CDT may be associated with reduced risk of developing RPVO after acute intermediate-risk PE, but further prospective studies are needed.

Author Contributions: Conceptualization, T.-A.A.H., J.P., P.R., G.C. and S.G.; methodology, T.-A.A.H., J.P. and S.G.; data curation, T.-A.A.H., J.P. and K.U.L.; writing—original draft preparation, T.-A.A.H. and J.P.; writing—review and editing, P.R., G.C. and S.G. All authors have read and agreed to the published version of the manuscript.

Funding: This research received no external funding.

Institutional Review Board Statement: This study was conducted in accordance with the Declaration of Helsinki and was approved by the Institutional Review Board (or Ethics Committee) of Temple University (protocol # TEMP-9448).

Informed Consent Statement: Patient consent was waived due to minimal risk and approval via a waiver from the Institutional Review Board.

Data Availability Statement: The data that support the findings of this study are available from the corresponding author upon reasonable request.

Conflicts of Interest: We have no conflicts of interest to disclose.

Abbreviations

RPVO, Residual Pulmonary Vascular Obstruction); PE, pulmonary embolism; CTEPH, chronic thromboembolic pulmonary hypertension; CTED, chronic thromboembolic disease; VTE, Venous Thromboembolism; CDT, catheter-directed therapies; DVT, deep vein thrombosis; AC, anticoagulation; BMI, body mass index; COPD, chronic obstructive pulmonary disease; sPESI, simplified pulmonary embolism severity index; BNP, brain natriuretic peptide; RV, right ventricular; CT, computed tomography; ECHO, echocardiogram; TTE, transthoracic echocardiogram; CTA, computed tomography angiography; DVT, deep vein thrombosis.

References

1. Simonneau, G.; Torbicki, A.; Dorfmüller, P.; Kim, N. The pathophysiology of chronic thromboembolic pulmonary hypertension. *Eur. Respir. Rev.* **2017**, *26*, 160112. [CrossRef] [PubMed]
2. Meneveau, N.; Ider, O.; Seronde, M.-F.; Chopard, R.; Davani, S.; Bernard, Y.; Schiele, F. Long-term prognostic value of residual pulmonary vascular obstruction at discharge in patients with intermediate- to high-risk pulmonary embolism. *Eur. Heart J.* **2013**, *34*, 693–701. [CrossRef]
3. Bonnefoy, P.B.; Margelidon-Cozzolino, V.; Catella-Chatron, J.; Ayoub, E.; Guichard, J.B.; Murgier, M.; Bertoletti, L. What's next after the clot? Residual pulmonary vascular obstruction after pulmonary embolism: From imaging finding to clinical consequences. *Thromb. Res.* **2019**, *184*, 67–76. [CrossRef] [PubMed]
4. Tromeur, C.; Sanchez, O.; Presles, E.; Pernod, G.; Bertoletti, L.; Jego, P.; Duhamel, E.; Provost, K.; Parent, F.; Robin, P.; et al. Risk factors for recurrent venous thromboembolism after unprovoked pulmonary embolism: The PADIS-PE randomised trial. *Eur. Respir. J.* **2018**, *51*, 1701202. [CrossRef]
5. Planquette, B.; Ferré, A.; Peron, J.; Vial-Dupuy, A.; Pastre, J.; Mourin, G.; Emmerich, J.; Collignon, M.-A.; Meyer, G.; Sanchez, O. Residual pulmonary vascular obstruction and recurrence after acute pulmonary embolism. A single center cohort study. *Thromb. Res.* **2016**, *148*, 70–75. [CrossRef] [PubMed]

6. Pesavento, R.; Filippi, L.; Palla, A.; Visonà, A.; Bova, C.; Marzolo, M.; Porro, F.; Villalta, S.; Ciammaichella, M.; Bucherini, E.; et al. Impact of residual pulmonary obstruction on the long-term outcome of patients with pulmonary embolism. *Eur. Respir. J.* **2017**, *49*, 1601980. [CrossRef]
7. Raj, L.; Robin, P.; Le Mao, R.; Presles, E.; Tromeur, C.; Sanchez, O.; Pernod, G.; Bertoletti, L.; Jego, P.; Leven, F.; et al. Predictors for Residual Pulmonary Vascular Obstruction after Unprovoked Pulmonary Embolism: Implications for Clinical Practice—The PADIS-PE Trial. *Thromb. Haemost.* **2019**, *119*, 1489–1497. [CrossRef] [PubMed]
8. Sanchez, O.; Helley, D.; Couchon, S.; Roux, A.; Delaval, A.; Trinquart, L.; Collignon, M.A.; Fischer, A.M.; Meyer, G. Perfusion defects after pulmonary embolism: Risk factors and clinical significance. *J. Thromb. Haemost.* **2010**, *8*, 1248–1255. [CrossRef]
9. Pietrasik, A.; Gasecka, A.; Kotulecki, A.; Karolak, P.; Araszkiewicz, A.; Darocha, S.; Grabowski, M.; Kurzyna, M. Catheter-directed therapy to treat intermediateand high-risk pulmonary embolism: Personal experience and review of the literature. *Cardiol. J.* **2023**, *30*, 462–472. [CrossRef]
10. Kucher, N.; Boekstegers, P.; Müller, O.J.; Kupatt, C.; Beyer-Westendorf, J.; Heitzer, T.; Tebbe, U.; Horstkotte, J.; Müller, R.; Blessing, E.; et al. Randomized, Controlled Trial of Ultrasound-Assisted Catheter-Directed Thrombolysis for Acute Intermediate-Risk Pulmonary Embolism. *Circulation* **2014**, *129*, 479–486. [CrossRef]
11. Piazza, G.; Hohlfelder, B.; Jaff, M.R.; Ouriel, K.; Engelhardt, T.C.; Sterling, K.M.; Jones, N.J.; Gurley, J.C.; Bhatheja, R.; Kennedy, R.J.; et al. A Prospective, Single-Arm, Multicenter Trial of Ultrasound-Facilitated, Catheter-Directed, Low-Dose Fibrinolysis for Acute Massive and Submassive Pulmonary Embolism. *JACC Cardiovasc. Interv.* **2015**, *8*, 1382–1392. [CrossRef] [PubMed]
12. Bashir, R.; Foster, M.; Iskander, A.; Darki, A.; Jaber, W.; Rali, P.M.; Lakhter, V.; Gandhi, R.; Klein, A.; Bhatheja, R.; et al. Pharmacomechanical Catheter-Directed Thrombolysis with the Bashir Endovascular Catheter for Acute Pulmonary Embolism. *JACC Cardiovasc. Interv.* **2022**, *15*, 2427–2436. [CrossRef] [PubMed]
13. Sedhom, R.; Megaly, M.; Elbadawi, A.; Elgendy, I.Y.; Witzke, C.F.; Kalra, S.; George, J.C.; Omer, M.; Banerjee, S.; Jaber, W.A.; et al. Contemporary National Trends and Outcomes of Pulmonary Embolism in the United States. *Am. J. Cardiol.* **2022**, *176*, 132–138. [CrossRef] [PubMed]
14. Konstantinides, S.V.; Meyer, G.; Becattini, C.; Bueno, H.; Geersing, G.-J.; Harjola, V.-P.; Huisman, M.V.; Humbert, M.; Jennings, C.S.; Jiménez, D.; et al. 2019 ESC Guidelines for the diagnosis and management of acute pulmonary embolism developed in collaboration with the European Respiratory Society (ERS): The Task Force for the diagnosis and management of acute pulmonary embolism of the European Society of Cardiology (ESC). *Eur. Respir. J.* **2019**, *54*, 1901647. [CrossRef] [PubMed]
15. Fink, M.A.; Mayer, V.L.; Schneider, T.; Seibold, T.; Stiefelhagen, R.; Kleesiek, J.; Weber, T.F.; Kauczor, H.-U. CT Angiography Clot Burden Score from Data Mining of Structured Reports for Pulmonary Embolism. *Radiology* **2022**, *302*, 175–184. [CrossRef]
16. Choi, K.-J.; Cha, S.-I.; Shin, K.-M.; Lim, J.-K.; Yoo, S.-S.; Lee, J.; Lee, S.-Y.; Kim, C.-H.; Park, J.-Y.; Lee, W.-K. Factors determining clot resolution in patients with acute pulmonary embolism. *Blood Coagul. Fibrinolysis* **2016**, *27*, 294–300. [CrossRef] [PubMed]
17. Aranda, C.; Gonzalez, P.; Gagliardi, L.; Peralta, L.; Jimenez, A. Prognostic factors of clot resolution on follow-up computed tomography angiography and recurrence after a first acute pulmonary embolism. *Clin. Respir. J* **2021**, *15*, 949–955. [CrossRef]
18. Sun, Z.-T.; Hao, F.-E.; Guo, Y.-M.; Liu, A.-S.; Zhao, L. Assessment of Acute Pulmonary Embolism by Computer-Aided Technique: A Reliability Study. *Med. Sci. Monit.* **2020**, *26*, e920239-1. [CrossRef]
19. Batra, K.; Xi, Y.; Al-Hreish, K.M.; Kay, F.U.; Browning, T.; Baker, C.; Peshock, R.M. Detection of Incidental Pulmonary Embolism on Conventional Contrast-Enhanced Chest CT: Comparison of an Artificial Intelligence Algorithm and Clinical Reports. *Am. J. Roentgenol.* **2022**, *219*, 895–902. [CrossRef]
20. Cheikh, A.B.; Gorincour, G.; Nivet, H.; May, J.; Seux, M.; Calame, P.; Thomson, V.; Delabrousse, E.; Crombé, A. How artificial intelligence improves radiological interpretation in suspected pulmonary embolism. *Eur. Radiol.* **2022**, *32*, 5831–5842. [CrossRef]
21. Jiménez, D.; Aujesky, D.; Díaz, G.; Monreal, M.; Otero, R.; Martí, D.; Marín, E.; Aracil, E.; Sueiro, A.; Yusen, R.D. Prognostic Significance of Deep Vein Thrombosis in Patients Presenting with Acute Symptomatic Pulmonary Embolism. *Am. J. Respir. Crit. Care Med.* **2010**, *181*, 983–991. [CrossRef] [PubMed]
22. Becattini, C.; Cohen, A.T.; Agnelli, G.; Howard, L.; Castejón, B.; Trujillo-Santos, J.; Monreal, M.; Perrier, A.; Yusen, R.D.; Jiménez, D. Risk Stratification of Patients with Acute Symptomatic Pulmonary Embolism Based on Presence or Absence of Lower Extremity DVT. *Chest* **2016**, *149*, 192–200. [CrossRef] [PubMed]
23. Nishiwaki, S.; Morita, Y.; Yamashita, Y.; Morimoto, T.; Amano, H.; Takase, T.; Hiramori, S.; Kim, K.; Oi, M.; Akao, M.; et al. Impact of no, distal, and proximal deep vein thrombosis on clinical outcomes in patients with acute pulmonary embolism: From the COMMAND VTE registry. *J. Cardiol.* **2021**, *77*, 395–403. [CrossRef] [PubMed]
24. Quezada, C.A.; Bikdeli, B.; Barrios, D.; Morillo, R.; Nieto, R.; Chiluiza, D.; Barbero, E.; Guerassimova, I.; García, A.; Yusen, R.D.; et al. Assessment of coexisting deep vein thrombosis for risk stratification of acute pulmonary embolism. *Thromb. Res.* **2018**, *164*, 40–44. [CrossRef] [PubMed]
25. Stevens, S.M.; Woller, S.C.; Kreuziger, L.B.; Bounameaux, H.; Doerschug, K.; Geersing, G.-J.; Huisman, M.V.; Kearon, C.; King, C.S.; Knighton, A.J.; et al. Antithrombotic Therapy for VTE Disease. *Chest* **2021**, *160*, e545–e608. [CrossRef] [PubMed]
26. Gayen, S.; Upadhyay, V.; Kumaran, M.; Bashir, R.; Lakhter, V.; Panaro, J.; Criner, G.; Dadparvar, S.; Rali, P. Changes in Lung Perfusion in Patients Treated with Percutaneous Mechanical Thrombectomy for Intermediate-Risk Pulmonary Embolism. *Am. J. Med.* **2022**, *135*, 1016–1020. [CrossRef]

27. Chernysh, I.N.; Nagaswami, C.; Kosolapova, S.; Peshkova, A.D.; Cuker, A.; Cines, D.B.; Cambor, C.L.; Litvinov, R.I.; Weisel, J.W. The distinctive structure and composition of arterial and venous thrombi and pulmonary emboli. *Sci. Rep.* **2020**, *10*, 5112. [CrossRef]
28. Czaplicki, C.; Albadawi, H.; Partovi, S.; Gandhi, R.T.; Quencer, K.; Deipolyi, A.R.; Oklu, R. Can thrombus age guide thrombolytic therapy? *Cardiovasc. Diagn. Ther.* **2017**, *7*, S186–S196. [CrossRef]

Disclaimer/Publisher's Note: The statements, opinions and data contained in all publications are solely those of the individual author(s) and contributor(s) and not of MDPI and/or the editor(s). MDPI and/or the editor(s) disclaim responsibility for any injury to people or property resulting from any ideas, methods, instructions or products referred to in the content.

MDPI AG
Grosspeteranlage 5
4052 Basel
Switzerland
Tel.: +41 61 683 77 34

Journal of Clinical Medicine Editorial Office
E-mail: jcm@mdpi.com
www.mdpi.com/journal/jcm

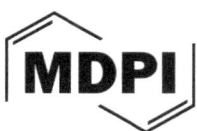

Disclaimer/Publisher's Note: The statements, opinions and data contained in all publications are solely those of the individual author(s) and contributor(s) and not of MDPI and/or the editor(s). MDPI and/or the editor(s) disclaim responsibility for any injury to people or property resulting from any ideas, methods, instructions or products referred to in the content.

www.ingramcontent.com/pod-product-compliance
Lightning Source LLC
LaVergne TN
LVHW070000100526
838202LV00019B/2587